T0212505

Lecture Notes in Computer Science   **10019**

Commenced Publication in 1973
Founding and Former Series Editors:
Gerhard Goos, Juris Hartmanis, and Jan van Leeuwen

More information about this series at http://www.springer.com/series/7412

Li Wang · Ehsan Adeli
Qian Wang · Yinghuan Shi
Heung-Il Suk (Eds.)

Machine Learning in Medical Imaging

7th International Workshop, MLMI 2016
Held in Conjunction with MICCAI 2016
Athens, Greece, October 17, 2016
Proceedings

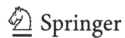 Springer

Editors
Li Wang
University of North Carolina
Chapel Hill, NC
USA

Ehsan Adeli
University of North Carolina
Chapel Hill, NC
USA

Qian Wang
Shanghai Jiaotong University
Shanghai
China

Yinghuan Shi
Nanjing University
Nanjing
China

Heung-Il Suk
Korea University
Seoul
Korea (Republic of)

ISSN 0302-9743   ISSN 1611-3349   (electronic)
Lecture Notes in Computer Science
ISBN 978-3-319-47156-3   ISBN 978-3-319-47157-0   (eBook)
DOI 10.1007/978-3-319-47157-0

Library of Congress Control Number: 2016953329

LNCS Sublibrary: SL6 – Image Processing, Computer Vision, Pattern Recognition, and Graphics

Printed on acid-free paper

This Springer imprint is published by Springer Nature
The registered company is Springer International Publishing AG
The registered company address is: Gewerbestrasse 11, 6330 Cham, Switzerland

Preface

The 7th International Workshop on Machine Learning in Medical Imaging (MLMI 2016) was held in the Intercontinental Athenaeum, Athens, Greece, on October 17, 2016, in conjunction with the 19th International Conference on Medical Image Computing and Computer-Assisted Intervention (MICCAI).

Machine learning plays an essential role in the medical imaging field, including computer-assisted diagnosis, image segmentation, image registration, image fusion, image-guided therapy, image annotation, and image database retrieval. With advances in medical imaging, new imaging modalities and methodologies, such as cone-beam CT, tomosynthesis, electrical impedance tomography, as well as new machine-learning algorithms/applications come to the stage for medical imaging. Owing to large inter-subject variations and complexities, it is generally difficult to derive analytic formulations or simple equations to represent objects such as lesions and anatomy in medical images. Therefore, tasks in medical imaging require learning from patient data for heuristics and prior knowledge, in order to facilitate the detection/diagnosis of abnormalities in medical images.

The main aim of the MLMI 2016 workshop was to help advance scientific research in the broad field of machine learning in medical imaging. The workshop focused on major trends and challenges in this area, and presented works aimed at identifying new cutting-edge techniques and their use in medical imaging. We hope that the MLMI workshop becomes an important platform for translating research from the bench to the bedside.

The range and level of submissions for this year's meeting were of very high quality. Authors were asked to submit full-length papers for review. A total of 60 papers were submitted to the workshop in response to the call for papers. Each of the 60 papers underwent a rigorous double-blinded peer-review process, with each paper being reviewed by at least two (typically three) reviewers from the Program Committee, composed of 81 well-known experts in the field. Based on the reviewing scores and critiques, the 38 best papers (63 %) were accepted for presentation at the workshop and chosen to be included in this Springer LNCS volume. The large variety of machine-learning techniques applied to medical imaging were well represented at the workshop.

We are grateful to the Program Committee for reviewing the submitted papers and giving constructive comments and critiques, to the authors for submitting high-quality papers, to the presenters for excellent presentations, and to all the MLMI 2016 attendees coming to Athens from all around the world.

August 2016

Li Wang
Ehsan Adeli
Qian Wang
Yinghuan Shi
Heung-Il Suk

Organization

Steering Committee

Dinggang Shen   University of North Carolina at Chapel Hill, USA
Pingkun Yan   Philips Research North America, USA
Kenji Suzuki   University of Chicago, USA
Fei Wang   AliveCor Inc., USA

Program Committee

Le An   UNC-Chapel Hill, USA
Siamak Ardekani   Johns Hopkins University, USA
Wenjia Bai   Imperial College London, UK
Heang-Ping Chan   University of Michigan Medical Center, USA
Hanbo Chen   The University of Georgia, USA
Pierrick Coupé   University of Bordeaux, France
Marleen de Bruijne   University of Copenhagen, Denmark
Emad Fatemizadeh   Sharif University of Technology, Iran
Jing Feng   Shanghai Jiao Tong University, China
Qianjin Feng   Southern Medical University, China
Jurgen Fripp   CSIRO, Australia
Yaozong Gao   Apple
Laura Gui   University of Geneva, Switzerland
Yanrong Guo   UNC-Chapel Hill, USA
Ghassan Hamarneh   Simon Fraser University, Canada
Ivana Isgum   University Medical Center Utrecht, The Netherlands
Zexuan Ji   Nanjing University of Science and Technology, China
Xi Jiang   The University of Georgia, USA
Yan Jin   UNC-Chapel Hill, USA
Nico Karssemeijer   Radboud University Nijmegen Medical Centre,
     The Netherlands
Jeremy Kawahara   Simon Fraser University, Canada
Minjeong Kim   UNC-Chapel Hill, USA
Simon Koppers   RWTH Aachen University, Germany
Elizabeth Krupinski   Emory University, USA
Cuijin Lao   UNC-Chapel Hill, USA
Byung-Uk Lee   Ewha W. University, South Korea
Gang Li   UNC-Chapel Hill, USA
Kaiming Li   West China Hospital of Sichuan University, China
Xiang Li   The University of Georgia, USA

Shu Liao	Siemens
Mingxia Liu	UNC-Chapel Hill, USA
Le Lu	NIH, USA
Dwarikanath Mahapatra	IBM Research, Australia
Antonios Makropoulos	Imperial College London, UK
Adriënne Mendrik	University Medical Center Utrecht, The Netherlands
Pim Moeskops	University Medical Center Utrecht, The Netherlands
Brent Munsell	College of Charleston, UK
Dong Nie	UNC-Chapel Hill, USA
Philip Ogunbona	University of Wollongong, Australia
Kazunori Okada	San Francisco State University, USA
Emanuele Olivetti	Fondazione Bruno Kessler, Italy
Jinah Park	KAIST, South Korea
Kilian Pohl	SRI International, Singapore
Bisser Raytchev	Hiroshima University, Japan
Xuhua Ren	Shanghai Jiao Tong University, China
Mert R. Sabuncu	Harvard University, USA
Clarisa Sanchez	Radboud University Nijmegen Medical Center, The Netherlands
Gerard Sanroma	Universitat Pompeu Fabra, Barcelona, Spain
Yeqin Shao	Nantong University, China
Li Shen	Indiana University School of Medicine, USA
Feng Shi	UNC-Chapel Hill, USA
Hamid Soltanian-Zadeh	University of Tehran, Iran
Kenji Suzuki	Illinois Institute of Technology, USA
Hotaka Takizawa	University of Tsukuba, Japan
Tolga Tasdizen	University of Utah, USA
Tatiana Tommasi	UNC-Chapel Hill, USA
Tong Tong	Harvard University, USA
Gozde Unal	Sabanci University, Turkey
Chunliang Wang	KTH Royal Institute of Technology, Sweden
Lei Wang	University of Wollongong, Australia
Yaping Wang	Zhengzhou University, China
Simon Warfield	Boston Children's Hospital, USA
Guorong Wu	UNC-Chapel Hill, USA
Lei Xiang	Shanghai Jiao Tong University, China
Jun Xu	Nanjing University of Information Science and Technology, China
Yiqiang Zhan	Siemens Medical Solutions, USA
Daoqiang Zhang	Nanjing University of Aeronautics and Astronautics, China
Jinpeng Zhang	Shanghai Jiao Tong University, China
Jun Zhang	UNC-Chapel Hill, USA
Lichi Zhang	UNC-Chapel Hill, USA
Shaoting Zhang	UNC Charlotte, USA
Guoyan Zheng	University of Bern, Switzerland
Yefeng Zheng	Siemens

Yuanjie Zheng   University of Pennsylvania, USA
Kevin Zhou   San Francisco State University, USA
Luping Zhou   University of Wollongong, Australia
Sean Zhou   Siemens Medical Solutions, USA
Xiaofeng Zhu   UNC-Chapel Hill, USA
Yingying Zhu   UNC-Chapel Hill, USA
Xiahai Zhuang   Shanghai Jiao Tong University, China

Contents

Identifying High Order Brain Connectome Biomarkers via Learning on Hypergraph

Chen Zu[1,2], Yue Gao[3], Brent Munsell[4], Minjeong Kim[1],
Ziwen Peng[5], Yingying Zhu[1], Wei Gao[6], Daoqiang Zhang[2],
Dinggang Shen[1], and Guorong Wu[1(✉)]

[1] Department of Radiology and BRIC,
University of North Carolina at Chapel Hill, Chapel Hill, NC, USA
grwu@med.unc.edu
[2] Department of Computer Science and Technology,
Nanjing University of Aeronautics and Astronautics, Nanjing, China
[3] School of Software, Tsinghua University, Beijing, China
[4] Department of Computer Science, College of Charleston, Charleston, SC, USA
[5] Centre for Studies of Psychological Application, School of Psychology,
South China Normal University, Guangzhou, China
[6] Biomedical Imaging Research Institute (BIRI),
Department of Biomedical Sciences and Imaging,
Cedars-Sinai Medical Center, Los Angeles, CA, USA

Abstract. The functional connectome has gained increased attention in the neuroscience community. In general, most network connectivity models are based on correlations between discrete-time series signals that only connect two different brain regions. However, these bivariate region-to-region models do not involve three or more brain regions that form a subnetwork. Here we propose a learning-based method to explore subnetwork biomarkers that are significantly distinguishable between two clinical cohorts. Learning on hypergraph is employed in our work. Specifically, we construct a hypergraph by exhaustively inspecting all possible subnetworks for all subjects, where each hyperedge connects a group of subjects demonstrating highly correlated functional connectivity behavior throughout the underlying subnetwork. The objective function of hypergraph learning is to jointly optimize the weights for all hyperedges which make the separation of two groups by the learned data representation be in the best consensus with the observed clinical labels. We deploy our method to find high order childhood autism biomarkers from rs-fMRI images. Promising results have been obtained from comprehensive evaluation on the discriminative power and generality in diagnosis of Autism.

1 Introduction

The brain can be partitioned into different regions according to various functions, and connectivity networks can be composed where information is continuously processed between these functionally linked brain regions [1]. In order to understand the pathological underpinnings of neurological disorder, many functional neuroimaging studies have been developed to investigate abnormal alternations among these brain

© Springer International Publishing AG 2016
L. Wang et al. (Eds.): MLMI 2016, LNCS 10019, pp. 1–9, 2016.
DOI: 10.1007/978-3-319-47157-0_1

connections. Recently, researchers have also used functional connectivity networks for diagnosing brain disease at individual level [2].

The brain is complex and oscillatory activities behind cognition are essentially the large-scale collaborative work among millions of neurons through multiple brain regions. The bivariate region-to-region interactions do not capture high order network architecture patterns that involve three or more brain regions in a subnetwork architecture. Recently, there is overwhelming evidence that brain network displays hierarchical modularity, making the investigation of high order network patterns more attractive to neuroscience and clinical practice than ever before.

Here, we propose a novel learning-based method to discover high order network connectome biomarkers that can be used to distinguish two clinical cohorts. Without doubt, there are thousands of high order connectome patterns varying from the number and combination of the involved brain regions. Considering the computational cost, we propose the following criteria to promote one high order network connectome to the biomarker: (a) *Small subnetwork architecture.* Since a triangle is one of the simplest types of subnetwork, we take a first step to discover high order connectome patterns that end up in the functional connectivity throughout the triangle cliques. (b) *Entire functional connectivity flow.* We examine the functional connectivity behavior throughout the subnetwork. Therefore, the connectome pattern is considered as a biomarker only if the entire functional connectivity flow inside the subnetwork, instead of particular predominant connection link, shows significant difference between two clinical cohorts.

To achieve it, we first construct a subnetwork repository that consists of all possible triangle cliques. The native solution is to measure and sort the significance of each triangle cliques via the independent statistical t-test. Since the subnetworks are highly correlated (e.g., large amount of overlap of edges among triangle cliques), independent statistical test can hardly be effective in looking for the critical subnetworks.

We utilize hypergraph technique to jointly find a set of the most significant high order connectome biomarkers by investigating subject-to-subject relationships based on functional connectivity flows in all possible subnetwork architectures. Specifically, each individual subject is treated as a vertex in the hypergraph. For each subnetwork architecture, a hyperedge is formed for each subject at a time that includes other subjects with similar functional connectivity flows throughout the same subnetwork architecture. Thus, the hypergraph eventually encodes a wide spectrum of high order connectome patterns in the population. The next step is to find the most significant biomarkers hiding behind thousands of subnetworks. Since each subject has the clinical label, the problem of seeking for high order biomarkers turns to the optimization of the weights on hyperedges such that the separation of subjects by the learned data representation (encoded by hypergraph) maximally agrees with the observed clinical labels. Intuitively, the learned weights reflect the significance in distinguishing two clinical cohorts. We have applied our learning-based method to discover the high order functional connectome patterns for childhood autism spectrum disorders (ASDs) and identify ASD individuals from ABIDE dataset. Promising classification results have been achieved which demonstrate the power of learned high order connectome patterns.

2 Method

Method Overview. Figure 1 illustrates the intuition behind our proposed learning-based method. For clarity, we assume there are three subjects in one cohort (top left in Fig. 1) and two subjects in anther cohort (bottom left in Fig. 1). Only two possible subnetworks (triangle cliques in purple and red) are under investigation. The goal is to find out which subnetwork is able to separate subjects from two groups more accurately than the other, based on the functional connectivity flow inside the sub-network. Eventually, the selected subnetworks are considered as biomarkers to identify other individual subjects.

Hypergraph is employed to measure the high order subject-wise relationships based on the functional connectivity flow running inside each subnetwork. Specifically, subjects are considered as vertices (v_1–v_5 in Fig. 1) in the hypergraph. In general, a set of subjects fall into the same hyperedge only if their functional connectivity flows in the same subnetwork show high correlations. Thus, hyperedge can accommodate high order relationship that is beyond two subjects in the conventional graph technique. For example, subject v_2 and v_3 stay in the same hyperedge e_1 with v_1 since their functional connectivity flows (designated by the black arrows) are very similar inside the purple triangle clique. The standard way to construct hyperedges is to exhaustively visit each subject per each subnetwork. As the example shown in Fig. 1, we obtain four hyperedges (e_1–e_4) that are displayed by curves. Note, the identical hyperedges are discarded and the color on each hyperedge indicates the associated subnetwork.

A hypergraph learning technique is used to jointly quantify the significance of each subnetwork based on the ground truth clinical label on each subject. Intuitively, the more label discrepancies occur within the hyperedges related to the underlying sub-network, the lower the significance of that particular subnetwork becomes. Finally, the subnetworks with high overall significance value across related hyperedges are regarded as the biomarkers from rs-fMRI image. As shown in the left panel of Fig. 1, the labels in e_1 and e_2 (purple curves) are highly consistent, suggesting that the functional connectivity flow running on the purple triangle clique is a good biomarker to separate the subjects from two different groups. On the contrary, the functional

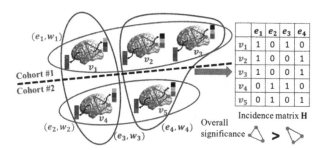

Fig. 1. The overview of our learning-based method to discover high order brain connectome patterns by hypergraph inference. (Color figure online)

connectivity flow inside the red triangle clique fails to be the biomarker since there are hyperedges built on the red triangle clique having subjects with different clinical labels, e.g., v_1 and v_4 are both in the hyperedge e_3.

2.1   Encode Subject-Wise Relationship in Hypergraph

Given a training set of N subjects $\{v_n | n = 1, \ldots, N\}$, where each subject has already been partitioned to R anatomical regions. Without loss of generality, we use '+1' and '−1' to distinguish the label for two clinical groups, and thus form a column vector $\mathbf{y} = [y_1, y_2, \ldots, y_N]^T$. Considering the computational cost and efficiency, we first construct the pool of all possible subnetworks $\Delta = \{\Delta_j | j = 1, \ldots, C\}$, where each triangle clique Δ_j is formed by three brain regions randomly picking up from totally R regions. Therefore, there are $C = \begin{pmatrix} R \\ 3 \end{pmatrix}$ combinations in total. Given subject v_n and particular subnetwork Δ_j, we can obtain a three-element vector of functional connectivity flow $\alpha_{n,j} = [\alpha_{n,j}^1, \alpha_{n,j}^2, \alpha_{n,j}^3]$, where each element in $\alpha_{n,j}$ is eventually the Pearson's correlation degree of the mean rs-fMRI signals, from subject v_n, between any two brain regions within the triangle clique Δ_j.

Construct Hypergraph. Next, we construct hypergraph, as denoted by $G = (V, E)$, where the hypergraph vertex set $V = \{v_n | n = 1, \ldots, N\}$ includes all subjects in the population. We use star-expansion algorithm to build a set of hyperedges by exhaustively visiting each vertex v_n for particular subnetwork Δ_j, thus forming the hyperedge set $E = \{e_{n,j} | n = 1, \ldots, N, j = 1, \ldots, C\}$. For each hyperedge $e_{n,j}$, we examine the similarity between functional connectivity flow $\alpha_{n,j}$ at current vertex v_n and $\alpha_{n'j}$ ($n' = 1, \ldots, N, n' \neq n$) at all others vertices. The criteria of allowing $v_{n'}$ be in the hyperedge $e_{n,j}$ (i.e., $v_{n'} \in e_{n,j}$) are (a) the Euclidian distance $d_j(n, n') = ||\alpha_{n,j} - \alpha_{n'j}||_2^2$ between $\alpha_{n,j}$ and $\alpha_{n'j}$ should be smaller than certain threshold; and (b) $\alpha_{n'j}$ should be within the k-nearest neighborhood in terms of $d_j(n, n')$.

Encode Hypergraph in Incidence Matrix. In a conventional graph based method, the relationships among graph vertices are encoded in a $N \times N$ affinity matrix. In hyper-graph, instead, the relationships between vertices are encoded using an incidence matrix $\mathbf{H}$, with the row and column denoting the vertices and hyperedges, respectively. Since each hyperedge $e_{n,j}$ is related with both vertex v_n and subnetwork Δ_j, we use the column index θ to delegate the bivariate index (n, j), i.e., $\theta \leftrightarrow (n, j)$, where θ ranges from 1 to $\Theta = N \cdot C$. Thus, $\mathbf{H}$ is a $N \times \Theta$ matrix. For each entry $h(n, \theta)$, we set $h(n, \theta) = 1$ if the vertex v_n is in hyperedge $e(n, j)$. Otherwise, $h(n, \theta) = 0$. The example of incidence matrix is shown in the right panel of Fig. 1. Apparently, the incidence matrix conveys more information than the affinity matrix used in conventional approaches based on simple graphs.

Hyperedge Weights. For convenience, we use e_θ denote the particular hyperedge in the following text, instead of $e_{n,j}$. Each hyperedge e_θ has a non-negative weight w_θ.

Furthermore, we construct a $\Theta \times \Theta$ diagonal matrix $\mathbf{W}$ where each diagonal element is the hyperedge weight w_θ. Given $\mathbf{H}$ and $\mathbf{W}$, we can define the vertex degree $d(n) = \sum_{\theta=1}^{\Theta} w_\theta h(n, \theta)$ for each v_n and the hyperedge degree $\delta(\theta) = \sum_{n=1}^{N} h(n, \theta)$ for each e_θ.

2.2 Discover High Order Brain Connectome Patterns by Hypergraph Learning

Our learning-based method aims to find out the biomarkers by inspecting the performance of each hyperedge in separating subjects from two groups. To that end, we first assume the label on each subject is not known yet. Thus, we use hypergraph learning technique to estimate the likelihood f_n for each subject v_n, which is driven by (a) the minimization of discrepancies between ground truth label vector $\mathbf{y}$ and the estimated likelihood vector $\mathbf{f} = [f_1, f_2, \ldots, f_N]^T$, and (b) the consistency of clinical labels within each hyperedge. The consistency requirement can be defined as:

$$\Omega_{\mathbf{f}}(\mathbf{W}) = \sum_{\theta=1}^{\Theta} \sum_{n,n'=1}^{N} \frac{w_\theta h(n, \theta) h(n', \theta)}{\delta(\theta)} \left(\frac{f_n}{\sqrt{d(n)}} - \frac{f_{n'}}{\sqrt{d(n')}} \right)^2. \quad (1)$$

The regulation term $\Omega_{\mathbf{f}}(\mathbf{W})$ penalizes the label discrepancy by encouraging the difference between the normalized likelihoods $f_n / \sqrt{d(n)}$ and $f_{n'} / \sqrt{d(n')}$ to be as small as possible if v_n and $v_{n'}$ are in the same hyperedge e_θ. It is clear that the regularization term $\Omega_{\mathbf{f}}(\mathbf{W})$ is a function of both $\mathbf{W}$ and $\mathbf{f}$, *which eventually makes the optimization of $\mathbf{W}$ reflect the quality of each hyperedge being the biomarker.* In order to avoid overfitting, we use Frobenius norm on the weighting matrix $\mathbf{W}$. Therefore, the objective function to look for high order connectome patterns is:

$$\arg\min_{\mathbf{W}, \mathbf{f}} \Omega_{\mathbf{f}}(\mathbf{W}) + \lambda ||\mathbf{y} - \mathbf{f}||_2^2 + \mu ||\mathbf{W}||_F^2. \quad (2)$$

where λ and μ are two scalars controlling the strength of data fitting term and Frobenius norm on the weighting matrix $\mathbf{W}$, respectively.

Optimization. $\Omega_{\mathbf{f}}(\mathbf{W})$ in Eq. (2) is called as hypergraph balance term in [3] and can be reformulated into a matrix form: $\Omega_{\mathbf{f}}(\mathbf{W}) = \mathbf{f}^T (\mathbf{I} - \Lambda) \mathbf{f} = \mathbf{f}^T \mathcal{L} \mathbf{f}$, where $\mathcal{L}$ is the normalized hypergraph Laplacian, $\mathbf{I}$ is the identity matrix, and $\Lambda = \mathbf{D}_v^{-\frac{1}{2}} \mathbf{H} \mathbf{W} \mathbf{D}_e^{-1} \mathbf{H}^T \mathbf{D}_v^{-\frac{1}{2}}$. Note, $\mathbf{D}_v = diag(d(n))$ and $\mathbf{D}_e = diag(\delta(\theta))$ are the diagonal matrices of the vertex degrees and the hyperedge degrees, respectively. It is clear that the objective function in Eq. (2) is not jointly convex with respect to $\mathbf{W}$ and $\mathbf{f}$. Hence, we propose the following solution to find $\mathbf{W}$ and $\mathbf{f}$, alternatively.

Solve Likelihood Vector f. Fixing $\mathbf{W}$, the objective function becomes:

$$\arg\min_{\mathbf{f}} \phi(\mathbf{f}) = \mathbf{f}^T \mathcal{L} \mathbf{f} + \lambda ||\mathbf{y} - \mathbf{f}||_2^2. \quad (3)$$

Conventional hypergraph inference method can be used to estimate $\mathbf{f}$ by letting $\frac{\partial \phi}{\partial \mathbf{f}} = 0$, which leads to the deterministic solution: $\widehat{\mathbf{f}} = \left(\mathbf{I} + \frac{1}{\lambda}\mathcal{L}\right)^{-1}\mathbf{y}$.

Optimize the Hypergraph Weight W. After discarding unrelated terms w.r.t. $\mathbf{W}$ in Eq. (2), we derive the objective function for hypergraph weight as:

$$\arg\min_{\mathbf{W}} \varphi(\mathbf{W}) = \mathbf{f}^T \mathcal{L} \mathbf{f} + \mu \sum\nolimits_{\theta=1}^{\Theta} (w_\theta)^2. \tag{4}$$

Since each w_θ in $\mathbf{W}$ is independent, we can yield the optimized hyperedge weight as $\widehat{w}_\theta = \max\left(\frac{\mathbf{f}^T \mathbf{D}_v^{-\frac{1}{2}} \mathbf{H} \mathbf{I}_\theta \mathbf{D}_e^{-1} \mathbf{H}^T \mathbf{D}_v^{-\frac{1}{2}} \mathbf{f}}{2\mu}, 0\right)$ by letting the derivative $\frac{\partial \varphi}{\partial w_\theta} = 0$ and projecting $\widehat{w}_\theta$ to meet the non-negative constraint. Note, $\mathbf{I}_\theta$ is the $\Theta \times \Theta$ selection matrix which is zero everywhere except at entry (θ, θ).

Discover High Order Connectome Biomarkers. Since $\mathbf{W}$ and $\mathbf{f}$ are coupled in Eq. (2), the estimated hypergraph weights in $\mathbf{W}$ is driven to achieve (a) the least discrepancy between ground truth $\mathbf{y}$ and estimated likelihood $\mathbf{f}$, and (b) highest label consistency within each hyperedge, which exactly matches with the important properties of imaging biomarkers. In our method, we sort the significance of the subnetworks according to the mean hyperedge weight over all subjects, i.e., $\widehat{w}_j = \sum_{n=1}^{N} \widehat{w}(n, j)$. After that, a set of the critical subnetworks $P = \{\Delta_j | j = 1, \ldots, C, \widehat{w}_j > \varepsilon\}$, as long as their mean hyperedge weights beyond certain threshold ε, are considered as the biomarkers where the functional connectivity flows running inside have significant difference between two clinical cohorts.

3 Experiments

3.1 Critical Subnetworks Learned by Hypergraph Inference

In this section, we applied our learning-based method to find critical subnetworks P based on 45 ASD and 47 typical control (TC) subjects from the NYU site of Autism Brain Imaging Data Exchange (ABIDE) database [4]. The first 10 obtained rs-fMRI images of each subject are removed to ensure magnetization equilibrium. After slice timing and head motion correction, the images are normalized into MNI space and then segmented into 116 regions-of-interest (ROIs) according to Automated Anatomical Labeling (AAL) template. Following this, the images underwent signal detrending and bandpass filtering (0.01–0.08 Hz). For each subject, the mean time series of each ROI is obtained by averaging the rs-fMRI time series over all voxels in that particular ROI. Note, the total number of possible subnetworks is $\binom{116}{3} = 253,460$. We jointly find the best parameters for λ and μ in Eq. (2) using the line search strategy with range from 0.1 to 10.0.

Figure 2 shows the top 10 most critical subnetworks (white triangle cliques) out of 253,460 candidates between ASD and TC cohorts. The color on each vertex differentiates the functions in human brain. It is clear (a) most of the brain regions involved

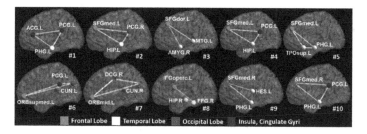

Fig. 2. The top 10 selected subnetworks (white triangle cliques) where the functional connectivity flow running inside has significant difference between ASD and TC cohorts. (Color figure online)

in the selected top 10 critical subnetworks locate the key areas related with ASD, such as amygdala, middle temporal gyrus, superior frontal gyrus; and (b) most of the selected subnetworks travel cross the subcortical and cortical regions, which is in consensus with the recent discover of autism pathology in neuroscience community [5].

3.2 Identification of ASD Subjects with the Learned Subnetwork

In the following experiments, we use functional connectivity flows on top 200 critical subnetworks as the feature representation (feature dimension: 200×3) to classify ASD and TC subjects. Then traditional Support Vector Machine (SVM) [6] is adopted to train the classifier directly based on the concatenated feature vector, denoted as *Subnetwork-SVM*. Since the functional connectivity flow comes from each subnetwork, it is straightforward to organize them to a tensor representation and use advanced Support Tensor Machine (STM) [7] to take advantage of the structured feature representation, denoted as *Subnetwork-STM* in the following experiments. In order to demonstrate the advantage of subnetwork over the conventional region-to-region connection in brain network, we compare with two counterpart methods *Link-SVM* (use the Pearson's correlations on each link as the feature) and *Toplink-SVM* (select top 600 links by *t*-test and use the Pearson's correlation on the selected links to form the feature vector).

Evaluation on Discrimination Power. In this experiment, we use 10-fold cross validation strategy to evaluate the classification accuracy (ACC), sensitivity (SEN), specificity (SPE), positive predictive value (PPV), and negative predictive value (NPV) on 45 ASD and 47 TC subjects from NYU site in ABIDE database. As the classification performance plots and the ROC curves shown in Fig. 3, the classifiers trained on connectome features from our learned subnetworks have achieved much higher classification performance than those trained by the same classification tool but based on the connectome features from the conventional region-to-region connection links. Also, the substantial classification improvements by *Subnetwork-STM* over *Subnetwork-SVM* indicate the benefit of using structured data presentation in classification where such high order information is clearly delivered in the learned subnetworks.

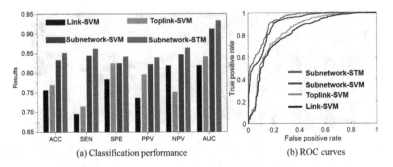

(a) Classification performance   (b) ROC curves

Fig. 3. Classification performance of four different classification methods.

Evaluation on Generality. To verify the generality of learned subnetworks, we directly apply the subnetworks learned on the NYU dataset to the classification of 44 ASD and 53 TC subjects from the UM (University of Michigan) site in ABIDE database. The accuracies obtained by Link-SVM and Toplink-SVM are 0.6086 and 0.6253, respectively, which is comparable to that in reference [8]. Our Subnetwork-SVM and Subnetwork-STM can improve the accuracy up to 0.6469 and 0.6610, respectively. Again, the classification methods using the features extracted from the learned top subnetworks achieve much higher classification accuracy than the counterpart *Link-SVM* and *Toplink-SVM* methods.

4 Conclusion

In this paper, we propose a novel learning method to discover high order brain connectome biomarkers which are beyond the widely used region-to-region connections in conventional brain network analysis. Hypergraph technique is introduced to model complex subject-wise relationships in terms of various subnetworks and quantify the significance of each subnetwork based on the discrimination power across clinical groups and consistency within each cohort. We apply our learning-based method to find the subnetwork biomarkers between ASD and TC subjects. The learned top subnetworks are not only in consensus with the recent clinical findings, but also able to significantly improve accuracy in identifying ASD subjects, strongly supporting their potential use and impact in neuroscience study and clinic practice.

References

1. Van Den Heuvel, M.P., Pol, H.E.H.: Exploring the brain network: a review on resting-state fMRI functional connectivity. Eur. Neuropsychopharmacol. **20**(8), 519–534 (2010)
2. Zeng, L.L., Shen, H., Liu, L., Wang, L., Li, B., Fang, P., Zhou, Z., Li, Y., Hu, D.: Identifying major depression using whole-brain functional connectivity: a multivariate pattern analysis. Brain **135**(5), 1498–1507 (2012)

3. Zhou, D., Huang, J., Schölkopf, B.: Learning with hypergraphs: clustering, classification, and embedding. In: Advances in Neural Information Processing Systems, vol. 19, pp. 1601–1608 (2006)
4. Di Martino, A., Yan, C.G., Li, Q., Denio, E., Castellanos, F.X., Alaerts, K., Anderson, J.S., Assaf, M., Bookheimer, S.Y., Dapretto, M., et al.: The autism brain imaging data exchange: towards a large-scale evaluation of the intrinsic brain architecture in autism. Mol. Psychiatry **19**(6), 659–667 (2014)
5. Minshew, N.J., Williams, D.L.: The new neurobiology of autism: cortex, connectivity, and neuronal organization. Arch. Neurol. **64**(7), 945–950 (2007)
6. Cortes, C., Vapnik, V.: Support-vector networks. Mach. Learn. **20**(3), 273–297 (1995)
7. Tao, D., Li, X., Wu, X., Hu, W., Maybank, S.J.: Supervised tensor learning. Knowl. Inf. Syst. **13**(1), 1–42 (2007)
8. Nielsen, J.A., Zielinshi, B.A., Fletcher, P.T., Alexander, A.L., Lange, N., Bigler, E.D., Lainhart, J.E., Anderson, J.S.: Multisite functional connectivity MRI classification of autism: abide results. Frontiers Hum. Neurosci. **7**(1), 599 (2013)

Bilateral Regularization in Reproducing Kernel Hilbert Spaces for Discontinuity Preserving Image Registration

Christoph Jud$^{(\boxtimes)}$, Nadia Möri, Benedikt Bitterli, and Philippe C. Cattin

Department of Biomedical Engineering, University of Basel, Switzerland
Gewerbestrasse. 14, 4123 Allschwil, Switzerland
christoph.jud@unibas.ch
http://dbe.unibas.ch

Abstract. The registration of abdominal images is an increasing field in research and forms the basis for studying the dynamic motion of organs. Particularly challenging therein are organs which slide along each other. They require discontinuous transform mappings at the sliding boundaries to be accurately aligned. In this paper, we present a novel approach for discontinuity preserving image registration. We base our method on a sparse kernel machine (SKM), where reproducing kernel Hilbert spaces serve as transformation models. We introduce a bilateral regularization term, where neighboring transform parameters are considered jointly. This regularizer enforces a bias to homogeneous regions in the transform mapping and simultaneously preserves discontinuous magnitude changes of parameter vectors pointing in equal directions. We prove a representer theorem for the overall cost function including this bilateral regularizer in order to guarantee a finite dimensional solution. In addition, we build direction-dependent basis functions within the SKM framework in order to elongate the transformations along the potential sliding organ boundaries. In the experiments, we evaluate the registration results of our method on a 4DCT dataset and show superior registration performance of our method over the tested methods.

1   Introduction

The image-based analysis of organ motion has attracted increasing attention in medical image analysis. Applications range from statistical motion modelling for motion compensation [4] over dynamic treatment planning [6] through to disease progression monitoring of the lung [1] to mention a few. Image registration of 4d datasets turned out to be the beating heart of a successful estimation of motion, where correspondence among temporal states is recovered by finding a meaningful spatial alignment of the image sequence. In contrast to classical registration approaches where smooth transformations are preferred, in the analysis of organ motion the spatial transform mappings are required to contain discontinuous transforms in between the organs along the sliding boundaries. Hence, if

© Springer International Publishing AG 2016
L. Wang et al. (Eds.): MLMI 2016, LNCS 10019, pp. 10–17, 2016.
DOI: 10.1007/978-3-319-47157-0_2

these boundaries are not explicitly considered, the registration usually fails due to misalignments near organ boundaries.

In this paper, we present a new *bilateral* regularization which prefers transformations which are locally homogeneous while preserving discontinuous changes in magnitude of neighboring parameter vectors having equal and opposite directions. This has the effect that non-smooth transformations across organ boundaries stay admissible, with minor influence to the regularization penalty, and simultaneously regions within organs are transformed similarly. Hand in hand with this bilateral regularizer, we construct anisotropic basis functions which consider the structure tensor of the reference image. Thus, we align the transformations tangential to the potential organ boundaries which favours displacements along the boundaries and hinders them to evolve orthogonal to the boundaries.

Our method builds upon a recently presented sparse kernel machine (SKM) [3] for discontinuous registration. Our contribution is threefold: (1) we add bilateral regularization terms which *need not to be norms* and prove the corresponding representer theorem. (2) We integrate anisotropy into the spatially varying kernel of the SKM. Finally, (3) we provide a GPU accelerated implementation which we will make publicly available[1]. We evaluate our method on the 4DCT dataset of the POPI model [13].

The parametric approach to non-rigid image registration has been studied for more than two decades. After the introduction of the free-form deformations into registration [9], a lot of advanced registration approaches have been applied successfully to medical images. A comprehensive overview over non-rigid image registration methods, including non-parametric and discrete approaches, can be found in [11].

Discontinuity preserving attempts appeared increasingly in the past few years [5,8,10,14]. In [10], an anisotropic regularization has been introduced into a Demons like [12] framework, where the regularization has been splitted into tangential and normal directions of the image gradients. In [8], the Demons framework has been extended with an anisotropic *and* a bilateral filtering. Both approaches are non-parametric and specify the transformation properties indirectly through differential operators or smoothing filters and therefore are conceptually rather rigid. Parametric approaches for discontinuity preserving registration are less common [3,14]. In [14], discontinous basis functions are used jointly with a total-variation regularization. They have not explicitly considered organ boundaries and do not explicitly preserve discontinuous changes in the regularizer.

2   Background

In this section, we provide a brief overview over the SKM for image registration originally introduced in [3]. We especially pay attention to the representer theorem which allows for the discretization of the transformation model, having the

---

[1] https://github.com/ChristophJud/SKMImageRegistration.git.

guarantee of a finite dimensional minimizer. We will stick to the notation used in [3].

Let the reference and target image $I_R, I_T : \mathcal{X} \to \mathbb{R}$ map the d-dimensional input domain $\mathcal{X} \subset \mathbb{R}^d$ to scalar values. Given a spatial transform mapping $f : \mathcal{X} \to \mathbb{R}^d$ image registration can be formulated as a regularized functional minimization problem

$$\min_{f} \mathcal{D}[I_R, I_T, f] + \eta \mathcal{R}[f]. \tag{1}$$

The dissimilarity measure $\mathcal{D}$ integrates over a loss function $\mathcal{L} : \mathbb{R} \times \mathbb{R} \to \mathbb{R}$ to indicate how good the target and the transformed reference image match

$$\mathcal{D}[I_R, I_T, f] := \int_{\mathcal{X}} \mathcal{L}(I_R(x + f(x)), I_T(x)) dx. \tag{2}$$

The regularization term $\mathcal{R}$ enforces certain properties of the transformation. A reproducing kernel Hilbert space (RKHS) is defined as transformation model

$$\mathcal{H} := \left\{ f \middle| f(x) = \sum_{i=1}^{\infty} c_i k(x_i, x), \quad x_i \in \mathcal{X}, \quad c_i \in \mathbb{R}^d, \quad \|f\|_{\mathcal{H}} < \infty \right\}, \tag{3}$$

where $k : \mathcal{X} \times \mathcal{X} \to \mathbb{R}$ is a positive definite kernel. For a comprehensive introduction to kernel methods and RKHS we refer to [2]. The RKHS norm $\|f\|_{\mathcal{H}} = \sqrt{\langle f, f \rangle}$, with the inner product $\langle \cdot, \cdot \rangle$ of $\mathcal{H}$, measures the magnitude of f and can be defined as regularization term. Thus, functions within $\mathcal{H}$ which have smaller magnitude are preferred. For the SKM, a sparsity inducing l_1-type norm was introduced as regularization

$$\|f\|_1 := \sum_{i=1}^{N} \|c_i\|_1 + \|v_f\|_{\mathcal{H}}, \tag{4}$$

where $v_f \in \mathcal{H}$ is orthogonal to $\mathcal{H}_0$ and

$$\mathcal{H}_0 = \left\{ f_0 \in \mathcal{H} \middle| f_0(\cdot) = \sum_{i=1}^{N} c_i k(x_i, \cdot), \quad c_i \in \mathbb{R} \right\} \tag{5}$$

is a finite dimensional linear subspace of $\mathcal{H}$ with pair-wise distinct sampled points $\{x_i\}_{i=1}^{N}, x_i \in \mathcal{X}$.

Theorem 1. *Let the training data $\{(x_i, y_i) \in \mathcal{X} \times \mathbb{R} | i = 1, \ldots, N\}$, a loss function $\mathcal{L} : \mathcal{X} \times \mathbb{R} \times \mathbb{R}^d \to \mathbb{R} \cup \{\infty\}$ and two functions $g : \mathbb{R} \to \mathbb{R}$ and $h : \mathbb{R} \to \mathbb{R}$ be given. If one of the two functions g or h is strictly increasing and the other one is nondecreasing, the minimization problem*

$$\min_{f \in \mathcal{H}} \sum_{i=1}^{N} \mathcal{L}(x_i, y_i, f(x_i)) + g(\|f\|_{\mathcal{H}}) + h(\|f\|_1) \tag{6}$$

has a minimizer taking the form

$$f(x) = \sum_{i=1}^{N} c_i k(x_i, x), \quad c_i \in \mathbb{R}^d. \tag{7}$$

In [3] it was proven that each f can be decomposed as

$$f(x) = \sum_{i=1}^{N} c_i k(x_i, x) + v_f \tag{8}$$

for *unique* c_i. Moreover, they showed that $\mathcal{L}$ is independent of v_f and v_f has to be zero for minimizing $g(\|f\|_{\mathcal{H}}) + h(\|f\|_1)$. Hence, each minimizer of (6) lies within $\mathcal{H}_0$. In the following, we will introduce an additional regularization term which will fulfill an extended representer theorem.

3   Method

Both of the above mentioned regularization terms consider the magnitude of the function f. Hence, functions which deviate from the zero transformation are penalized and the smoothness is implicitly given by the basis functions $k(x_i, \cdot)$. In addition, for the sliding organ boundaries, we have the following requirements on the regularization: (1) nearby transform parameters should be locally homogeneous (within organs), (2) they should be admissible if they are pointing in opposite direction (sliding organ boundaries) and (3) they should also be admissible if they have different magnitudes as long as they point in similar directions (moving tissue next to still structure).

3.1   Bilateral Regularizer

Let us start with the following regularization on f

$$\mathcal{B}(f) := \sum_{i,j=1}^{N} \|c_i - c_j\|^2 k(x_i, x_j) + \|v_f\|_{\mathcal{H}}. \tag{9}$$

Dependent on the proximity of the parameters c_i, c_j indicated by $k(x_i, x_j)$ their radiometric difference is penalized. We extend the representer theorem as follows:

Theorem 2. *Let the training data $\{(x_i, y_i) \in \mathcal{X} \times \mathbb{R} | i = 1, \ldots, N\}$ and a loss function $\mathcal{L} : \mathcal{X} \times \mathbb{R} \times \mathbb{R}^d \to \mathbb{R} \cup \{\infty\}$ be given. Furthermore, let the functions $g_i : \mathbb{R} \to \mathbb{R}$ and $p_i : \mathcal{H}_0 \to \mathbb{R}, i = 1 \ldots l$ be weakly lower semicontinuous and bounded from below. If at least one of the functions $g_{i=j}$ is strictly increasing and the other ones $g_{i \neq j}$ are nondecreasing, the minimization problem*

$$\min_{f \in \mathcal{H}} \sum_{i=1}^{N} \mathcal{L}\left(x_i, y_i, f(x_i)\right) + \sum_{i=1}^{l} g_i(p_i(f_0) + \|v_f\|_{\mathcal{H}}) \tag{10}$$

has a minimizer taking the form

$$f(x) = \sum_{i=1}^{N} c_i k(x_i, x), \quad c_i \in \mathbb{R}^d. \tag{11}$$

Proof. Since c_i are unique for a particular f, each summand $g_i(p_i(f_0) + \|v_f\|_{\mathcal{H}})$ is well-defined. As already proved in [3], $\mathcal{L}$ is independent of v_f. The following inequalities hold as g_i are nondecreasing

$$g_i(p_i(f_0) + \|v_f\|_{\mathcal{H}}) \geq g_i(p_i(f_0)) \quad \forall i. \tag{12}$$

For the functions g_i which are strictly increasing, we have that equality holds iff $v_f = 0$. As for the other functions the value does not increase when setting $v_f = 0$, we conclude that (10) can be minimized iff $v_f = 0$.   □

For the bilateral regularizer $\mathcal{B}$ as an example, we set the corresponding p_i to $p_i(f_0) = \sum_{i,j=1}^{N} \|c_i - c_j\|^2 k(x_i, x_j)$. Note that p_i need *not* to be a norm.

With the regularizer $\mathcal{B}$, we meet the first of our requirements. For the specific case of discontinuity preserving registration we want to integrate the two remaining properties as well. Consider the regularizer

$$\mathcal{B}_p(f) := \sum_{i,j=1}^{N} \frac{s^2}{2} \log\left(1 + \frac{1}{s}\mathcal{P}(c_i, c_j)^2\right) k(x_i, x_j) + \|v_f\|_{\mathcal{H}}, \tag{13}$$

where $\mathcal{P} : \mathbb{R}^d \times \mathbb{R}^d \to \mathbb{R}_{\geq 0}$ measures the area of the parallelogram[2] which is spanned by c_i and c_j and a positive scaling s. With this regularizer, nearby parameters which are aligned in direction can discontinuously vary in magnitude and even in pointing in opposite direction without influencing the value of $\mathcal{B}_p$. Thus, $\mathcal{B}_p$ does meet all the above mentioned requirements. The proof of the representer theorem including $\mathcal{B}_p$ is now straight forward. The effect of applying $\mathcal{B}_p$ is shown in Fig. 1.

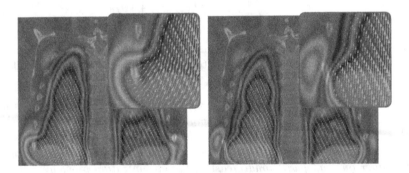

Fig. 1. Coronal slice of an example registration result applying $\mathcal{B}_p$ as regularizer once only slightly (left) and once very strongly (right). The over regularization (right) results in region-wise aligned transformations.

---

[2] Note that for $d = 3$, $\mathcal{P}$ is the magnitude of the cross-product $\|c_i \times c_j\|$.

3.2   Anisotropic Kernel

In addition to the introduced bilateral regularizers we further tailor the framework to sliding organ boundaries by introducing an anisotropic transformation model. We elongate the transformations along potential organ boundaries given a positive definite matrix-valued function Σ. Using Σ, we construct an *anisotropic* and *nonstationary* kernel as it has been proposed in [7]. Thus, we only need an appropriate Σ-function.

We assume, that high gradients in the image indicate potential sliding organ boundaries. Given a guidance image $I : \mathcal{X} \to \mathbb{R}$ (in our case the reference image) we derive the principal directions of intensity changes by performing eigen analysis on the structure tensor S, where $S(x) = U_x \Lambda_x \Lambda_x U_x^T$, U_x contains the eigenvectors column-wise and Λ_x is a diagonal matrix containing the eigenvalues λ_i of $S(x)$ on the diagonal. We use the largest eigenvalue to narrow the kernel in orthogonal direction to the sliding boundaries, while we stretch it in the remaining directions. We scale the eigenvalues

$$\tilde{\lambda}_1 = \frac{1}{1 + \lambda_1^\alpha}, \quad \tilde{\lambda}_i = 1 + \frac{\lambda_1^\alpha}{1 + \lambda_1^\alpha}, \quad i = \{2 \ldots d\}, \tag{14}$$

where α is a positive constant (e.g. $\alpha = 1.5$). The final covariances become $\Sigma(x) = U_x \tilde{\Lambda}_x \tilde{\Lambda}_x U_x^T$. As we assume, that the main motion induced by respiration is aligned with the z-axis, we scale λ_1 with $d^{-1/2}\mathcal{P}(u_1, e_z)^2$ where u_1 is the first eigenvector and e_z is the unit vector in z direction. Thus, the anisotropic distortion is damped, if the direction is not aligned to the respiratory motion.

4   Results

We evaluate our kernel machine with the $l1$-type regularizer (4) for a sparse transform mapping (sKM). Furthermore, denoted as pKM, we apply the parallelogram regularizer $\mathcal{B}_p$. We run sKM and pKM using the isotropic (iso) as well as the anisotropic (ani) transformation model. We used the combined *Wendland* kernel proposed in [3] and always apply the squared loss function.

As dataset, we used the 4DCT POPI model [13] containing a respiratory cycle of a patients thorax including ground truth landmarks. We manually optimized the parameters for image 7 and used the same configuration for all other time steps. The target image was image number 1. We performed gradient descent on three scales with an isotropic control point grid spacing of $\{16, 8, 4\}$ resulting in $\{25\,k, 189\,k, 1.5\,m\}$ parameters and uniformly sampled $\{133\,k, 258\,k, 619\,k\}$ image points. We compare our results to the free-form deformation method FFD [9] and an isotropic variant of the parametric total variation method pTV [14]. For the FFD, we took the transformations from the POPI homepage[3]. For pTV the authors of [14] have kindly provided their TRE[4] values. The expected target registration errors are listed in Table 1. On average (cf. Ø in Table 1), our

---

[3] http://www.creatis.insa-lyon.fr/rio/popi-model.

[4] Target registration error: Euclidean distance between ground truth landmarks and reference landmarks which have been warped by the resulting f.

Table 1. Expected TRE [mm] of the first 40 landmarks with respect to image 1.

Method	0	2	3	4	5	6	7	8	9	Ø	Ø*
No reg.	0.34	0.07	2.15	4.72	5.81	6.25	4.87	4.16	2.11	3.39	5.41
FFD [9]	0.87	0.56	1.01	1.05*	1.06*	1.02*	1.11*	0.76*	0.86	0.92	1.06
pTV [14]	0.64	0.73	1.08	0.99*	0.93*	0.94*	1.08*	0.82*	0.71	0.88	0.98
SKM [3]	0.65	0.50	1.14	0.97*	0.96*	0.90*	0.93*	0.73*	0.66*	0.83	0.94
sKM iso	0.67	0.55	1.00	0.94*	1.03*	0.92*	0.80*	0.69*	0.71	0.81	0.92
sKM ani	0.68	0.53	1.00	0.96*	0.93*	0.93*	0.89*	0.75*	0.71	0.82	0.93
pKM iso	0.69	0.54	0.96	0.94*	1.00*	0.92*	0.81*	0.69*	0.72	0.81	0.92
pKM ani	0.68	0.54	1.05	0.96*	0.93*	0.92*	0.88*	0.76*	0.71	0.83	0.92

The target registration errors have been fitted to the Maxwell-Boltzmann distribution where the derived mean values are listed in the table. In the last two columns, the average mean Ø and a significant average mean Ø* are provided.

methods perform similarly and outperform the tested methods FFD and pTV in terms of TRE. In addition, we highlight the cases 4 to 8, where all methods have a higher probability[5] than 0.95 to beat the non-registered TRE. Their average mean is listed as Ø*. These cases are in the exhalation phase and differ most from the reference image 1, which is in the inhalation state. In Fig. 2, we show qualitative improvements when applying the anisotropic methods.

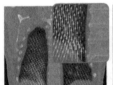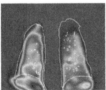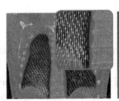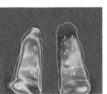

Fig. 2. Registration results (CT slice and corresponding transformation magnitudes) of pKM iso (left) and pKM ani (right). One can see, that with the anisotropic version the lower vertebra is not distorted and the ground truth outline (white) of the lung is better represented in the transformations.

5   Conclusion

We presented a novel method to approach discontinuity preserving image registration. With the introduction of bilateral regularization in a reproducing kernel Hilbert space we opened new possibilities to enforce certain neighborhood

---

[5] We defined the probability of a method H_a to beat the baseline H_0 as $P(X < Y)$, where the *independent* random variables X and Y are distributed according to the Maxwell-Boltzmann distribution of the respective method H_a and H_0.

properties of the transform mapping. By design, the parallelogram regularizer $\mathcal{B}_p$ allows discontinuous changes in neighboring transform parameters as long as they are aligned in direction while it prefers locally homogeneous parameters otherwise. We additionally integrated an anisotropic transformation model into the SKM framework to align the transformations with potential sliding organ boundaries. Our method outperforms the tested approaches on the POPI dataset which was shown in the experiments. However, a thorough evaluation on further datasets is needed and planned in near future.

References

1. Gorbunova, V., Lo, P., Ashraf, H., Dirksen, A., Nielsen, M., de Bruijne, M.: Weight preserving image registration for monitoring disease progression in lung CT. In: Axel, L., Fichtinger, G., Metaxas, D., Székely, G. (eds.) MICCAI 2008, Part II. LNCS, vol. 5242, pp. 863–870. Springer, Heidelberg (2008)
2. Hofmann, T., Schölkopf, B., Smola, A.J.: Kernel methods in machine learning. Ann. Stat. **36**, 1171–1220 (2008)
3. Jud, C., Möri, N., Cattin, P.C.: Sparse kernel machines for discontinuous registration. In: 7th International Workshop on Biomedical Image Registration (2016)
4. Jud, C., Preiswerk, F., Cattin, P.C.: Respiratory motion compensation with topology independent surrogates. In: Workshop on Imaging and Computer Assistance in Radiation Therapy (2015)
5. Kiriyanthan, S., Fundana, K., Majeed, T., Cattin, P.C.: A primal-dual approach for discontinuity preserving image registration through motion segmentation. Int. J. Comput. Math. Methods Med. (2016, in press)
6. Möri, N., Jud, C., Salomir, R., Cattin, P.C.: Leveraging respiratory organ motion for non-invasive tumor treatment devices: a feasibility study. Phys. Med. Biol. **61**(11), 4247–4267 (2016)
7. Paciorek, C.J., Schervish, M.J.: Spatial modelling using a new class of nonstationary covariance functions. Environmetrics **17**(5), 483–506 (2006)
8. Papież, B.W., Heinrich, M.P., Fehrenbach, J., Risser, L., Schnabel, J.A.: An implicit sliding-motion preserving regularisation via bilateral filtering for deformable image registration. Med. Image Anal. **18**(8), 1299–1311 (2014)
9. Rueckert, D., Sonoda, L.I., Hayes, C., Hill, D.L.G., Leach, M.O., Hawkes, D.J.: Nonrigid registration using free-form deformations: application to breast MR images. IEEE Trans. Med. Imaging **18**(8), 712–721 (1999)
10. Schmidt-Richberg, A.: Sliding motion in image registration. Registration Methods for Pulmonary Image Analysis, pp. 65–78. Springer, Wiesbaden (2014)
11. Sotiras, A., Davatzikos, C., Paragios, N.: Deformable medical image registration: a survey. IEEE Trans. Med. Imaging **32**(7), 1153–1190 (2013)
12. Thirion, J.-P.: Image matching as a diffusion process: an analogy with Maxwell's demons. Med. Image Anal. **2**(3), 243–260 (1998)
13. Vandemeulebroucke, J., Sarrut, D., Clarysse, P.: The POPI-model, a point-validated pixel-based breathing thorax model. In: International Conference on the Use of Computers in Radiation Therapy, vol. 2, pp. 195–199 (2007)
14. Vishnevskiy, V., Gass, T., Székely, G., Goksel, O.: Total variation regularization of displacements in parametric image registration. In: Yoshida, H., Näppi, J.J., Saini, S. (eds.) ABDI 2014. LNCS, vol. 8676, pp. 211–220. Springer, Heidelberg (2014)

Do We Need Large Annotated Training Data for Detection Applications in Biomedical Imaging? A Case Study in Renal Glomeruli Detection

Michael Gadermayr[1]([✉]), Barbara Mara Klinkhammer[2], Peter Boor[2], and Dorit Merhof[1]

[1] Aachen Center for Biomedical Image Analysis, Visualization and Exploration
(ACTIVE), Institute of Imaging and Computer Vision,
RWTH Aachen University, Aachen, Germany
`Michael.Gadermayr@lfb.rwth-aachen.de`
[2] Institute of Pathology, University Hospital Aachen, RWTH Aachen University,
Aachen, Germany

Abstract. Approaches for detecting regions of interest in biomedical image data mostly assume that a large amount of annotated training data is available. Certainly, for unchanging problem definitions, the acquisition of large annotated data is time consuming, yet feasible. However, distinct practical problems with large training corpi arise if variability due to different imaging conditions or inter-personal variations lead to significant changes in the image representation. To circumvent these issues, we investigate a classifier learning scenario which requires a small amount of positive annotation data only. Contrarily to previous approaches which focus on methodologies to explicitly or implicitly deal with specific classification scenarios (such as one-class classification), we show that existing supervised classification models can handle a changed setting effectively without any specific modifications.

1 Introduction

The detection of regions of interest is a highly relevant field in biomedical image analysis. Some specific applications comprise the detection of cells [11] in microscopic image data and the localization of intracranial aneurysms [5].

Depending on intra- and inter-class variations in image data sets, for effective training of classification models large amounts of annotated training data have to be acquired in order to precisely estimate the decision boundaries [7]. For unchanging problem definitions, the acquisition and annotation of large training data is time consuming, but acceptable. However, issues with large training data arise if variations due to different imaging conditions or due to manual acquisition [4] lead to distinct changes in the image representation. This inflexibility of learning-based systems constitutes a severe obstacle for realistic application scenarios.

In recent literature, several strategies to deal with variations in the image domain were identified. Specific variations can be compensated by means of

L. Wang et al. (Eds.): MLMI 2016, LNCS 10019, pp. 18–26, 2016.
DOI: 10.1007/978-3-319-47157-0_3

image normalization. The proposed methods reach from simple contrast normalization to more sophisticated and specific methods such as stain normalization [2]. Another approach to compensate variability such as scale-, rotation- and illumination-variations is given by invariant image descriptors [3]. Finally, variations can be modeled and compensated by learning a transformation between training and test data [9]. Whereas domain adaptation methods [9] are explicitly developed to deal with slight domain shifts only, methods claimed to be invariant [3] not necessarily outperform conventional ones in real-world applications. Normalization is only sensibly applicable for some specific kinds of variations such as changes in color-intensity.

In order to circumvent issues arising due to distinct variability in the image data, we pose the question if we can elude the requirement of large expert-annotated training data in the detection scenario. Our further considerations are based on two observations which apply to many biomedical detection applications [11]: (1) Target objects (samples of positive class) in the detection scenario constitute a small area compared to the overall image and (2) intra-class variations within the positive class are generally smaller than variations within the negative class.

For traditional supervised machine learning, experts would either need to extract significant amounts of positive and negative class patches in several images, or they would need to fully detect all target objects per image (so that the rest is negative). Both procedures are time consuming and thereby represent obstacles for real world application of computer-aided detection systems in practical scenarios. In order to circumvent the necessity of large training data, we consider a learning scenario with few annotated positive samples only, which can be quickly and interactively labeled by the user. For classifier training, these positive samples are combined with randomly chosen negative samples which thereby contain noise due to overlaps with positive class regions.

Detection approaches from literature dealing with learning scenarios that deviate from the traditional supervised dichtomizing classification include learning from positive and unlabeled samples [12], one-class learning [8] as well as learning with noisy labels [10]. All of these well-known approaches consider training scenarios which are not based on reliable label data of all classes. To compensate the modified requirement, they rely on separate pre-processing steps [10,12] or on algorithms which can handle the changed setting implicitly [8]. Recent work [7] also addressed the question whether expert annotation can be circumvented by substantially larger training data labeled by non-experts. For a different classification application, evidence is available that negative effects of label noise can actually be compensated by large training corpi without any modifications of the underlying classification model.

Similarly, in this work we do not propose a novel learning approach to handle specific anomalies within the image data. Instead, we study the fundamental question whether a robust discriminative classification model can handle the changed scenario without any further adjustments, which has not been investigated so far.

1.1   Contribution

In this work, we investigate whether learning could be effectively performed based on few user labeled positive samples as well as a large number of randomly selected negative samples. The small number of positive training samples can be easily and efficiently obtained by user interaction for each individual image being totally independent from large training corpi as well as inter-image similarities. The negative training samples are automatically and randomly extracted from the images. Thereby these samples contain noise due to random overlaps with positive class regions. Our case study especially investigates the task of glomeruli detection from whole slide images of kidneys [4,6]. Due to high-resolution image data, a manual annotation is extremely time consuming. Traditional supervised methods suffer from distinct inter-slide variations caused by the preparation of slides, the staining process as well as histopathological variations. Relying on a standard classification model as well as four image representation approaches, we show that the investigated setting performs well and outperforms the traditional supervised classification protocol based on a similar amount of annotated training data.

2   Experimental Study

In this experimental study, the focus is on detecting renal glomeruli based on histological whole-slide image data [4,6]. In mammalian kidneys, glomeruli are the first segment of nephrons, the microscopical functional unit of kidneys, and consist of a tuft of small blood vessels (capillaries), where blood is filtered and primarily urine is produced. Several kidney diseases affect and damage the glomeruli, which results in a loss of the filter function. The diagnosis, and thereby the decision on adequate treatment is currently based on renal biopsies. Due to clinical needs there is also a strong research focus on renal diseases and specifically on the analyses of glomerular damage. Since such manual identification and quantification of morphological glomerular alterations is extremely time consuming, supporting automated glomeruli detection would greatly facilitate the analyses of glomerular diseases in both clinical and experimental settings.

Methods for detecting renal glomeruli have to deal with inconveniences: Due to strong variability especially in the negative class (non-glomerulus), large amounts of labeled training data have to be acquired in order to obtain reliable classification models. Additionally, variations due to different staining protocols so far require separate training sets per imaging protocol. These variations do not only occur between whole slide images prepared with different stains, but also in case of similar ones which is due to the manual image acquisition process. Finally, detection has to cope with variations due to pathological changes. In spite of these difficult circumstances, the two observations (from Sect. 1) generally drawn from many detection applications are assumed to apply because: (1) Glomeruli cover insignificant areas of the kidney and thereby the introduced noise level is assumed to be low. Whereas the kidney covers approximately $10^5 \times 10^5$ pixels, one glomerulus typically has a size of about 250×250 pixels. As a whole slide

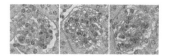 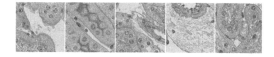

Fig. 1. Example patches of positive (glomeruli, left) and negative class (right).

image contains typically 200 glomeruli, these structure covers approximately 10^7 pixels, which is a fraction of only 0.1 %. (2) Whereas texture outside of regions to be detected shows strong variations, texture of the target objects visually exhibits a rather low degree of intra-class variability as exemplarily illustrated in Fig. 1.

2.1   Image Dataset

The image data was obtained from resected mice kidneys (showing high similarity to human kidneys). Kidneys were processed as previously described [1], in short they were fixed in methyl Carnoy's solution and embedded in paraffin. Paraffin sections ($1 \mu m$) were stained with periodic acid-Schiff reagent and counterstained with hematoxylin. Whole slides were digitalized with a Hamamatsu NanoZoomer 2.0HT digital slide scanner and a 20× objective lens. For evaluation, three renal whole slide images showing significant variations with a size of 53248×40704 pixels are evaluated containing 147 (image 1), 183 (image 2) and 199 renal glomeruli (image 3), respectively. The background of the whole slide image data, is not considered during processing.

2.2   Proposed Architecture

First, for classifier training, patches of a fixed size are extracted in the center of annotated glomeruli, representing the positive class. Negative class patches are randomly selected from the whole slide image without considering the positive class samples. The patch size depends on the utilized image representation (Sect. 2.3). We specifically investigate varying numbers of labeled overall training samples s with $s \in \{2, 4, 8, 16, 32\}$ and three different scenarios: First, we investigate traditional classifier training with $\frac{s}{2}$ labeled samples of both classes (referred to as BASE). The two further approaches rely on s labeled positive samples and $10s$ randomly selected samples (Tx10) or 1000 randomly selected samples as negative class sample data (T1000), respectively. For classification, a linear C-SVM[1] is trained with four different image representations. This model is furthermore utilized to evaluate probabilities of evaluation set patch data by applying the sliding window approach with a step size of 50 pixels [6]. The matrix representing the positive class probabilities is convolved with a Laplacian-of-Gaussian operator to delineate punctually high probabilities in the midst of

---

[1] We use the MATLAB C-SVM implementation.

low probabilities. The Gaussian σ is set in a way that the radius of zeros corresponds to the expected glomeruli size which is generally relatively constant (128 pixels). Finally, these values are thresholded and the maxima of each connected component are extracted representing the detected glomeruli centers. In order to avoid any bias, the threshold for one image is evaluated based on the maximization of the balanced F-score of the other whole slide images. Training and evaluation is performed on the same images to focus on a realistic interactive learning scenario independent of any stored training data.

2.3 Image Representations and Evaluation Details

For image representation, two methods which have been successfully applied in glomerulus detection (Rectangular histogram of oriented gradients (HOG) [6], 3D Color Histograms (I1H2H3) [4] consisting of 10^3 bins) have been deployed as well as two further, more compact and straightforward representations (MS, MSD), which are supposed to be suitable in combination with few training data. MS is a simple descriptor consisting of the means and the standard deviations for each of the three color channels of the RGB image. Thereby, the color distribution in the images which is Gaussian-like is efficiently captured. MSD consists of mean gray values after binarization (setting the threshold to the median of the image) and erosion as well as dilation with disks of variable radii. Specifically, radii between one and six pixels are chosen corresponding to typical sizes of structures in the histopathological images. Applying this procedure separately to each color channel, a 36-dimensional vector is obtained $(3 \cdot (6 + 6))$. Thereby, statistical information of the shapes obtained after binarization is extracted. The latter two methods are deployed due to their compactness, because high dimensional methods such as HOG with 128 dimensions are supposed to be vulnerable to small training data sets. As proposed, the patch size is set to 800×800 pixels (HOG [6]) and 200×200 pixels in case of the other descriptors [4], respectively. All descriptors are L^2 normalized.

The SVM's c-values (one per class) are evaluated during cross-validation. However, the ratio between the c-values of the two classes is fixed according to the ratio of utilized training data. Thereby, a false sample in the negative class training data (which has a lower weight due to the larger amount of data) only marginally influences the evaluated decision hyperplane. In order to obtain stable results, classifier training and evaluation is performed 16 times. In each iteration, the random selection of training set samples is repeated. Finally, in the results section we report the mean F-scores as well as standard-deviations. To assess whether improvements are statistically significant a left-tailed Wilcoxon rank-sum test is applied.

2.4 Fraction of Mislabeled Training Data

Before assessing the performance of the proposed training scenario, we estimate the amount of false training samples in the negative class (Sect. 2, observation (1)). As extracted patches are not necessarily located completely inside or outside

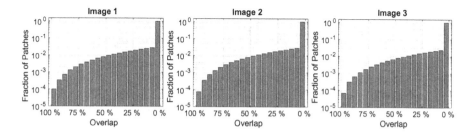

Fig. 2. Overlaps (Jaccard index) of negative class training data with positive class.

of glomeruli, we differentiate with regard to the area of overlap between negative class samples and positive class image regions. Figure 2 shows for varying overlap fractions the cumulative density of the thus distorted negative class training data. For a certain overlap fraction, the bar represents the fraction of negative class data which is at least affected by this overlap. Considering the second bar from the right (per plot), it can be observed that approximately 2 % of patches contain any overlap with data corresponding to the false class. Regarding only distinct overlaps ($\geq$50 %), less than 1 % of patches are affected.

2.5 Variability in Positive and Negative Class

Next, we experimentally evaluate if observation (2) can be confirmed quantitatively. We compute the mean between all pairwise Euclidean feature distances within the two classes. In Fig. 3, the fraction between the mean of the positive and the negative class is reported. Thereby, a small value indicates a high difference and a value close to one indicates a low difference. We notice that (apart form HOG), the assumption definitely holds as the fractions are generally low ($<$0.25).

2.6 Detection Results

In our main experiment, we study the performance obtained with the proposed protocol compared to traditional supervised training based on correct positive

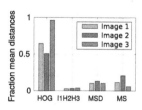

Fig. 3. Fraction of mean distances of positive and mean distances of negative class.

and negative samples (referred to as BASE). We evaluate varying overall training set sizes as well as two settings of the novel protocol. Setting Tx10 considers ten times more negative training data compared to positive class training data. Setting T1000 collects a fixed amount of 1000 samples of the negative class. Figure 4 shows the balanced F-scores obtained with the proposed protocol (Tx10 and T1000) as well as traditional supervised training (BASE) combined with all image description methods. The large symbols (see legend) connected by the solid lines show the mean F-scores whereas the small symbols connected by vertical dashed lines present the standard deviations. On the horizontal axis, the number of overall labeled training samples is provided. Asterisks (see legend) indicate a statistically significant improvement of both new protocols (Tx10 and T1000) compared to traditional classification. Regarding the outcomes with image descriptors which have already been investigated with respect to glomeruli

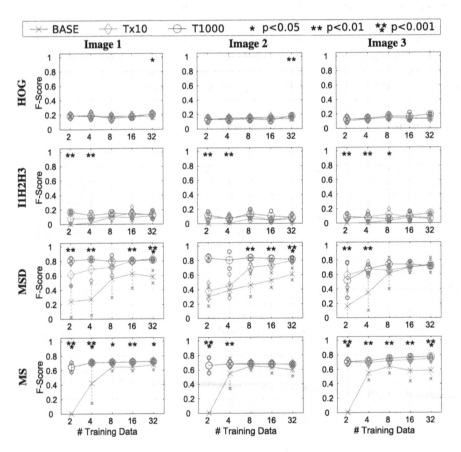

Fig. 4. Performance comparison of renal glomeruli detection protocols: These plots present F-scores obtained with the proposed protocol (Tx10 and T1000) compared to traditional supervised learning (BASE) for varying training set sizes. Asterisks indicate significant improvements of both new methods compared to the traditional approach.

detection, it can be observed that these methods do not perform well. Similarly for HOG and I1H2H3, even with 32 labeled samples for classifier training, an appropriate classification model cannot be estimated. Regardless of the training protocol, F-scores remain below 0.25. Considering the outcomes of the more compact MSD descriptor, a significantly improved performance can be observed. With the standard protocoll (BASE), F-scores between 0.44 and 0.62 are achieved with only eight training data images. With the proposed technique these performances can be even increased further and detection rates of up to 0.84 are obtained. The setting based on more (fixed) training data (T1000) mostly delivers superior outcomes. Similar results are observed in case of the very simple and efficient MS descriptor. Traditional supervised classification can be clearly outperformed by the new protocol and even with only two annotated samples F-scores up to 0.70 can be reached. The standard-deviations generally decrease in case of the proposed technique.

3   Discussion

In this work, an effective learning protocol is proposed which can be practically applied to manifold detection scenarios as it is not based on large training data and can be combined with traditional supervised classification models. Here, we specifically investigated a linear SVM which is known to be robust to label noise, however, other models could be considered in future work as well. We showed that the fraction of overlaps between negative training data and positive image regions is small and that variability within the positive class is smaller than in the negative class. Considering the main experiments, even with very few manually labeled training samples, the proposed protocol delivers excellent outcomes. Additionally, we notice that the novel protocol corresponds to distinctly decreased standard-deviations which means that the impact of the selection of the training data virtually vanishes. Methods extracting high dimensional features cannot be effectively applied in combination with few training data. Even with the new protocol, only subtle performance gains are achieved. This is supposedly due to larger intra-class variations in the feature space of positive class samples in combination with the higher dimensional descriptors (especially with HOG). Considering the distribution of false-negative samples in the training data (Fig. 2), image 3 seems to be most appropriate containing the lowest number of false training samples. Although the overlap differences are quite small, most distinct improvements considering the detection performance (Fig. 4) in case of this image could indicate a correlation.

In summary, this work shows that an existing supervised machine learning method has not necessarily to be modified to deal with the investigated learning scenario. Our results indicate that related detection scenarios with comparable distributions of regions of interest can benefit in a similar way from the proposed protocol.

Acknowledgments. This work was supported by the German Research Foundation (DFG), grant number ME3737/3-1.

References

1. Boor, P., et al.: Role of platelet-derived growth factor-CC in capillary rarefaction in renal fibrosis. Am. J. Pathol. **185**, 2132–2142 (2015)
2. Dauguet, J., Mangin, J.-F., Delzescaux, T., Frouin, V.: Robust inter-slice intensity normalization using histogram scale-space analysis. In: Barillot, C., Haynor, D.R., Hellier, P. (eds.) MICCAI 2004. LNCS, vol. 3216, pp. 242–249. Springer, Heidelberg (2004). doi:10.1007/978-3-540-30135-6_30
3. Hegenbart, S., Uhl, A., Vécsei, A., Wimmer, G.: Scale invariant texture descriptors for classifying celiac disease. Med. Image Anal. **17**(4), 458–474 (2013)
4. Herve, N., Servais, A., Thervet, E., Olivo-Marin, J.C., Meas-Yedid, V.: Statistical color texture descriptors for histological images analysis. In: ISBI, pp. 724–727. IEEE press, New York (2011)
5. Jerman, T., Pernuš, F., Likar, B., Špiclin, Ž.: Computer-aided detection and quantification of intracranial aneurysms. In: Navab, N., Hornegger, J., Wells, W.M., Frangi, A.F. (eds.) MICCAI 2015. LNCS, vol. 9350, pp. 3–10. Springer, Heidelberg (2015). doi:10.1007/978-3-319-24571-3_1
6. Kato, T., Relator, R., Ngouv, H., Hirohashi, Y., Takaki, O., Kakimoto, T., Okada, K.: Segmental HOG: new descriptor for glomerulus detection in kidney microscopy image. BMC Bioinform. **16**(1), 316 (2015)
7. Kwitt, R., Hegenbart, S., Rasiwasia, N., Vécsei, A., Uhl, A.: Do we need annotation experts? A case study in celiac disease classification. In: Golland, P., Hata, N., Barillot, C., Hornegger, J., Howe, R. (eds.) MICCAI 2014. LNCS, vol. 8674, pp. 454–461. Springer, Heidelberg (2014). doi:10.1007/978-3-319-10470-6_57
8. Liu, W., Hua, G., Smith, J.R.: Unsupervised one-class learning for automatic outlier removal. In: CVPR, pp. 3826–3833. IEEE press, New York (2014)
9. Mirrashed, F., Rastegari, M.: Domain adaptive classification. In: ICCV, pp. 2608–2615. IEEE press, New York (2013)
10. Vahdat, A., Mori, G.: Handling uncertain tags in visual recognition. In: ICCV, pp. 737–744. IEEE press, New York (2013)
11. Xie, Y., Xing, F., Kong, X., Su, H., Yang, L.: Beyond classification: structured regression for robust cell detection using convolutional neural network. In: Navab, N., Hornegger, J., Wells, W.M., Frangi, A.F. (eds.) MICCAI 2015. LNCS, vol. 9351, pp. 358–365. Springer, Heidelberg (2015). doi:10.1007/978-3-319-24574-4_43
12. Zuluaga, M.A., Hush, D., Delgado Leyton, E.J.F., Hoyos, M.H., Orkisz, M.: Learning from only positive and unlabeled data to detect lesions in vascular CT images. In: Fichtinger, G., Martel, A., Peters, T. (eds.) MICCAI 2011. LNCS, vol. 6893, pp. 9–16. Springer, Heidelberg (2011). doi:10.1007/978-3-642-23626-6_2

Building an Ensemble of Complementary Segmentation Methods by Exploiting Probabilistic Estimates

Gerard Sanroma[1]([✉]), Oualid M. Benkarim[1], Gemma Piella[1],
and Miguel Ángel González Ballester[1,2]

[1] Univ. Pompeu Fabra, Barcelona, Spain
gerard.sanroma@upf.edu
[2] ICREA, Barcelona, Spain

Abstract. Two common ways of approaching atlas-based segmentation of brain MRI are (1) intensity-based modelling and (2) multi-atlas label fusion. Intensity-based methods are robust to registration errors but need distinctive image appearances. Multi-atlas label fusion can identify anatomical correspondences with faint appearance cues, but needs a reasonable registration. We propose an ensemble segmentation method that combines the complementary features of both types of approaches. Our method uses the probabilistic estimates of the base methods to compute their optimal combination weights in a spatially varying way. We also propose an intensity-based method (to be used as base method) that offers a trade-off between invariance to registration errors and dependence on distinct appearances. Results show that sacrificing invariance to registration errors (up to a certain degree) improves the performance of our intensity-based method. Our proposed ensemble method outperforms the rest of participating methods in most of the structures of the NeoBrainS12 Challenge on neonatal brain segmentation. We achieve up to ~10 % of improvement in some structures.

Keywords: Multi-atlas segmentation · Ensemble learning · Patch-based label fusion · Brain MRI

1 Introduction

Segmentation of brain tissues and structures is important for quantitative analysis of neuroimaging data. Two major trends of approaching this problem are multi-atlas label fusion and intensity-based modelling. Multi-atlas label fusion (MALF) consists of registering a set of atlases onto the target image, and then combining their labelmaps into a consensus target segmentation [4,10,13]. The label on each target point is usually computed as a weighted voting of the registered atlas labels in a neighborhood. Such weights, denoting the importance of each atlas decision, are usually computed by means of local image (i.e., patch) similarity. Patch similarity is highly effective at delimiting different structures,

© Springer International Publishing AG 2016
L. Wang et al. (Eds.): MLMI 2016, LNCS 10019, pp. 27–35, 2016.
DOI: 10.1007/978-3-319-47157-0_4

even when they share similar appearance characteristics. However, a reasonable registration is needed, since anatomical correspondence is based on a neighborhood search. This is partially alleviated by using multiple atlases, but it is a problem when using only a few atlases, especially in the case of convoluted structures. Also, enlarging the neighborhood search beyond certain limits actually degrades the performance due to false positives issues with the patch similarity criteria. Another kind of methods use image intensity-based models, either generative [3] or discriminative ones [1]. Most of these methods assume a global intensity model for each structure, so they are robust to registration errors to some extent (or do not require registration at all). This is an advantage for convoluted structures which are difficult to register, but it is a problem for the ones with weak appearance cues. As our first contribution, we propose a discriminative method that alleviates this problem by breaking down the modeling of the intensities in the image into different (automatically defined) regions. By building region-specific models, we improve the discrimination based on intensity at the cost of relying on a rough spatial localization of the regions in the image. A similar idea was explored in [8], although they used generative models and manually-defined regions.

The main contribution of this paper is an ensemble segmentation method that combines the complementary features of intensity-based and label fusion approaches. Following the idea of stacking [7], we learn the systematic combination of base methods that produces the best accuracy. Our method does not require any additional data besides the atlases already used by the base methods. To further limit the dependence on the number of atlases, we use the probabilistic estimates of the base methods (instead of the crisp segmentations), which improves the generalization abilities of stacking [7]. Although we focus on combining intensity-based and label fusion methods, the methodological framework described in this paper can be used to combine any kind of base methods as long as they provide probabilistic estimates. Figure 1 shows the pipeline of our

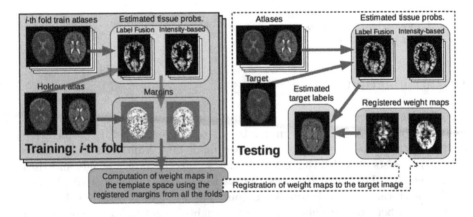

Fig. 1. Pipeline of the method. (Color figure online)

method. A related work by Ledig *et al.* [6] proposed to refine the results of label fusion by using intensity-based models. Such refinement was based on the variation of intensity distributions between the refined and non-refined segmentations. This heuristic is suitable for correcting errors that produce large variations in the intensity distributions (typically, merging csf-like with non-csf-like structures), whereas our method deals with learning a systematic combination of an arbitrary set of methods which is optimal given the set of available atlases.

2   Method

We denote the to-be-segmented target image as T, with T_i denoting the image intensity at voxel i. The atlases consist of a set of n images and labelmaps, where A_{ij} and $L_{ij} \in \{1, \dots, p\}$ denote, respectively, the intensity value and anatomical structure present at voxel i of j-th atlas (we assume that atlas images and labelmaps are registered to the target). We first present our regional learning-based method, as a representative of intensity-based methods, and then we move on to present our proposed ensemble method.

2.1   Regional Learning-Based Segmentation

Learning-based methods aim at finding a function $f : \mathbb{R}^d \to \{1, \dots, p\}$ mapping a set of image features with their corresponding anatomical label. In supervised learning, we use a training set drawn from the atlases, denoted as $\{\mathbf{x}_{ij}, y_{ij} | i \in \Omega\}_{j=1}^n$, using the whole image domain Ω, where $\mathbf{x}_{ij}$ and y_{ij} denote the image features and anatomical label from atlas j at position i, respectively. Note that this approach is invariant to registration, since the classifier is learned on the whole image domain, but it assumes stable appearance properties across the image. An option to roughly take into account the spatial information is to include the position i into the feature vector as done by [1]. Instead, we propose to partition the image into disjoint parcels, denoted as $\{\Gamma_r | \bigcup_r \Gamma_r = \Omega\}$, and learn a different classifier f_r for each region. In order to generate appropriate regions for the classifiers, we use the SLIC [11] algorithm to divide a template image into super-voxels. Note that we need the training images to be registered to a template in order to draw the samples from each region. Our goal is to learn a classifier f_r for each region Γ_r independently. In the case of SVM, we compute each regional classifier f_r by optimizing the following objective:

$$\min_{f_r} \; \text{reg}\,(f_r) + C \sum_j^n \sum_{i \in \Gamma_r} \xi_{ij} \quad \text{s.t.} \quad y_{ij} f_r(\mathbf{x}_{ij}) \geq 1 - \xi_{ij} \tag{1}$$

where $\text{reg}\,(\cdot)$ is the regularization term penalizing highly complex functions, ξ_{ij} indicates the error incurred by each training sample and C controls the trade-off between data fitting and regularization.

In the testing phase, the (crisp) label at position $i \in \Gamma_r$ on a new target image, denoted as F_i, is assigned using the corresponding regional classifier $F_i = f_r(\mathbf{x}_i)$, where $\mathbf{x}_i$ denotes the target image features at position i. In order to obtain probabilistic estimates to be used by our ensemble method, we apply the method by Wu *et al.* [15].

2.2   Ensemble Segmentation Based on Probabilistic Estimates

Based on the observation that label fusion and intensity-based segmentation methods have complementary features, we aim at finding the optimal combination at the different regions. We follow the idea of stacking which consists in combining the prediction of the base methods, in particular their probabilistic estimates, in an effective way. Formally, the target label at position i is computed as follows:

$$F_i = \arg \max_{s \in \{1,\ldots,p\}} \sum_k \omega_{ik} P_{is}^k, \tag{2}$$

where P_{is}^k is the probability of voxel i having label s according to the k-th segmentation method (yellow panels in Fig. 1) and ω_{ik} is the weight for method k at position i (red panels in Fig. 1).

The margin of a classifier is related to the distance of the samples to the classification boundary. The higher the value of the margin, the lower the risk of misclassification. The margin of a base method at point i can be defined as $m_i^k = \Lambda_{ik} P_{ic}^k$, where $\Lambda_{ik} \in \{1, -1\}$ denotes whether the predicted label by method k (say, c) is correct (1) or not (-1) and P_{ic}^k is the confidence of such prediction. The margin is positive in case of correct prediction and negative otherwise (proportionally to the confidence of the prediction). The green panels in Fig. 1 show the margins of the base methods. Here, the notion of complementarity is nicely captured by the fact that their margins should be uncorrelated.

We compute the weights of the ensemble in a leave-one-atlas-out fashion (gray panel in Fig. 1). That is, we use each method to segment the hold-out atlas using the rest of the atlases (yellow panel in Fig. 1). For each point i, the margin of the ensemble is defined as [7]:

$$m_i(\mathbf{w}) = \sum_k \omega_k \Lambda_{ik} P_{ic}^k \quad \text{s.t.} \quad \sum_k \omega_k = 1, \tag{3}$$

where $\omega_k \in \mathbf{w}$ is the weight of method k and $\Lambda_{ik} P_{ic}^k$ is its margin. To avoid the loss of precision, the margins of each method are computed in the native space of each hold-out atlas and then transformed to the template space to compute the weights (orange panel in Fig. 1). Instead of computing a weights $\mathbf{w}$ for each point, we use a certain step size and compute the weights for a neighborhood $\mathcal{N}$. We compute the weights that minimize the following quadratic loss:

$$\min_{\mathbf{w}} \sum_{i \in \mathcal{N}} (1 - m_i(\mathbf{w}))^2 + \lambda \|\mathbf{w}\|^2 = \min_{\mathbf{w}} \|U - M\mathbf{w}\|_2^2 + \lambda \|\mathbf{w}\|_2^2, \tag{4}$$

where U is a vector of ones, M is a matrix with each column M_k containing the margins of method k for all the neighborhood (i.e., $M_k = \left[m_1^k, \ldots, m_i^k, \ldots, m_{|\mathcal{N}|}^k\right]^\top$, $i \in \mathcal{N}$) and λ is a regularization parameter.

The computed weights can be used to segment any new target image using the same atlases and segmentation methods as used for training. Given a new target image T, first, the segmentation probabilities are obtained by each of the methods (yellow panel in Fig. 1). Then, the weight maps are registered to the target space and the target labels are obtained as denoted in Eq. (2) (blue panel in Fig. 1).

3   Experiments

We present tissue segmentation experiments in the IBSR dataset [14] and tissue/sub-cortical structure segmentation experiments in the NeoBrainS12 challenge dataset [5]. Prior to segmentation we correct inhomogeneities with the N4 algorithm [12] and match the histograms to a template image [9]. Template images have been built from the images of the respective datasets using the ANTs [2] script `buildtemplateparallel.sh`. Images have been non-rigidly registered to the template, and pairwise atlas-target registrations required by the base methods are obtained by concatenating the registrations through the template.

3.1   IBSR Dataset

The IBSR dataset [14] contains 18 images with manual annotations of several tissues. We evaluate the segmentation performance on white matter (WM), gray matter (GM) and ventricular cerebrospinal fluid (CSF). We use 4 images as atlases and the remaining 14 as targets. We try to select 4 representative atlases according to their distribution in the manifold.

We combine joint label fusion (JointLF) with the regional learning-based (RegLB) method proposed in Sect. 2.1. For RegLB, we use the following image features: image intensity, laplacian and magnitude of the gradient after convolution with a Gaussian kernels with $\sigma = 1, 2, 3$ (we did not find any improvement by including position as feature). We randomly pick 5 % of the data to train the classifier for each region.

First, in Fig. 2 (left) we show the boxplots of the Dice scores obtained by increasing the number of parcels in RegLB. As we can see, the accuracy increases by decreasing the size of the parcels until the top performance is reached at ~5000 parcels, thus confirming the hypothesis that better results are obtained with more local models. In Fig. 2 (middle) we show the boxplots of the Dice scores by JointLF, RegLB (5000 parcels) and their combination as described in Sect. 2.2. As we can see, results by JointLF and RegLB are similar in terms of Dice score. However, their combination improves considerably, thus confirming the advantages of combining complementary methods (we also tried to combine different RegLB at multiple parcellation levels, obtaining no improvement). Finally, Fig. 2 (right) shows a slice of the weight maps obtained for each of the base methods. As we can see, RegLB has higher weights in the cortical area (a highly convoluted area) whereas JointLF has higher weights in the interior.

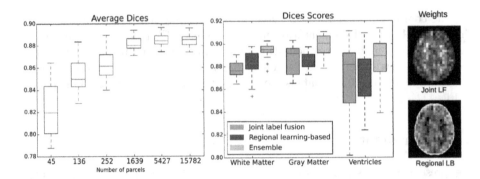

Fig. 2. Results in the IBSR dataset.

3.2   NeoBrainS12 Challenge

The NeoBrainS12 Challenge dataset contains T1 and T2 scans of neonates at
30 weeks and 40 weeks gestational age (GA), divided into training and testing
sets. Training images include manual annotations of the following 8 structures:
cortical gray matter, basal ganglia and thalami, unmyelinated white matter,
myelinated white matter, brainstem, cerebellum, ventricles and cerebrospinal
fluid in the extracerebral space. Participants have no access to the manual annotations on the testing set. There are 2 training and 5 testing images at 30 weeks
coronal, 2 training and 5 testing images at 40 weeks axial, and 5 remaining testing images at 40 weeks coronal. We use the 2 training images at each gestational
age as atlases in our method. Here, we combine joint label fusion [13] (JointLF)
and the intensity-based method Atropos [3]. We use the probabilistic results of
JointLF as spatial prior for Atropos. There is a parameter $0 \leq w \leq 1$ regulating
the importance of the prior in Atropos, with $w = 0$ resulting in segmentations
totally driven by image intensities and $w = 1$ resulting in segmentations very
similar to JointLF. The optimal value of this parameter, based on the results in
the training set, were $w = 0.2$ for 30 weeks GA and $w = 0.1$ for 40 weeks GA.
In Table 1 we show the average Dice scores obtained by our method over the
testing images (as reported by the organizers[1]) in each of the structures, along
with the best score obtained among *all* the rest of methods.

As we can see, our method obtains the best results in the majority of the
structures overall. It is worth noting that we are comparing our results with the
best performing method among the rest, which is usually different for each structure. Our method achieves improvements of up to ~10 % in some structures such
as the brainstem and the challenging myelinated white matter (MWM). Figure 3
shows some qualitative segmentation results on the testing images for 30 weeks
(top) and 40 weeks (bottom) gestational age. Yellow ellipses denote interior
structures where Atropos fails likely due to weak appearance cues. Blue ellipses

---

[1] Results should appear as "SIMBioSys_UPF" at http://neobrains12.isi.uu.nl/
mainResults.php.

denote cortical zones where JointLF fails likely due to registration artifacts. Our ensemble method obtains a satisfactory combination in all areas.

Table 1. Dice scores in the NeoBrainS12 Challenge.

30 weeks coronal

	Cb	MWM	BGT	Vent	UWM	BS	CoGM	CSF	U+M	CSF+V
Ensemble	**0.92**	0.66	**0.90**	**0.88**	**0.93**	**0.86**	**0.75**	**0.85**	**0.93**	**0.86**
Best score*	0.88	**0.69**	0.84	**0.88**	0.91	0.76	0.71	0.83	0.90	0.84

40 weeks axial

	Cb	MWM	BGT	Vent	UWM	BS	CoGM	CSF	U+M	CSF+V
Ensemble	**0.94**	**0.54**	**0.93**	0.83	**0.91**	**0.85**	0.85	**0.79**	0.90	0.79
Best score*	0.92	0.47	0.92	**0.86**	0.90	0.83	**0.86**	**0.79**	**0.92**	**0.80**

40 weeks coronal

	Cb	MWM	BGT	Vent	UWM	BS	CoGM	CSF	U+M	CSF+V
Ensemble	0.91	0.33	**0.89**	**0.85**	0.87	**0.76**	0.73	0.72	**0.86**	0.73
Best score*	**0.92**	**0.48**	0.88	0.84	**0.89**	0.75	**0.77**	**0.77**	0.84	**0.79**

*Best score obtained among the rest of participants.

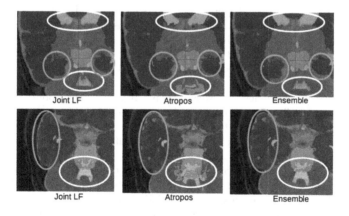

Joint LF   Atropos   Ensemble

Joint LF   Atropos   Ensemble

Fig. 3. Qualitative results, for 30 weeks (top) and 40 weeks (bottom) GA.

4   Conclusions

We presented an ensemble segmentation method to combine label fusion and intensity-based segmentation that uses probabilistic estimates of the base methods. We also proposed an intensity-based method with arbitrarily defined spatial domain. Results show that reducing the spatial domain of the intensity-based models considerably improves the segmentation performance. Results also show that the combination of complementary methods, such as label fusion and intensity-based, using the proposed ensemble framework considerably improves the results. We outperform the rest of the methods in the segmentation of the majority of the structures in neonatal images from the NeoBrainS12 Challenge.

Acknowledgements. The first author is co-financed by the Marie Curie FP7-PEOPLE-2012-COFUND 462 Action. Grant agreement no: 600387.

References

1. Anbeek, P., Isgum, I., van Kooij, B.J.M., Mol, C.P., Kersbergen, K.J., Groenendaal, F., Viergever, M.A., de Vries, L.S., Benders, M.J.N.L.: Automatic segmentation of eight tissue classes in neonatal brain MRI. PLoS ONE **8**(12) (2013)
2. Avants, B.B., Epstein, C.L., Grossman, M., Gee, J.C.: Symmetric diffeomorphic image registration with cross-correlation: evaluating automated labeling of elderly and neurodegenerative brain. Med. Image Anal. **12**(1), 26–41 (2008)
3. Avants, B.B., Tustison, N.J., Wu, J., Cook, P.A., Gee, J.C.: An open source multivariate framework for n-tissue segmentation with evaluation on public data. Neuroinformatics **9**(4), 381–400 (2011)
4. Coupé, P., Manjón, J.V., Fonov, V., Pruessner, J., Robles, M., Collins, D.L.: Patch-based segmentation using expert priors: application to hippocampus and ventricle segmentation. NeuroImage **54**(2), 940–954 (2011)
5. Isgum, I., Benders, M.J.N.L., Avants, B., Cardoso, M.J., Counsell, S.J., Gomez, E.F., Gui, L., Hüppi, P.S., Kersbergen, K.J., Makropoulos, A., Melbourne, A., Moeskops, P., Mol, C.P., Kuklisova-Murgasova, M., Rueckert, D., Schnabel, J.A., Srhoj-Egekher, V., Wu, J., Wang, S., de Vries, L.S., Viergever, M.A.: Evaluation of automatic neonatal brain segmentation algorithms: the neobrains12 challenge. Med. Image Anal. **20**(1), 135–151 (2015)
6. Ledig, C., Heckemann, R.A., Hammers, A., Lopez, J.C., Newcombe, V.F.J., Makropoulos, A., Lötjönen, J., Menon, D.K., Rueckert, D.: Robust whole-brain segmentation: application to traumatic brain injury. Med. Image Anal. **21**, 40–58 (2015)
7. Li, L., Hu, Q., Wu, X., Yu, D.: Exploration of classification confidence in ensemble learning. Pattern Recogn. **47**, 3120–3131 (2014)
8. Makropoulos, A., Gousias, I.S., Ledig, C., Aljabar, P., Serag, A., Hajnal, J.H., Edwards, A.D., Counsell, S.J., Rueckert, D.: Automatic whole brain MRI segmentation of the developing neonatal brain. IEEE TMI **33**(9), 1818–1831 (2014)
9. Nyúl, L.G., Udupa, J.K.: On standardizing the MR image instensity scale. Magn. Reson. Med. **42**(6), 1072–1081 (1999)
10. Sanroma, G., Benkarim, O.M., Piella, G., Wu, G., Zhu, X., Shen, D., Ballester, M.Á.G.: Discriminative dimensionality reduction for patch-based label fusion. In: Bhatia, K., et al. (eds.) MLMMI 2015. LNCS, vol. 9487, pp. 94–103. Springer, Heidelberg (2015). doi:10.1007/978-3-319-27929-9_10
11. Shaji, R.A.A., Smith, K., Lucchi, A., Fua, P., Susstrünk, S.: SLIC superpixels compared to state-of-the-art superpixel methods. IEEE Trans. Pattern Anal. Mach. Intell. **34**(11), 2274–2282 (2012)
12. Tustison, N.J., Avants, B.B., Cook, P.A., Zheng, Y., Egan, A., Yushkevich, P.A., Gee, J.C.: N4ITK: improved N3 bias correction. IEEE Trans. Med. Imaging **29**(6), 1310–1320 (2010)

13. Wang, H., Suh, J.W., Das, S.R., Pluta, J.B., Craige, C., Yushkevich, P.A.: Multi-atlas segmentation with joint label fusion. IEEE Trans. Pattern Anal. Mach. Intell. **35**(3), 611–623 (2013)
14. Worth, A.J.: The internet brain segmentation repository (ibsr)
15. Wu, T.F., Lin, C.J., Weng, R.C.: Probability estimates for multi-class classification by pairwise coupling. J. Mach. Learn. Res. **5**, 975–1005 (2004)

Learning Appearance and Shape Evolution for Infant Image Registration in the First Year of Life

Lifang Wei[1,4], Shunbo Hu[2,4], Yaozong Gao[4], Xiaohuan Cao[3,4],
Guorong Wu[4], and Dinggang Shen[4(✉)]

[1] College of Computer and Information Sciences,
Fujian Agriculture and Forestry University, Fuzhou 350002, China
[2] School of Information, Linyi University, Linyi 276005, China
[3] School of Automation, Northwestern Polytechnical University, Xi'an, China
[4] Department of Radiology and BRIC,
University of North Carolina at Chapel Hill, Chapel Hill, NC 27599, USA
dgshen@med.unc.edu

Abstract. Quantify dynamic structural changes in the first year of life is a key step in early brain development studies, which is indispensable to accurate deformable image registration. However, very few registration methods can work universally well for infant brain images at arbitrary development stages from birth to one year old, mainly due to (1) large anatomical variations and (2) dynamic appearance changes. In this paper, we propose a novel learning-based registration method to *not only* align the anatomical structures *but also* estimate the appearance difference between two infant MR images with possible large age gap. To achieve this goal, we leverage the random forest regression and auto-context model to learn the evolution of shape and appearance from a set of longitudinal infant images (with subject-specific temporal correspondences well determined) and then predict both the deformation pathway and appearance change between two new infant subjects. After that, it becomes much easier to deploy any conventional image registration method to complete the remaining registration since the above challenges for current state-of-the-art registration methods have been solved successfully. We apply our proposed registration method to align infant brain images of different subjects from 2-week-old to 12-month-old. Promising registration results have been achieved in terms of registration accuracy, compared to the counterpart registration methods.

1 Introduction

Many neuroscience studies are dedicated to understand the human brain development in the first year of life. Modern imaging, such as MRI (magnetic resonance imaging), provides a safe, non-invasive measurement of the whole brain. Hence, MRI has been increasingly used in many neuroimaging based studies for early brain development and developmental disorders [1].

L. Wang et al. (Eds.): MLMI 2016, LNCS 10019, pp. 36–44, 2016.
DOI: 10.1007/978-3-319-47157-0_5

In order to quantitatively measure brain development in such a dynamic period, accurate image registration method for different infant subjects with possibly large age gap is of high demand. However, it is difficult to register infant MR brain images, due to the following challenges: (**1**) Fast brain development *not only* on the expansion of whole brain volume, *but also* on cortical folding patterns from birth to 1 year old. Hence, infant image registration is required to have the capability of dealing with this rapid brain growth. (**2**) Dynamic and non-linear appearance changes across different brain development stages due to white matter myelination.

To address the above two challenges, we propose a novel learning-based registration framework to accurately register any two infant subjects (even with possibly large age gap) to a pre-defined template image. Since volumetric image is in the high dimension, random forest regression [2, 3] is applied to learning two complex mappings in a patch-wise manner: (**1**) Patch-wise *appearance-displacement model* that can characterize the mapping from patch-wise image appearance to voxel-wise displacement vector, where the displacement locates at the patch center and points to the corresponding position in the template image space. (**2**) Patch-wise *appearance-appearance model* that encodes the evolution of patch-wise appearance from one particular brain development stage to the corresponding stage in the template space. In the application, before registering the new infant brain image to the template, we *first* visit each point in the new infant brain image and predict its initial displacement to the template by the learned patch-wise *appearance-displacement model*. In this way, we can obtain a dense deformation field to initialize the registration of the new infant brain image to the template. *Then*, we further apply the learned patch-wise *appearance-appearance model* to predict the template-like appearance for the new infant image. With this initialized deformation and also estimated appearance for the new infant image under registration, the conventional registration method can be applied to further estimating the remaining *small* deformation between new infant brain image and the template.

In this paper, we have comprehensively evaluated the registration performance of our proposed method for infant images, with comparison to the state-of-the-art deformable registration methods, including Demons registration method [4] (http://www.insight-journal.org/browse/publication/154), 3D-HAMMER [5] using the segmented images obtained with iBEAT software (http://www.nitrc.org/projects/ibeat/) [6], and a sparse representation based registration method (SR-based) [7]. Through both quantitative measurement and visual inspection, our proposed learning-based registration method outperforms all other deformable registration methods under comparison.

2 Methods

2.1 Integrated Random Forest Regression and Auto-Context Model

In the training stage, N MR image sequences $\left\{ I_n^t | n = 1, \ldots, N, t = 1, \ldots M \right\}$, each with $M = 5$ time points (scanned at 2-week-old, 3-month-old, 6-month-old, 9-month-old, and 12-month-old), are used as the training data. Note that, although in the application stage only *either* T1 *or* T2 weighted MR images will be used for registration, in the training stage we use multimodality images, such as T1-weighted MRI, T2-weighted MRI, and DTI (diffusion tensor imaging), for helping training. Thanks for the complete longitudinal image information and also the complementary multimodality imaging information, we first deploy the state-of-the-art longitudinal multi-modality image segmentation method [6] to accurately segment each infant image to WM (white matter), GM (gray matter), and CSF (cerebrospinal fluid). Since there are no any appearance changes in these segmented images, we can directly use longitudinal image registration method [8] to simultaneously estimate temporal deformation pathways from every time point to a pre-defined template image T, with the temporal consistency also enforced along the estimated spatial deformation fields over time. Thus, we can obtain the deformation pathway $\boldsymbol{\Phi}_n^t = \{\boldsymbol{\varphi}_n^t(v)|v \in \boldsymbol{\Omega}_T\}$ for each image $\boldsymbol{I}_n^t$. It is worth noting that our goal of training patch-wise appearance-displacement model is to predict the displacement vector for the center of subject image patch (prior to image registration) in the application stage. Therefore, we need to reverse each deformation pathway $\boldsymbol{\Phi}_n^t$ to make the deformation field defined in each training image domain, i.e., $\boldsymbol{\Psi}_n^t = \{\boldsymbol{\Psi}_n^t(u)|u \in \boldsymbol{\Omega}_{I_n^t}\}$. We follow the diffeomorphism principle in [9] to reverse $\boldsymbol{\Phi}_n^t$ by integrating the reversed velocity field of $\boldsymbol{\Phi}_n^t$. Thus, for each voxel u in the training image $\boldsymbol{I}_n^t$, its corresponding location in the template image space is $u + \boldsymbol{\Psi}_n^t(u)$.

Since human brain develops dramatically in the first year, we train both the patch-wise *appearance-displacement* and patch-wise *appearance-appearance* regression models from 2-week-old to 12-month-old domain (used as template time-point) separately, as detailed below.

Patch-Wise *Appearance-Displacement Model*. Training samples for learning patch-wise *appearance-displacement model* consist of pairs of the randomly-sampled local image patch $\boldsymbol{P}_n^t(u)$ extracted at voxel u of training image $\boldsymbol{I}_n^t$ and its displacement vector $\boldsymbol{\Psi}_n^t(u)$. Random forest regression [2, 3] is here used to learn the relationship between local image patch $\boldsymbol{P}_n^t(u)$ and displacement vector $\boldsymbol{\Psi}_n^t(u)$. Specifically, we calculate several patch-wise image features from $\boldsymbol{P}_n^t(u)$, including intensity (the intensity of the patch), 3-D Haar-like feature (a kind of two-block Haar-like features, which calculate the average intensity difference between two locations within the local patch), and coordinates (the coordinates of the center of an image patch in the common space to provide the spatial information). In addition, we use a multi-scale strategy by extracting Haar-like features in a set of nested neighborhoods with different scales by down-sampling in order to capture both global and local characteristics. To train a tree in the random forest, the parameters of each node are learned recursively, starting at the root node. Then, the training samples are recursively split into left and right nodes by selecting the optimal feature and threshold. Suppose Θ denotes a node in the random forest, its optimal feature and threshold are determined by maximizing the following objective function:

$$E = \sigma(\Theta) - \sum_{i \in \{L,R\}} \frac{N_i}{N} \sigma(\Theta_i) \qquad (1)$$

where Θ_i $(i \in \{L, R\})$ denotes the left/right children node of node Θ. N_i denotes the number of training samples at left/right children node. N is the number of training samples at node Θ. $\sigma(\Theta)$ denotes a function that measures variance of training samples at node Θ, which is defined as below:

$$\sigma(\Theta) = \frac{1}{|Z(\Theta)|} \sum_{(u,n) \in Z(\Theta)} ||\Psi_n^t(u) - \overline{d}||_2^2 \tag{2}$$

where $Z(\Theta)$ is the training set at node Θ, and $\overline{d}$ is the mean displacement vector of all training samples at node Θ. After determining the optimal feature and threshold for the node Θ by maximizing Eq. (1), the training samples are split into left and right children nodes by using the selected optimal feature and threshold. The same splitting process is recursively conducted on the left and right children nodes until the maximal tree depth is reached *or* the number of training samples at one node is less than a certain amount. When the splitting stops, we regard the current node as a leaf node and store the mean displacement there for future prediction.

Given a new image patch $P_s(u)$ $(u \in \Omega_s)$ from a testing subject S, we first extract the same patch-wise image features from $P_s(u)$. Then, based on the learned optimal feature and threshold at each node, the testing image patch $P_s(u)$ is guided towards leaf node. When it reaches a leaf node, the mean displacement vector stored there is used as the predicted displacement vector. For robustness, we train multiple regression trees independently using the idea of bagging. Thus, the final prediction is the average of predicted displacement vectors from all decision trees.

Patch-Wise Appearance-Appearance Model. Training samples for learning patch-wise *appearance-appearance model* consist of randomly-sampled local image patch $P_n^t(u + \Psi_n^t(u))$ extracted at voxel $u + \Psi_n^t(u)$ of the training image I_n^t and the corresponding image patch $P_T(u + \Psi_n^t(u))$ extracted at the location $u + \Psi_n^t(u)$ of the template T. We use the same random forest regression learning procedure (as described above) to train patch-wise *appearance-appearance model*, except that the mean displacement vector in the above is now replaced with the mean template-like image patch from all samples stored at leaf node. Specifically, to estimate the template-like patch appearance for the patch $P_s(u)$ $(u \in \Omega_s)$ of the new subject image S, we regard the mean image patch stored at destination leaf node after depth-first traverse as the prediction/estimation.

Integration of Random Forest with Auto-Context Model. It is obvious that the above two learning models use only the low-level image appearance features. Since the image contrast in infant brain images is poor, high-level feature representation is of high necessity to further improve the prediction of deformation pathway and patch-wise appearance, respectively. In the following, we take the *appearance-displacement* as example to explain the integration with auto-context model.

Specifically, we employ the context features that can describe spatial relationship of displacement vector in one local region to the displacement vectors in other brain regions. It is worth noting that the context features are extracted from the currently estimated displacement map for *appearance-displacement model* and the currently estimated appearance for *appearance- appearance model*. Then, we can use the context features as additional feature representations to train the random forest in the next layer. Since the high-level context features are used to refine the random forest regression, the predicted displacement can be improved, as shown in the red box in Fig. 1. By repeating these steps (i.e., re-calculate context features and train the random forest for the next layer), we can iteratively improve the prediction accuracy. Also, it is straightforward to apply the same strategy to enhance the predicted patch-wise *image appearance* by integrating the context into patch-wise *appearance-to-appearance model*.

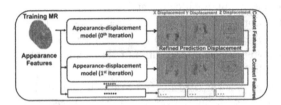

Fig. 1. The schematic illustration of the integration with auto-context model. (Color figure online)

2.2 Register New Infant Image with Two Learned Models

We register the new infant subject S to the template T (that sits in the same domain as in the training stage) in three steps, as also illustrated in Fig. 2.

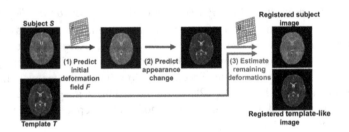

Fig. 2. The schematic illustration of the proposed registration process.

(1) We first visit each voxel u of the new infant subject S ($u \in \Omega_s$) and use the learned patch-wise *appearance-displacement model* to predict its displacement $h(u)$, pointing to the template image, based on the image patch $P_s(u)$ extracted at u. In this way, we can obtain the dense deformation field $H = \{h(u)|u \in \Omega_s\}$ and further calculate the initial deformation field F by reversing the dense deformation field H, since the deformation pathway (deforming subject image S to the template space Ω_T) should be defined in the template image space, i.e., $F = \{f(v)|v \in \Omega_T\}$.

(2) After deforming subject image S from its native space Ω_S to the template space Ω_T, we can further use the learned patch-wise *appearance-appearance model* to convert local image appearance $P_s(u)$ from the time point where subject image S was scanned to $Q(u)$ at the time point where the template image T was scanned. Thus, we can finally obtain a roughly-aligned subject image with also its template-like appearance, which can be denoted as $\widehat{S}$.

(3) Since the anatomical shape and appearance of $\widehat{S}$ are almost similar to the template image T, we can employ classic diffeomorphic Demons [4] to complete the estimation of the remaining deformation G. Finally, the whole deformation pathway Φ from subject image S to the template image T can be achieved by $\Phi = F \circ G$, where 'o' stands for deformation composition [9].

3   Experiments

Totally, 24 infant subjects are included in the following experiments, where each subject has T1- and T2-weighted MR images at 2-week-old, 3-, 6-, 9-, 12-month-old. The T1-weighted images were acquired with a Siemens head-only 3T MR scanner and had 144 sagittal slices at resolution $1 \times 1 \times 1$ mm^3. The T2-weighted images were obtained with 64 axial slices at resolution $1.25 \times 1.25 \times 1.95$ mm^3. For each subject, the T2-weighted image was linearly aligned to its T1-weighted image at the same time-point using FLIRT [10] and then further isotropically up-sampled to $1 \times 1 \times 1$ mm^3 resolution. The image preprocessing includes: skull-stripping, bias correction, and image segmentation.

Parameters Setting. The input patch size is 7 * 7 * 7 and output patch size is 1 * 1 * 1. The number of candidate thresholds is 100, the number of the tree is 50, the depth is 100, the number of random feature is 1000, and the minimum number for training samples in each leaf node is 8 and 32 for *appearance-displacement model* and *appearance-appearance model*, respectively. The multi-resolution is 3, and the number of auto-context iterations is 3.

Inter-Subject Brain Images. We compare the registration accuracy of our proposed learning-based infant brain registration method with several state-of-the-art deformable registration methods under the following three categories. **(1)** Intensity based image registration. We employ diffeomorphic Demons deformable image registration method [4]. **(2)** Feature-based image registration. HAMMER [5] is one of typical feature-based registration methods, which computes geometric moments for all tissue types as morphological signature at each voxel. Apparently, the registration performance of this method is highly dependent of segmentation quality. In the following experiment, we assume the to-be-registered new infant image has been well segmented, which is, however, not practical in real application since segmentation of infant image at single time point is difficult without complementary longitudinal and multi-modal information. **(3)** Other learning based registration. A sparse representation based registration method (SR-based) [7] is compared, which leverages the known temporal correspondences in the training subjects to tackle the appearance gap between the two different time-point images under registration.

It is more challenging to register infant images of different subjects with possibly large age gap. Here, the longitudinal scans of 12 infant subjects are used as the training dataset to train both the *appearance-displacement* and *appearance-appearance models*. The 1-year-old image of one remaining infant subject is treated as template. Then, we register the 2-week-old of another remaining infant subject to the template. We first can visually check the registration results in Fig. 3. The 2-week-old subject (the preprocessing is done) and 1-year-old template with T2 weighted images are shown in the first column. We show the registration results by directly using diffeomorphic Demons (2nd column top), 3D-HAMMER (2nd column bottom), and our proposed method (last column; including the aligned subject image and the aligned template-like image), respectively. It is apparent that: **(1)** our learning-based registration method achieves much better registration results than directly using diffeomorphic Demons and 3D-HAMMER, **(2)** patch-wise *appearance-appearance* can predict the appearance change and covert the subject image with template-like appearance, and **(3)** patch-wise *appearance-displacement model* can predict the initial deformation/displacement for warping the subject image close to the template's shape.

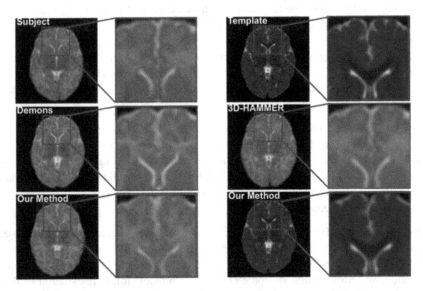

Fig. 3. Inter-subject registration results on infant brain images. 1-year-old template with T2 weighted image is shown in the right of the first row. We show the registration results using Demons directly (2nd row, left), 3D-HAMMER (2nd row, right), and our proposed method (last row, including the aligned subject image and the aligned *template-like* image), respectively.

Iterative Refinement by Auto-Context Model. We further show the gradually refined appearance estimation, displacement prediction accuracy, and Dice ratios for registration results in Figs. 4 and 5, respectively. As shown in Fig. 4, the quality of learned appearance becomes more and more similar to the template image (right end) as the more and more layers of random forest model are used with context features. In

Table 1. The mean and standard deviation of the combined WM and GM Dice ratios, obtained for registering 2-week-old and 3-month-old images to the 12-month-old image by 4 different methods. The best Dice ratio is shown in bold.

Method	Demons	3D-HAMMER	SR-based	Our method
2-week-old to 12-month-old	0.550 ± 0.050*	0.662 ± 0.023*	0.673 ± 0.016*	**0.707 ± 0.013**
3-month-old to 12-month-old	0.573 ± 0.033*	0.642 ± 0.026*	0.665 ± 0.017*	**0.703 ± 0.018**

We report the averaged Dice ratio of WM and GM in Table 1, where '*' indicates the statistically significant improvement of our method over the counterpart method according to the paired t-test ($p < 0.05$). It is also apparent that our learning-based registration method achieves much better registration results than directly using *either* intensity-based *or* feature-based registration method.

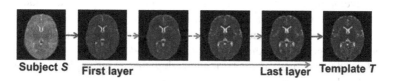

Subject S **First layer** ——————————▶ **Last layer** **Template T**

Fig. 4. Demonstration of contribution of auto-context model in learning appearance changes. Subject S and template T are the 2-week-old and 1-year-old T2-weighted images, respectively. The middle images show the results of learned appearance changes with iterative auto-context model.

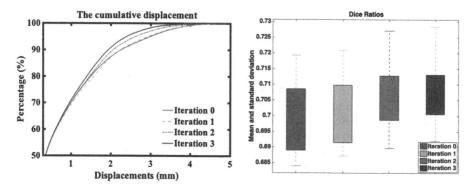

Fig. 5. Demonstration of contribution of auto-context model in improving the quality of learned displacements (left) and registration accuracy (right). The left panel shows the cumulative deformation prediction errors, compared to ground-truth deformations, by different number of iterations (from 0 to 3) in the auto-context model. The right panel shows the Dice ratios obtained by registering the subject and template images, with different number of iterations in auto-context model for learning appearance-appearance relationship in the testing stage.

Fig. 5, the left panel shows the cumulative deformation prediction errors, compared to ground-truth deformations (obtained by multimodal longitudinal segmentation and 4D registration), by different numbers of iterations (from 0 to 3) in the auto-context model. The right panel shows the Dice ratio (of combined WM and GM) obtained by registering the subject and template images under each iteration of auto-context model for enhancing appearance-appearance relationship in the testing stage. It is apparent that (1) the auto-context model is very useful in improving the quality of predicting both appearance and displacement, and (2) the auto-context model can further assist in refining the registration accuracy.

4   Conclusion

In this paper, a novel learning-based registration method has been presented to tackle the challenging infant brain image registration in the first year of life. To address the rapid brain development and dynamic appearance change, we deploy the random forest regression and auto-context model to learn both the deformation pathway and appearance change at different time points. Specifically, to register a new infant image with the possibly large age gap, the learned *appearance-displacement* and *appearance-appearance models* are first applied to initializing the image registration and also making the local image appearance similar to the template image. Then, we use a conventional image registration method to estimate the remaining deformation field, which is often small and thus much easier to estimate, compared to direct estimation of deformation field from the original image. We have extensively evaluated registration accuracy of our proposed method with longitudinal scans, and achieved the highest registration accuracy compared with other counterpart registration methods.

References

1. Giedd, J.N., et al.: Structural MRI of pediatric brain development: what have we learned and where are we going? Neuron **67**, 728–734 (2010)
2. Breiman, L.: Random forests. Mach. Learn. **45**, 5–32 (2001)
3. Criminisi, A., et al.: Regression forests for efficient anatomy detection and localization in computed tomography scans. Med. Image Anal. **17**, 1293–1303 (2013)
4. Vercauteren, T., et al.: Diffeomorphic demons: efficient non-parametric image registration. Neuroimage **45**, S61–S72 (2009)
5. Shen, D.G., et al.: HAMMER: hierarchical attribute matching mechanism for elastic registration. IEEE Trans. Med. Imaging **21**, 1421–1439 (2002)
6. Dai, Y.K., et al.: iBEAT: a toolbox for infant brain magnetic resonance image processing. Neuroinformatics **11**, 211–225 (2013)
7. Wu, Y., et al.: Hierarchical and symmetric infant image registration by robust longitudinal-example-guided correspondence detection. Med. Phys. **42**, 4174–4189 (2015)
8. Shen, D.G., et al.: Measuring temporal morphological changes robustly in brain MR images via 4-dimensional template warping. Neuroimage **21**, 1508–1517 (2004)
9. Ashburner, J.: A fast diffeomorphic image registration algorithm. Neuroimage **38**, 95–113 (2007)
10. Jenkinson, M., et al.: Fsl. Neuroimage **62**, 782–790 (2012)

Detecting Osteophytes in Radiographs of the Knee to Diagnose Osteoarthritis

Jessie Thomson[1,2(✉)], Terence O'Neill[2,3], David Felson[2,3,4], and Tim Cootes[1]

[1] Centre for Imaging Sciences, University of Manchester, Manchester, UK
Jessie.Thomson@postgrad.man.ac.uk
[2] NIHR Manchester Musculoskeletal BRU,
Central Manchester NHS Foundation Trust, MAHSC, Manchester, UK
[3] Arthritis Research UK Centre for Epidemiology, University of Manchester,
Manchester, UK
[4] Boston University, Boston, MA, USA

Abstract. We present a fully automatic system for identifying osteophytes on knee radiographs, and for estimating the widely used Kellgren-Lawrence (KL) grade for Osteoarthritis (OA). We have compared three advanced modelling and texture techniques. We found that a Random Forest trained using Haar-features achieved good results, but the optimal results are obtained by combining shape modelling and texture features. The system achieves the best reported performance for identifying osteophytes (AUC: 0.85), for measuring KL grades and for classifying OA (AUC: 0.93), with an error rate half that of the previous best method.

Keywords: Medical image analysis · Computer-aided diagnosis

1 Introduction

Osteoarthritis is one of the leading causes of disability today. It is a degenerative disease that effects the entire joint. The disease is associated with pain, disability and substantial care costs each year [1]. Current clinical diagnosis relies on manually analysing images using semi-quantitative measurements, which are time consuming and suffer from inter-rater variability. One of the main features associated with OA of the knee is the formation of osteophytes - bony spurs that form from the articular surfaces around the joint. Despite their relevance very few automated methods specifically measure osteophytes. The KOACAD [2] algorithm measures the area of the medial tibial osteophytes, whereas other methods capture osteophytes through shape of the entire joint [3]. The aim of this work is to detect marginal osteophytes (found along the medial and lateral sides of the tibia and femur) from radiographs of the knee, and to use the resulting features to grade signs of OA. We describe a fully automated system that finds the outline of the bones and analyses regions where osteophytes are known to develop. We explored three advanced modelling techniques for evaluating marginal osteophytes: two which explicitly attempt to measure the shape of the

© Springer International Publishing AG 2016
L. Wang et al. (Eds.): MLMI 2016, LNCS 10019, pp. 45–52, 2016.
DOI: 10.1007/978-3-319-47157-0_6

contour around the osteophytes and one which analyses the texture pattern in regions where osteophytes may form. In addition we trained classifiers to discriminate knees with OA from those without, and to estimate the Kellgren-Lawrence grades. We show that using each osteophyte measure alone gives encouraging results when in diagnosing knee OA from radiographs, but that the best performance was obtained when combining all three measures. Marginal osteophytes are the clearest locations in AP radiographs, and are used in the experiments to compare to OARSI scores that grade these areas specifically. The key novel factors of this work are: (i) A method for detecting marginal osteophytes using shape and appearance features, (ii) a method for diagnosing OA and the associated KL grade using osteophyte features which yields the best yet reported performance for an automated system.

2   Background

2.1   Osteoarthritis Grading

Kellgren-Lawrence Grading. The most widely used OA grading is the Kellgren-Lawrence (KL) method [7], which splits disease development into five classes: normal (KL0), doubtful (KL1), minimal (KL2), moderate (KL3) and severe (KL4). Onset of the disease is usually taken to be KL2 and above. The definition of each grade relies on the degree of osteophyte development, with each stage containing at least some further progression in the osteophytes from the one before. KL grading is performed by visual inspection by a clinician, so is subjective and prone to inter-rater variability, especially when distinguishing between the central grades (KL 1–3). Due to this there is a variability of inter-rater reliability with papers reporting kw (weighted kappa) in the range 0.36–0.8 [10] in comparison to the gold standard, where 0 means agreement equivalent to chance, [0.9–1.0] near perfect agreement.

OARSI Grading. To assess osteophytes independently, the manual OARSI [12] grading method is often used. This uses reference images to grade the relevant features of OA. The development is split into four stages: normal (0), mild (1), moderate (2) and severe (3). The method is again semi-quantitative with inter-reader reliability kw 0.72 (CI 0.64–0.8) [11].

2.2   Automated Methods

There are few published methods for fully automated analysis of knee osteophytes. The KOACAD algorithm [2] analyses knee radiographs for signs of OA through Joint Space Narrowing (JSN), osteophyte area, and femorotibial angle. For the osteophytes, they focus on the region of the medial tibial margin. This is done by finding the medially prominent edge of the osteophytes extending from the tibial plateau. The area is taken between the outline of the osteophyte and the outline of the medial tibial side. The classification accuracy (AUC) of the osteophyte area is 0.646. This result could be due to the method analysing only one of the regions in which osteophytes develop.

Thomson et al. [3] describe a system combining bone shape and trabecular texture measures to discriminate OA from non-OA. They report an AUC of 0.845 in two-class OA classification (split KL0,1 vs KL2,3,4). However, this method doesn't explicitly analyse osteophytes, instead implicitly including them in the overall shape and appearance information.

2.3   Shape Modelling and Matching

Statistical Shape Models [6] are widely used for studying the contours of bones. They encode the contour with a set of model points, whose variation is described using:

$$x = T(\hat{x} + Pb) \tag{1}$$

Where T is a global similarity transform applied to the points, x is a vector of point coordinates representing the shape in a reference frame, $\hat{x}$ is the mean shape, P is a set of eigenvectors describing the modes of variation, and b is a vector of shape parameters.

One of the most effective algorithms for locating the outline of bones in radiographs is the RFCLM [8], which has been applied to study OA in the hip [4] and the knee [3]. This uses a collection of Random Forests (RFs) to predict the most likely location of each point based on nearby image patches. A shape model is then used to constrain the points and encode the result.

3   Methods

Following [3] we used an RFCLM to find the outline of the bones in the knee. We trained a 74 point shape model and RFCLM with 500 images. After a global search for the approximate joint location we used a sequence of four models with increasing resolution to find the bone contours. We then analysed shape and texture across regions around the bones where osteophytes typically occur.

3.1   Osteophyte Features

We used two different methods of finding the outline of osteophytes and one method relying only on patterns of intensities within the region of interest. In each case we trained three separate random forests, to identify (i) osteophytes (or not), (ii) KL grade, (iii) OA vs no-OA.

Contour Shape from RFCLM. The basic knee model represents the normal shape of the femur and tibia using 74 points, ignoring osteophytes (which cause irregular bony material beyond the normal outline). We augment this with an additional 11 points placed evenly between start and end points placed on either

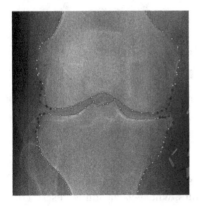

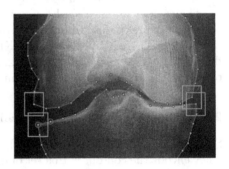

Fig. 1. Annotated 118 points. 74 blue points for shape outline, and 44 osteophyte points in red (Color figure online)

Fig. 2. Locations of the four marginal texture ROIs

side of the margins, these define contours around the osteophytes (where present) in each of four regions (44 points in total) - see Fig. 1.

We trained a new 2 stage coarse-to-fine RFCLM using this model. For the analysis, we extracted the osteophyte points from the 118 found points. We built shape models on the 44 points alone and trained RF classifiers on the shape parameters of the osteophyte detail only. The shape model had 50 modes, sufficient to explain 99 % of the variation in the training set. The shape parameters, corresponding to elements of b in Eq. (1), were then used as features in Random Forest classifiers.

Contour Shape from Dynamic Programming. The 74 point RFCLM finds the outline of the normal bone. Osteophytes tend to extend out from this contour. An alternative way of locating them is to search for strong edges along profiles normal to the main bone contour (see Fig. 3). The profiles are defined as the lines $x_i + d_i.u_i$, where x_i is a point on the main bone contour, u_i is the unit normal to the curve at that point and d_i is the distance along the profile. To find the best continuous contour we find the points at distance d_i along each profile from the bone model contour, which minimise the following cost function

$$Q = \sum_{i=1}^{n} -|g_i(d_i)| + \alpha \sum_{i=1}^{n-1} (d_i - d_{i+1})^2 \tag{2}$$

where $g_i(d_i)$ is the intensity gradient at distance d_i along the profile i and the second term encourages a smooth shape. This can be solved efficiently using the dynamic programming algorithm. We use 12 profiles for each region, leading to 12 points defining the shape of the osteophytic region. The parameter α was chosen by pilot experiments on a subset of the data. We trained shape models on the resulting points and encoded each example using the resulting shape parameters. The shape model had 98 % variation, equating to 22 shape modes.

Texture Analysis. Rather than explicitly finding the bone contour, we identified signs of disease by training a classifier on image texture in areas where osteophytes occur. We defined four regions of interest (ROIs) using points from the base RFCLM object detection stage, the points chosen were close to the four respective regions (medial tibial, lateral tibial, lateral femur and medial femur - see Fig. 2) and trained an RF classifier for each. We used Haar features to split at each tree node. The output of the RF is an estimate of the probability of each class. The classification score for the whole knee was taken as the mean of the response for each of the four regions.

4   Experiments

4.1   Data

To compare our methods we take data from the OsteoArthritis Initiative [5] dataset. The study is an observational prospective study of OA, taking participants across four sites across USA. The study began with 4796 participants, ranging between the ages of 45–79. All images have been independently graded with KL [7] and osteophyte grades (0–3) using the OARSI scale [12]. For this study we have taken two samples of PA radiographs, the first set is for osteophyte detection and uses 640 knees with a range of OARSI osteophyte grades across the four sites (lateral femur, medial femur, lateral tibia, medial tibia): 0–44.7 % (368, 303, 301, 173), 1–30 % (114, 95, 231, 327), 2–11.3 % (70, 73, 57, 90), 3–14 % (88, 169, 51, 50). The second set consists of 747 knee images with a range of KL grades: KL0–169 (22.7 %), KL1–203 (27.2 %), KL2–134 (18 %), KL3–176 (23.6 %), KL4–64 (8.5 %). For the two-class OA classification experiments we split the grades to distinguish either OA or non-OA (KL 0, 1 vs. KL 2, 3, 4).

4.2   Classification Experiments

To test the accuracy of the methods, we ran various experiments using Random Forest [9] classifiers trained on the osteophyte features. The methods are combined by taking the mean output from the separate classifiers. The experiments are

(i) Detecting osteophytes via OARSI grades (0, 1 vs. 2, 3)
(ii) Classification of OA and non-OA images (374/372)
(iii) Multi-class classification of the images into the respective grades (KL0-4)

Table 1. Osteophyte detection performance

Analysis method	Mean AUC (std.)
SSM-RS	0.756(0.056)
SSM-DP	0.663 (0.072)
Haar features	0.771 (0.053)
SSM-RS + SSM-DP	0.769 (0.065)
SSM-RS + Haar	0.826 (0.015)
SSM-DP + Haar	0.806 (0.015)
All methods	**0.846 (0.014)**

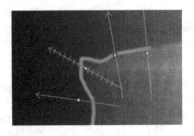

Fig. 3. Interpolated points with normals. The red line indicates the desired edge. (Color figure online)

We report independent and combined results for each method: Statistical Shape Model - RFCLM Search (SSM-RS), Statistical Shape Model - Dynamic Programming contours (SSM-DP), and texture analysis using Haar-features (Haar). For each experiment we used 5-fold cross validation and permutated the data for 2 repeats, taking the mean accuracy and Area under the ROC (AUC) to assess each algorithm.

4.3 Osteophyte Detection

We ran each method over the four marginal regions detecting osteophytes in each region separately. We then took the mean AUC from each region per method for the results in Table 1 below. The best independent classifier is the RF based on Haar-features with AUC 0.77. By combining all methods we achieve AUC 0.85.

4.4 OA vs Non-OA

The cross validation mean AUC results are shown in Table 2. The best independent method is that using Haar features, with an AUC of 0.92. Combining this method with both the DP and SSM method does slightly improve the AUC to 0.931. Adding the full shape from the 74 point model did not significantly improve the performance (multi-class: 48.8 %, AUC: 0.932).

4.5 Multi-class Experiments

We then tested how well the methods identify KL grades. Table 2 shows the per-class accuracy and the overall probability that the correct class is chosen. All methods have difficulty identifying KL2, with Haar features achieving the best accuracy (21.9 %). The Haar features achieve the best results (47.8 %), and the combination of all the methods improves the overall accuracy (All) to 50.2 %. The reliability (kw) and confidence interval (CI) in the table show the reliability in comparison to the gold standard to be moderate (kw 0.565), but within the range exhibited by human observers (0.36–0.8).

Table 2. Accuracy of the KL grading, and AUC of the OA vs non-OA experiments

	Accuracy (%)						kw (CI 95%)	AUC (std.)
Analysis method	KL0	KL1	KL2	KL3	KL4	All (std.)	Multi-class	Two-class
SSM-RS	44.1	47.5	18.9	46	**68.8**	43 (0.8)	0.44 (0.39–0.49)	0.85 (0.001)
SSM-DP	**46.5**	41.9	21.3	43.2	55.5	40.7 (0.5)	0.42 (0.37–0.48)	0.86 (0.003)
Haar features	43.5	49.8	**21.9**	64	63	47.8 (0.3)	0.51 (0.47–0.56)	0.92 (<0.001)
SSM-RS + SSM-DP	39.4	41.7	18.7	47	57.8	39.7 (0.7)	0.41 (0.36–0.45)	0.87 (0.002)
SSM-RS + Haar	42	51.6	19.4	**68**	63.5	48.5 (1.5)	0.56 (0.51–0.59)	0.926 (0.002)
SSM-DP + Haar	42.9	50.2	19.2	67.4	65.1	48.3 (1.6)	0.54 (0.49–0.58)	0.926 (0.001)
All methods	45.9	**53.5**	20.1	**68**	65.6	**50.2 (0.5)**	**0.56 (0.52–0.6)**	**0.931 (0.002)**

5 Discussion and Conclusion

Experiments show that a Random Forests based on Haar features give the best individual results, probably because they do not rely on identifying a particular bone contour. The DP contour detection will find the edges with the highest gradient differences, this can often ignore less well defined osteophytes in the radiograph caused through under-exposed regions. Over and under-exposed images were not removed from the set unless in extreme cases where the overall bone outline could not be found. Shape models can be biased towards the mean shape within images missing the osteophytes which can exhibit a wide range of shapes. Combining all methods together marginally improves the accuracy in all three experiments showing that texture can be improved by added shape information.

Our algorithm performs significantly better (AUC 0.93) than the previously best reported accuracy for the two-class problem [3] (AUC 0.845). This demonstrates the advantages of focusing on osteophytes, a main feature of OA ([3] uses shape information from the overall outline).

The proposed method achieves a better result than the KOACAD [2] algorithm. To perform a fair comparison, we tested the shape of the medial tibia osteophytes to classify the data, and found our method achieved an AUC of 0.895, compared to 0.646 KOACAD. This may be because there is important information in the texture on and surrounding the osteophytes. However, there may also be some bias towards our algorithm which will inherently measure some joint space narrowing information (which tends to be correlated with OA progression) in the extreme cases of OA, through overlapping texture regions.

The multi-class experiments have achieved a reliability of kw 0.565, which is within the range achieved by human grading (0.36–0.8) [10]. The experiments have also shown that all methods are relatively poor at detecting KL2 grades. This may be due to the osteophytes being too similar to the other grades (KL1 and KL 3). The descriptions for each grade are that KL1 has "osteophytes", KL2 has "definite osteophytes" and KL3 has "multiple osteophytes". This will be reliant on osteophytes being visible at a certain size, meaning the automated method could have detected multiple smaller features where only one would be recognised. This is supported by the Haar-feature method results, which estimated the majority of the KL2 images (79.8%) to be in the grades KL1–3 (34.8% KL1, 21.9% KL2 and 23.1% KL3).

In this paper we have analysed different methods for automatically measuring osteophytes. The independent and combined features were compared using two- and multi-class OA detection experiments. In future work we will: examine the correlation between osteophytes and clinical symptoms of Osteoarthritis (such as pain and functionality); analyse relation between osteophytes and future onset OA or pain; and compare our 2D analysis to 3D osteophyte measures.

Acknowledgements. This report includes independent research funded by the National Institute for Health Research Biomedical Research Unit Funding Scheme. The views expressed in this publication are those of the author(s) and not necessarily those of the NHS, the NIHR or the Department of Health.

References

1. Chen, A., Gupte, C., Akhtar, K., Smith, P., Cobb, J.: The global economic cost of osteoarthritis: how the UK compares. Arthritis **2012**, Article ID 698709, 6 (2012). doi:10.1155/2012/698709
2. Oka, H., Muraki, S., Akune, T., Nakamura, K., Kawaguchi, H.: Normal and thresh- old values of radiographic parameters for knee osteoarthrits using a computer- assisted measuring system (KOACAD): the ROAD study. J. Orthop. Sci. **15**, 781– 789 (2010)
3. Thomson, J., O'Neill, T., Felson, D., Cootes, T.: Automated shape and texture analysis for detection of osteoarthritis from radiographs of the knee. In: Navab, N., Hornegger, J., Wells, W.M., Frangi, A.F. (eds.) MICCAI 2015. LNCS, vol. 9350, pp. 127–134. Springer, Heidelberg (2015). doi:10.1007/978-3-319-24571-3_16
4. Lindner, C., Thiagarajah, S., Wilkinson, J.M., Wallis, G.A., Cootes, T.F.: Accurate bone segmentation in 2D radiographs using fully automatic shape model matching based on regression-voting. In: Mori, K., Sakuma, I., Sato, Y., Barillot, C., Navab, N. (eds.) MICCAI 2013. LNCS, vol. 8150, pp. 181–189. Springer, Heidelberg (2013). doi:10.1007/978-3-642-40763-5_23
5. Lester, G.: Clinical research in OA. The NIH osteoarthritis initiative. J. Muscu- loskelet. Neuronal Interact. **8**(4), 313–314 (2008)
6. Cootes, T.F., Taylor, C.J.: Statistical models of appearance for computer vision. Technical report, University of Manchester (2004)
7. Kellgren, J.H., Lawrence, J.S.: Radiological assessment of osteo-arthrosis. Ann. Rheum. Dis. **16**(4), 494–502 (1957)
8. Cootes, T.F., Ionita, M.C., Lindner, C., Sauer, P.: Robust and accurate shape model fitting using random forest regression voting. In: Fitzgibbon, A., Lazebnik, S., Perona, P., Sato, Y., Schmid, C. (eds.) ECCV 2012. LNCS, vol. 7578, pp. 278– 291. Springer, Heidelberg (2012). doi:10.1007/978-3-642-33786-4_21
9. Breiman, L.: Random forests. Mach. Learn. **45**(1), 5–32 (2001)
10. Riddle, D.I., Jiranek, W.A., Hull, J.R.: Validity and reliability of radiographic knee osteoarthritis measures by arthroplasty surgeons. Orthopedics **36**(1), e25– e32 (2013)
11. Hayashi, D., Gusenburg, J., Roemer, F.W., Hunter, D.J., Li, L., Guermazi, A.: Reliability of semiquantitative assessment of osteophytes and subchondral cysts on tomosynthesis images by radiologists with different levels of expertise. Diagn. Interv. Radiol. **20**, 353–359 (2014)
12. Altman, R.D., Hochberg, M., Murphy Jr., W.A., Wolfe, F., Lequesne, M.: Atlas of individual radiographic features in osteoarthritis. Osteoarthritis Cartilage **3**, A3–A70 (1995)

Direct Estimation of Fiber Orientations Using Deep Learning in Diffusion Imaging

Simon Koppers$^{(\boxtimes)}$ and Dorit Merhof

Institute of Imaging and Computer Vision,
RWTH Aachen University, Aachen, Germany
Simon.Koppers@lfb.rwth-aachen.de

Abstract. An effective technique for investigating human brain connectivities, is the reconstruction of fiber orientation distribution functions based on diffusion-weighted MRI. To reconstruct fiber orientations, most current approaches fit a simplified diffusion model, resulting in an approximation error. We present a novel approach for estimating the fiber orientation directly from raw data, by converting the model fitting process into a classification problem based on a convolutional Deep Neural Network, which is able to identify correlated diffusion information within a single voxel. We evaluate our approach quantitatively on realistic synthetic data as well as on real data and achieve reliable results compared to a state-of-the-art method. This approach is even capable to relieable reconstruct three fiber crossing utilizing only 10 gradient acquisitions.

1 Introduction

Diffusion Tensor Imaging (DTI) makes it possible to non-invasively reconstruct fiber pathways of human white matter using only six gradient measurements. Since [3] showed that DTI is neither capable of estimating kissing nor crossing fibers, various approaches have been proposed [9] that are able to detect multiple of fiber directions in a voxel. This is crucial as voxels containing multiple fiber directions occur in 60 % to 90 % of human white matter [5]. These High Angular Resolution Diffusion Imaging techniques require a multitude of measured gradient directions per voxel for reconstruction of fiber orientation distribution functions (fODF) in order to achieve maximum accuracy, resulting in an increased MRI acquisition time.

As the number of gradient directions decreases, fitting these complex models result in an approximation error. To address this issue, we take a step back and formulate the task of deriving fiber directions directly from the signal as a classification problem. Recently proposed methods showed the strength of machine learning and especially Deep Learning (DL) to approximate complex functions using only a few input measurements [4,6].

In this work, we present a novel approach for direct estimating multiple fiber directions without any a-priori knowledge using convolutional Deep Neural Networks (CNN). For this purpose, we replace the reconstruction process by a

© Springer International Publishing AG 2016
L. Wang et al. (Eds.): MLMI 2016, LNCS 10019, pp. 53–60, 2016.
DOI: 10.1007/978-3-319-47157-0_7

classification approach. A CNN is applied to estimate the correct class, while each class defines a precise direction, using only raw data as input.

2   Material

The CNN is evaluated using real and synthetic diffusion data.

For this purpose 20 healthy volunteers are measured using a Siemens Tim Trio 3 T scanner using 200 gradient directions, a b-value of $b = 2700 \frac{s}{mm^2}$ and a voxel size of $2.5 \times 2.5 \times 2.5 \, mm^3$. Based on this setting, our SNR_0 [2] ranges from ≈ 23 to ≈ 42 and has a mean value of ≈ 33. Afterwards, each voxel is categorized according to its number of compartments [7] and sub-sampled based on Spherical Harmonics for 10, 15, 30, 60 and 120 directions. In order to generate a ground truth for classification purposes, the Ball-and-Stick model proposed in [8] creates a relative ground truth in each voxel based on the original raw data with 200 gradient directions. For training we randomly extract 5000 voxels for each combination of each of the five gradient sets and $k = \{1, 2, 3\}$ number of fibers per voxel using always the same 15 real datasets, resulting in a total of 225 000 voxels. Testing is performed on 5000 randomly extracted voxels per dataset from the remaining five datasets, resulting in a total of 75 000 voxels.

For quantitative evaluation, our database is generated based on synthetic simulated diffusion-weighted data for 10, 15, 30, 60 and 120 gradient directions utilizing the multi-tensor model proposed in [10]. The b-value is set to $b = 2700 \frac{s}{mm^2}$ and a Rician noise with $SNR_0 = \frac{1}{\sigma} = 30$ is added, which is chosen to be similar to the acquired real data. Eigenvalues are sampled based on real DW-MRI data according to [1] and the volume fraction f_i is chosen randomly with $f_i \in [0.2, 1]$, while f_0 is considered to be a completely isotropic tensor. Afterwards, $|f|$ is normalized to 1. Inter-fiber angles below $15°$ and fibers with $f_i < 0.2$ are rejected. Our training set consists of 25 000 random voxels and our test set of 5000 random voxels for each combination of directions and number of fibers, resulting in 225 000 random voxels for training and 75,000 random voxels for testing.

3   Deep Learning

Recently, representation learning techniques (e.g. Neural Networks) had a very big impact on the field of machine learning, due to their ability to automatically discover important features for classification from raw data. Important features are detected by applying different kinds of transformations to raw data, making them ideal in classification scenarios using very abstract data. Deep Learning creates a new classifier by stacking multiple "hidden" layers of representation learning algorithms, resulting in a network of connected transformations. These networks are able to describe even more abstract relations in the input data and represent more complex functions. After the last layer of each network a pseudo probability distribution is calculated, which has to be maximized for a corresponding class. Therefore, a loss function is utilized and the network is trained using a standard Stochastic Gradient Descent (SGD) algorithm training the whole network at once. Our constructed network is trained without pretraining, using a learning rate of 0.01 and a momentum of 0.9. In this work we focus on CNNs, which apply convolutional transformations in several layers of the network. For constructing our network we utilize the toolbox MatConvNet [11].

4 Using CNN for Estimating the fODF

In order to adapt a CNN to Diffusion Imaging we propose a new framework which is composed of two parts. The first part estimates the correct number of fiber directions in a voxel, based on a reliable method presented in [7], while the second part determines the fiber orientations, using three different CNNs according to the number of fiber directions. The following sections describe how the classes are defined, which kind of preprocessing is required and how the new network is structured. These parts are utilized for each of the three CNNs in the second part of the framework.

4.1 Class Definition

In case of Diffusion Imaging a fODF is a continuous function over a unit sphere. In order to transfer the fODF of a voxel into a classification problem, the fODF is assumed to be symmetric and can be discretized. For this purpose one hemisphere of the fODF is equidistantly sampled for 250 possible fiber directions, resulting in an angular quantization error of $\approx 4.5°$. Each sampled direction forms a class for the classification problem.

4.2 Pre-processing

Due to the fact that it is recommended for a CNN to use zero-mean data, the signals' mean is subtracted, resulting in a removal of its isotropic compartment leaving only the relative changes of the anisotropic parts. This can be explained using the multi-tensor model [3] that describes the signal S as

$$S = S_{\text{isotropic}} + S_{\text{anisotropic}}, \tag{1}$$

where $S_{\text{isotropic}}$ represents the isotropic part of the signal that remains unchanged for each gradient direction, and $S_{\text{anisotropic}}$ represents the anisotropic part, which differs for every gradient direction, respectively. Consequently, subtracting the signals' mean results in

$$S - \text{mean}(S) = S_{\text{anisotropic}} - \text{mean}(S_{\text{anisotropic}}). \tag{2}$$

In addition, to ensure that the CNN can be applied for 15 as well as for 120 gradient directions, the acquired signal vector is interpolated using Spherical Harmonics and resampled to 120 pre-defined gradient directions, which are equidistantly sampled over a hemisphere. After these preprocessing steps, the 1D signal vector

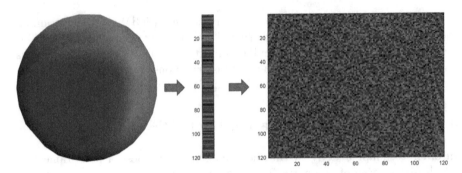

Fig. 1. Pre-processing workflow: a continuous 3D-spherical diffusion signal is transformed into a 2D-image to reconstruct neighboring information.

is converted, so that a CNN is able to learn neighboring information. For this purpose, the 1D-vector is transformed into a 2D-image by incremental cyclic shifting: The 1D-vector is inserted in the image's leftmost free column resulting in an image (see Fig. 1) and the algorithm stops as soon as the initial signal is repeated.

4.3   The Architecture

The CNN architecture in this work consists of five different kinds of layers. The most important one is the Convolutional Layer (CL), which convolutes the input image of size $W \times H \times C$, where W is the width, H the height and C the number of channels of the image with a kernel. The kernel size is $M \times N \times F \times K$, where $M \times N$ defines the area of convolution, F is the weighting function over all channels and K is the number of different kernels. Due to the weighting function, each CL is a fully-connected layer. In addition, a CL can reduce the input image size using a sub-sampling factor s. This layer identifies important relationships between different gradient signals within a voxel.

The second most important layer is the activation function called Rectified Linear Unit (ReLu), which applies $x_{\text{out}} = \max(x_{\text{in}}, 0)$ to each pixel value x on an image in each channel.

The third kind of utilized layers is the Maximal Pooling (MaxPool) operation, which reduces the image size by keeping only the maximal value in an area of $M \times N$ in an image. Similar to the CL a MaxPool can further reduce the image size using a sub-sampling factor s.

To use the network as a classifier for the fODF, a normalized exponential function (SoftMax) is applied as the last layer to calculate the pseudo probability of each class, i.e. its corresponding fiber direction. To train the network the common Logarithmic-Loss (LogLoss) function is extended for a multi-label problem to

$$\text{logloss} = \frac{1}{L} \cdot \sum_{i=1}^{L} \sum_{j=1}^{P} y_{i,j} \log(p_{i,j}), \tag{3}$$

where L is the number of labels per image, P is the number of possible classes, y is a binary label matrix, which contains true or false. p is the pseudo probability of each class after the SoftMax.

In addition, dropout layers (DL) are applied during training, which discard input pixels at random positions with a probability of p, to prevent the classifier from overfitting. In Table 1 the architecture is described.

Table 1. Architecture of the network.

#	Type	Parameters
1	DL	$p = 0.2$
2	CL	$7 \times 7 \times 1 \times 128$ and $s = 2$
3	ReLu	-
4	MaxPool	$3 \times 3 \times$ and $s = 2$
5	CL	$5 \times 5 \times 128 \times 32$ and $s = 2$
6	ReLu	-
7	MaxPool	$3 \times 3 \times$ and $s = 2$
8	CL	$3 \times 3 \times 32 \times 512$ and $s = 1$
9	ReLu	-
10	CL	$3 \times 3 \times 512 \times 368$ and $s = 1$
11	DL	$p = 0.5$
12	CL	$1 \times 1 \times 368 \times 250$ and $s = 1$
13	DL	$p = 0.5$
14	SoftMax LogLoss	-

5   Results

All computations are performed on a PC equipped with an Intel Core i5-4670 CPU, using 4 cores with 3.4 GHz each, 32 GB RAM and a NVIDIA GeForce GTX 980 Ti with 8 GB RAM for CUDA computations.

For comparison, a well-established state-of-the-art method proposed in [8], which combines the extremely fast spherical deconvolution with the very accurate ball-and-stick model (BS), is considered. This method proved to be one of the best methods to reconstruct diffusion data with only few gradient directions, which is even suitable for clinical scenarios [9]. The CNN is trained for each combination of measured direction and k fiber directions per voxel. The angular error of the known ground truth for synthetic data and the relative ground truth for real data ranges from 0° to 90° (with 0° being the optimal and 90° being the worst possible result).

Figure 2 presents the resulting angular errors for crossing fibers and 10, 15, 30, 60 and 120 gradient directions. The curves, representing the CNN approach in dashed lines and the BS model in solid lines, are plotted in blue for synthetic data and in red for real data.

It can be seen that the CNN approach achieves similar results on synthetic data in comparison to the BS model, while it achieves a lower angular error on real data. In addition, it can be seen that the resulting angular error increases significantly for the BS model if less than 30 gradient directions are acquired. More detailed results are presented in Table 2, which contains the mean angular errors of the BS model and CNN approach for synthetic and real data utilizing $k = \{1, 2, 3\}$ fiber directions, and the clinical most relevant 10, 15, 30 and 60 gradient directions.

Considering the single-fiber case ($k = 1$), the BS model achieves better results than the CNN model for 15 and more gradient directions on synthetic data and for 30 and more gradient directions on real data. For crossing fibers ($k = \{2, 3\}$) it shows the same trends as in Fig. 2. The CNN approach achieves much lower angular errors than the BS model if only a few gradient directions are acquired or if there are complex voxel structures such as three crossing fibers.

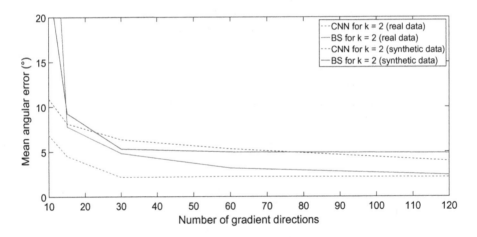

Fig. 2. The resulting error curves for real and synthetic data, $k = 2$ and different gradient directions. (Color figure online)

Regarding computational performance, the BS model achieves a computational speed of ≈ 3330 voxels per second for 120 directions and $k = 3$, while the CNN approach always achieves a higher computation speed of ≈ 4500 voxels per second, respectively.

6   Discussion

Regarding the mean angular error for crossing fibers in Fig. 2, it can be seen that the CNN model achieves similar results on synthetic data, while it outperforms

Table 2. Mean angular errors for $k = \{1, 2, 3\}$ in comparison to 10, 15, 30 and 60 gradient directions.

	\multicolumn{8}{c}{Mean angular error ($^\circ$) for synthetic data}							
	10 Dir		15 Dir		30 Dir		60 Dir	
k	CNN	BS	CNN	BS	CNN	BS	CNN	BS
1	**4.92**	16.99	3.86	1.51	2.75	0.79	2.58	0.75
2	**10.90**	24.30	**8.13**	9.26	6.36	5.32	5.33	4.97
3	**12.49**	42.20	**7.67**	19.85	**7.60**	13.29	**6.56**	10.52

	\multicolumn{8}{c}{Mean angular error ($^\circ$) for real data}							
	10 Dir		15 Dir		30 Dir		60 Dir	
k	CNN	BS	CNN	BS	CNN	BS	CNN	BS
1	**5.50**	45.00	**2.42**	2.87	2.48	0.74	2.72	0.42
2	**6.86**	45.00	**4.51**	6.51	**2.56**	4.83	**2.43**	3.19
3	**12.44**	45.00	**7.51**	15.55	**6.23**	11.20	**6.09**	8.47

the BS model on real data, respectively. This mean angular gap grows with increasing voxel complexity as it can be seen in Table 2. As expected, the BS model becomes unstable for 15 and less gradient directions for both synthetic and real data, due to a minimal number of required gradient directions, while the CNN approach achieves an acceptable stable angular error.

Considering the single-fiber case, the CNN approach converges for 15 and more gradient directions on synthetic data and for 30 gradient directions on real data, respectively. On the one hand, this may be a consequence of the quantization blur, while on the other hand it shows that the CNN is insensitive towards different number of gradient directions. The same effect can be seen for crossing fibers on real data in Fig. 2. Here, the CNN achieves almost the same mean angular error for 15 gradient directions and for 120 gradient directions.

In addition, the fact that the performance of the CNN converges suggests that it does not improve further when more gradient directions are available, while on the other hand it seems to improve for a higher SNR, as the synthetic data has a SNR_0 of 30, while our real data has a mean SNR_0 of ≈ 33. Utilizing this approach for estimating the fODF, an enhancement of SNR may be more important than increasing the number of gradient directions.

Taking a look at the computation time, both models show an equally fast performance, while the CNN approach is slightly ahead.

A limitation of this work is that it is evaluated using the same scanner as well as the same scanner protocol for training and testing. In order to make the CNN applicable for other scanner types or different scanning protocols, [7] proposed a method to simulate realistic training data for a specific scanner type and a specific scanning protocol. Utilizing this signal generation approach, the CNN may be applicable across multiple scanner types, which shall be investigated in future work. Furthermore, we will investigate other approaches for converting a 1D signal into a 2D image, in order to retrieve neighboring information.

7   Conclusion

We introduce a completely new, very fast and accurate way of deriving the fODF in a diffusion voxel, which achieves more stable and better results than the state-of-the-art BS model on real data and a comparable angular error on synthetic data. In addition, the presented CNN is insensitive with respect to different numbers of gradient directions and remains stable even for less than 15 gradient directions, while the BS model starts to deteriorate. To the best of our knowledge, this is the first time that a Deep Learning approach is used for reconstructing the fODF. In future work, we will investigate a quantization free approach, in order to eliminate the quantization blur.

References

1. Canales-Rodríguez, E.J., Melie-García, L., Iturria-Medina, Y.: Mathematical description of q-space in spherical coordinates: exact q-ball imaging. Magn. Reson. Med. **61**(6), 1350–1367 (2009)
2. Jones, D.K., Knösche, T.R., Turner, R.: White matter integrity, fiber count, and other fallacies: the do's and don'ts of diffusion MRI. NeuroImage **73**, 239–254 (2013)
3. Tuch, D.S., Reese, T.G., Wiegell, M.R., Makris, N., Belliveau, J.W., Wedeen, J.: High Angular resolution diffusion imaging reveals intravoxel white matter fiber heterogeneity. Magn. Reson. Med. **48**(4), 577–582 (2002)
4. Golkov, D., Sämann, P., Sperl, J.I., Sprenger, T., Czisch, M., Menzel, M.I., Gómez, P.A., Haase, A., Brox, T., Cremers, D.: Q-space deep learning: twelve-fold shorter and model-free diffusion MRI scans. IEEE Trans. Med. Imaging **35**(5), 1344–1351 (2016)
5. Jeurissen, B., Leemans, A., Tournier, J.D., Jones, D.K., Sijbers, J.: Investigating the prevalence of complex fiber configurations in white matter tissue with diffusion magnetic resonance imaging. Hum. Brain Mapp. **34**(11), 2747–2766 (2013)
6. Neher, P.F., Götz, M., Norajitra, T., Weber, C., Maier-Hein, K.H.: A machine learning based approach to fiber tractography using classifier voting. In: Navab, N., Hornegger, J., Wells, W.M., Frangi, A.F. (eds.) MICCAI 2015. LNCS, vol. 9349, pp. 45–52. Springer, Heidelberg (2015). doi:10.1007/978-3-319-24553-9_6
7. Schultz, T.: Learning a reliable estimate of the number of fiber directions in diffusion MRI. In: Ayache, N., Delingette, H., Golland, P., Mori, K. (eds.) MICCAI 2012. LNCS, vol. 7512, pp. 493–500. Springer, Heidelberg (2012). doi:10.1007/978-3-642-33454-2_61
8. Schultz, T., Westin, C.-F., Kindlmann, G.: Multi-diffusion-tensor fitting via spherical deconvolution: a unifying framework. In: Jiang, T., Navab, N., Pluim, J.P.W., Viergever, M.A. (eds.) MICCAI 2010. LNCS, vol. 6361, pp. 674–681. Springer, Heidelberg (2010). doi:10.1007/978-3-642-15705-9_82
9. Seunarine, K.K., Alexander, D.C.: Multiple fibers: beyond the diffusion tensor. In: Diffusion MRI: From Quantitative Measurement to In Vivo Neuroanatomy, vol. 1, pp. 55–72 (2009)
10. Tuch, D.S.: Q-ball imaging. Magn. Reson. Med. **52**(6), 1358–1372 (2004)
11. Vedaldi, A., Lenc, K.: MatConvNet: convolutional neural networks for MATLAB. In: Proceedings of 23rd ACM International Conference on Multimedia, pp. 689–692. ACM (2015)

Segmentation of Perivascular Spaces Using Vascular Features and Structured Random Forest from 7T MR Image

Jun Zhang[1], Yaozong Gao[1,2], Sang Hyun Park[1], Xiaopeng Zong[1], Weili Lin[1], and Dinggang Shen[1,3(✉)]

[1] Department of Radiology and BRIC, UNC at Chapel Hill, Chapel Hill, NC, USA
dgshen@med.unc.edu
[2] Department of Computer Science, UNC at Chapel Hill, Chapel Hill, NC, USA
[3] Department of Brain and Cognitive Engineering, Korea University, Seongbuk-gu, Republic of Korea

Abstract. Quantitative analysis of perivascular spaces (PVSs) is important to reveal the correlations between cerebrovascular lesions and neurodegenerative diseases. In this study, we propose a learning-based segmentation framework to extract the PVSs from high-resolution 7T MR images. Specifically, we integrate three types of vascular filter responses into a structured random forest for classifying voxels into PVS and background. In addition, we also propose a novel entropy-based sampling strategy to extract informative samples in the background for training the classification model. Since various vascular features can be extracted by the three vascular filters, even thin and low-contrast structures can be effectively extracted from the noisy background. Moreover, continuous and smooth segmentation results can be obtained by utilizing the patch-based structured labels. The segmentation performance is evaluated on 19 subjects with 7T MR images, and the experimental results demonstrate that the joint use of entropy-based sampling strategy, vascular features and structured learning improves the segmentation accuracy, with the Dice similarity coefficient reaching 66 %.

1 Introduction

Perivascular spaces (PVSs) are cerebrospinal fluid (CSF) filled spaces ensheathing small blood vessels as they penetrate the brain parenchyma. The clinical significance of PVSs comes primarily from their tendency to dilate in the abnormal cases. For example, normal brains show a few dilated PVSs, while an increase of dilated PVSs has been shown to correlate with the incidence of several neurodegenerative diseases, making the research of PVS a hot topic. Since most of the current studies require the segmentation of PVS to calculate quantitative measurements, the accurate and automatic segmentation of PVS is highly desirable.

So far, there are a few studies focusing on automatic PVS segmentation from MR images. For example, Descombes *et al.* enhanced the PVSs with filters and used a region-growing approach to get initial segmentation, followed

© Springer International Publishing AG 2016
L. Wang et al. (Eds.): MLMI 2016, LNCS 10019, pp. 61–68, 2016.
DOI: 10.1007/978-3-319-47157-0_8

by a geometry prior constraint for further improving the segmentation accuracy [1]. Uchiyama *et al.* adopted a gray-level thresholding technique to extract PVSs from the MR images after being enhanced by a morphological white top-hat transform [2]. However, the segmentation accuracies are often limited with these unsupervised techniques, since it is very challenging to distinguish PVSs from confounding tissue boundaries. Recently, it has been demonstrated that the supervised methods are superior on the vessel segmentation problem by learning powerful classifiers. For example, Ricci and Perfetti employed the support vector machine (SVM) for retinal vessel segmentation with a specially designed line detector [3]. Marín *et al.* adopted the neural network (NN) for retinal vessel segmentation with gray-level and moment invariants based features [4].

However, there are several challenges for directly applying these supervised learning methods to PVS segmentation: (1) Since PVSs are extremely narrow and have low contrast compared with the neighboring tissues, general features may not capture the discriminative characters of PVSs compared with confounding background. (2) Informative tubular structures of PVSs cannot be considered in the label space, thus often leading to discontinuous and unsmooth segmentations. However, using a simple global geometrical constraint may cause over-fitting, since PVSs can appear at any locations and also have large shape variations (*e.g.*, different lengths, widths and curvatures). (3) Since the number of PVS voxels is much smaller than that of background voxels and there are always a large number of uninformative voxels in the background, it is difficult to train a reliable classifier with the conventional sampling method.

To address these challenges, we propose a structured learning-based framework for PVS segmentation from high-resolution 7T MR images. We integrate three types of vascular features, based on steerable filters, optimally oriented flux (OOF), and Frangi filter, into a structured random forest for classifying voxels into positive (*i.e.*, PVS) and negative (*i.e.*, background) classes. In addition, we also propose a novel entropy-based sampling strategy to extract informative samples in the background. Since various vascular features can be extracted by these three vascular filters, even thin and low-contrast structures can be effectively extracted from the noisy background. Moreover, the continuous and smooth segmentation results can be obtained by utilizing the patch-based structured labels.

2   Method

As shown in Fig. 1, our method is comprised of two stages. In the *training stage*, we first extract a region-of-interest (ROI) for each MR image. Then, we sample training voxels according to the probabilities calculated with local entropies. Next, the vascular features from MR images to describe a voxel's local structure are extracted, and the patch-based structured labels are also extracted from the binary segmentation (PVS) images as multiple target labels. Finally, a structured random forest is trained. In the *testing stage*, features are similarly extracted for each voxel in the ROI, and then all voxels in the ROI are classified by the trained structured random forest model.

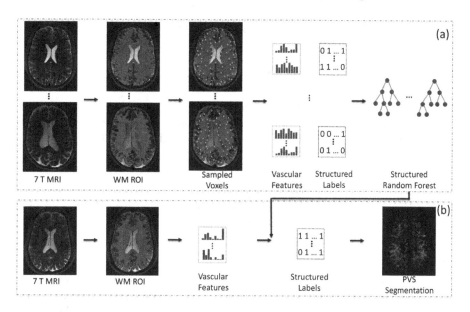

Fig. 1. Schematic diagram of the proposed method. (a) Training stage. (b) Testing stage.

2.1 Region-of-Interest Generation

PVSs only appear in the white matter (WM) tissue, and T2-weighted MRI is the best madality to identify all PVSs [5]. Therefore, we extract the WM tissue in the T2-weighted image as our ROI for PVS segmentation. Since image contrast between white matter and gray matter is clearer in the T1-weighted image, rather than the T2-weighted image, we rigidly align the T1-weighted image to the T2-weighted image, and then perform skull stripping and WM tissue segmentation in the aligned T1-weighted image. Therefore, we can obtain the WM segmentation in the T2-weighted image space.

2.2 Voxel Sampling Strategy

In general, the number of PVS voxels is much smaller (*i.e.*, ranging from several thousands to tens of thousands) than the total number of voxels in the WM (*i.e.*, millions). Therefore, we select all PVS voxels as positives samples for training. On the other hand, we extract negative samples from background, whose number is several times larger than that of the positive samples. Since the background includes a large number of uninformative (or less informative) voxels from the uniform regions but a relatively small number of informative voxels, it is inappropriate to randomly sample the negative voxels from background. In order to balance the proportions of uninformative and informative voxels, we propose to sample the voxels according to the probabilities calculated with the local entropies around voxels.

Specifically, for a region around a specific voxel $\mathbf{x}$, the local entropy $E(\mathbf{x})$ is defined as

$$E(\mathbf{x}) = -\sum_i p_i(s, \mathbf{x}) \log p_i(s, \mathbf{x}), \tag{1}$$

where i is a possible intensity value, and $p_i(s, \mathbf{x})$ is the probability distribution of intensity i within a spherical region $|\Omega(s, \mathbf{x})|$ centered at $\mathbf{x}$ with a radius of s.

Then, we sample the voxel $\mathbf{x}$ with the probability of $\mathcal{P}(\mathbf{x})$, which is defined as

$$\mathcal{P}(\mathbf{x}) = e^{-\frac{\alpha}{E(\mathbf{x})}}, \tag{2}$$

where α is a coefficient that directly affects the sampling probability and also controls the total number of sampled voxels.

2.3   Feature Extraction

For many vessel segmentation problems, the orientations of the vessels are generally irregular (*e.g.*, retinal vessels and pulmonary vessels). Therefore, the orientation invariance is an important property of features. However, unlike these vessel segmentation problems, PVSs have roughly regular orientations that point to ventricles filled with CSF, as shown in Fig. 1(b) (PVS segmentation). To consider the useful orientation information, we extract three types of vascular features based on steerable filters, OOF, and Frangi filter from T2-weighed images. For each type of these features, we also employ multi-scale representation to capture both coarse and fine structural features.

Steerable Filter-Based Features: Since Gaussian derivative filters are steerable, any arbitrary oriented responses of the first-order and second-order Gaussian derivative filters can be obtained by the linear combinations of some basis filter responses [6], and the steerable filters have been broadly used for feature extraction [7–9]. In this paper, we extract the 3D steerable filter-based features including the responses of a Gaussian filter, 9 oriented first-order Gaussian derivative filters and 9 orientated second-order Gaussian derivative filters. Therefore, there are 19 features for each scale of steerable filters (*i.e.*, the standard deviation of Gaussian/Gaussian derivative filters).

OOF-Based Features: The OOF has been proven to be effective for enhancing the curvilinear structures by quantifying the amount of projected image gradient flowing in or out of a local spherical region [10]. We extract 4 features based on the first two eigenvalues (λ_1, λ_2) of OOF Hessian matrix, which are $(\lambda_1, \lambda_2, \sqrt{max(0, \lambda_1\lambda_2)}, \lambda_1 + \lambda_2)$. Moreover, we extract 2 orientation features based on the eigenvector (x_1, y_1, z_1) corresponding to the maximum eigenvalue λ_1, which are $(\arccos(\frac{|z_1|}{\sqrt{x_1^2+y_1^2+z_1^2}}), \arctan(\frac{y_1}{x_1}))$. Therefore, there are 6 features for each scale of spherical region (*i.e.*, the radius of spherical region for calculating the flux).

Frangi-Based Features: The Frangi vesselness measurements are extracted based on the Hessian matrix of second order Gaussian derivative filter responses [11]. In our study, we extract 3 features based on the eigenvalues $(\gamma_1, \gamma_2, \gamma_3)$ of the Hessian matrix, which are $(\frac{|\gamma_1|}{|\gamma_2|}, \frac{|\gamma_1|}{\sqrt{|\gamma_2\gamma_3|}}, \sqrt{\gamma_1^2 + \gamma_2^2 + \gamma_3^2})$. We also extract 2 orientation features based on the eigenvector (x_1', y_1', z_1') corresponding to the maximum eigenvalue γ_1, which are $(\arccos(\frac{|z_1'|}{\sqrt{x_1'^2 + y_1'^2 + z_1'^2}}),$ $\arctan(\frac{y_1'}{x_1'}))$. Therefore, there are 5 features for each scale of Gaussian derivative filters (*i.e.*, the standard deviation of Gaussian derivative filters).

2.4   Structured Random Forest

Random forest classifier is a combination of tree predictors [12]. For a general segmentation task, the input space corresponds to the extracted features of each voxel, and the output space corresponds to the label of that voxel. As a matter of fact, the PVSs have line-like structures such that the neighborhood labels have certain structured coherence. Therefore, we perform the structured learning strategy in our task, which addresses the problem of learning a mapping where the input or output space may represent complex morphological structures.

In our task, the output space is structured, so that we utilize the structured patch-based labels (*i.e.*, the cubic patch with a size of $n \times n \times n$) in the output space. Specifically, in the training stage, we first extract vascular features for each voxel sampled from T2-weighted image, as well as a corresponding cubic label patch from manually segmented binary image. Then, a structured random forest (multi-label) model is trained using the features and labels. In the testing stage, we similarly extract the respective features for all voxels in the WM tissue from the testing T2-weighted images. Then, the features are fed to the trained model, and each voxel outputs a label patch. By assigning the patch-based labels to the neighboring voxels, each voxel receives n^3 label values, and we take the majority value as the label for each voxel. Eventually, by using the structured labels, the local structural constraint of PVSs in the label space can be naturally added to the random forest model.

As we know, most of PVSs point to the ventricles, thus PVSs within each hemisphere have roughly statistical regularity of orientations. Therefore, we separately train one model for the left hemisphere and another model for the right hemisphere, to reduce the divergence of PVSs' orientations. Finally, voxels from each hemisphere of the testing image are fed to the corresponding trained model for prediction.

3   Experiments, Results and Discussions

A 7T Siemens Scanner with a 32-channel head coil and a single-channel volume transmit coil (Nova Medical, Wilmington, MA) was used during our data acquisition. Both T1- and T2-weighted images were scanned for each subject with the spatial resolution of $0.65 \times 0.65 \times 0.65 \, \mathrm{mm}^3$ and $0.5 \times 0.5 \times 0.5 \, \mathrm{mm}^3$ (or $0.4 \times 0.4 \times 0.4 \, \mathrm{mm}^3$), respectively. In total, there were 19 subjects. The manual labels of PVSs were generated from the T2-weighted images using a thresholding-based semi-automatic method, and then manually corrected by two experts.

Two-fold cross validation is used to evaluate the segmentation performance. In order to expand the training dataset, each training image is further left-right flipped to generate one more training image. The parameters are set as follows: For extracting multi-scale steerable filters-based features, the standard deviations of Gaussian filters are set as [0.5, 1.5, 2.5, 3.5], thus obtaining 76 features in total. For extracting multi-scale OOF-based features, the flux radii are set as [0.5, 1, 1.5, 2, 2.5, 3, 3.5, 4], thus obtaining 48 features in total. For extracting Frangi-based features, the standard deviations of Gaussian filters are set as [0.5, 1, 1.5, 2, 2.5, 3, 3.5], thus obtaining 35 features in total. Here, we select slightly denser scales for generating OOF and Frangi-based features than steerable filter-based features, to decrease the imbalance for the numbers of different types of features. For extracting patch-based labels, the patch size is set as $3 \times 3 \times 3$. For voxel sampling, the radius s is set as 10, and the coefficient parameter α is set as 15 to keep the proportion between positive voxels and negative voxels to be roughly 1:5. For training the structured random forest, 10 independent trees are trained and the depth of each tree is set as 20.

In our experiment, the segmentation performance is measured by Dice similarity coefficient (DSC). As a comparison, the results of Frangi [11] and OOF [10] with the thresholding strategy are reported in Fig. 2(a). As can be seen, our method achieves the best result as compared to these two thresholding methods, thus demonstrating the effectiveness of our learning-based framework. Figure 2(a) also shows the results by random forest (not structured) and the vascular features. It can be seen that the use of structured random forest achieves roughly 6 % improvement in terms of DSC as compared to the standard random forest.

Sampling Strategy: In our method, we sample voxels from background with the probabilities in proportion to their local entropies. For comparison, we also show the result of random sampling voxels from background. As shown in Fig. 2(b), the proposed sampling strategy improves the segmentation performance by more than 8 % in terms of DSC for both random forest and structured random forest strategies. Figure 3(a) also shows an example of PVS segmentation of using different sampling strategies. As indicated, random sampling strategy has potential risk of wrongly classifying the confounding edge voxels as PVS. Specifically, if we sample the background voxels randomly, many voxels that are similar to PVS may not be sampled for training, since there are millions of uninformative voxels in background. The use of redundant unrepresentative sampled voxels for training may adversely affect the accuracy of classification model. As shown in Fig. 3(a), our method can distinguish the voxels that are similar to the PVS, but not PVS, compared with random sampling strategy.

Structured Random Forest: Figure 3(b) also compares a pair of segmentation results between random forest and structured random forest. As can be seen,

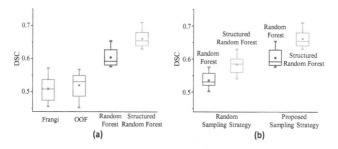

Fig. 2. Quantitative evaluation of segmentation results. (a) Results of different methods. (b) Results of using different voxel sampling strategies.

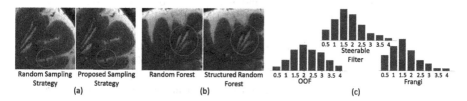

Fig. 3. Analysis of PVS segmentation. (a) Qualitative comparison between random sampling and our proposed sampling for obtaining the training voxels. (b) Qualitative comparison between random forest and the structured random forest. (c) Frequency of features being selected at each spatial scales.

the result by the random forest model is discontinuous and unsmooth, while the structured random forest improves such circumstance due to the use of local structural constraint in the label space.

Feature Scale Selection: One important parameter for feature extraction is the scale range for multi-scale representation. In our experiment, we define the scales of vascular features by their frequencies of being selected in all split nodes of a trained classification model. Specifically, we feed redundant features with many scales to train a classification model. Then, we count the frequencies of selected features in terms of scales. As shown in Fig. 3(c), the distribution demonstrates the importance of each scale in extracting vascular features. Finally, we only use the scales in the reasonable range for each feature type, as introduced in our parameter setting part.

4   Conclusion

In this paper, we propose a PVS segmentation method based on vascular features and structured random forest. In the input feature space, the vascular features can distinguish the PVSs from complex background. In the output label space, the patch-based structured labels preserve the local structure of PVS. Moreover, a novel voxel sampling strategy is also proposed to further improve the segmentation performance. The superior segmentation performance demonstrates the effectiveness of our structured learning-based framework for PVS segmentation.

References

1. Descombes, X., Kruggel, F., Wollny, G., Gertz, H.J.: An object-based approach for detecting small brain lesions: application to Virchow-Robin spaces. IEEE Trans. Med. Imaging **23**(2), 246–255 (2004)
2. Uchiyama, Y., Kunieda, T., Asano, T., Kato, H., Hara, T., Kanematsu, M., Iwama, T., Hoshi, H., Kinosada, Y., Fujita, H.: Computer-aided diagnosis scheme for classification of lacunar infarcts and enlarged virchow-robin spaces in brain MR images. In: Engineering in Medicine and Biology Society, pp. 3908–3911. IEEE (2008)
3. Ricci, E., Perfetti, R.: Retinal blood vessel segmentation using line operators and support vector classification. IEEE Trans. Med. Imaging **26**(10), 1357–1365 (2007)
4. Marín, D., Aquino, A., Gegúndez-Arias, M.E., Bravo, J.M.: A new supervised method for blood vessel segmentation in retinal images by using gray-level and moment invariants-based features. IEEE Trans. Med. Imaging **30**(1), 146–158 (2011)
5. Hernández, M., Piper, R.J., Wang, X., Deary, I.J., Wardlaw, J.M.: Towards the automatic computational assessment of enlarged perivascular spaces on brain magnetic resonance images: a systematic review. J. Magn. Reson. Imaging **38**(4), 774–785 (2013)
6. Freeman, W.T., Adelson, E.H.: The design and use of steerable filters. IEEE Trans. Pattern Anal. Mach. Intell. **9**, 891–906 (1991)
7. Zhang, J., Liang, J., Zhao, H.: Local energy pattern for texture classification using self-adaptive quantization thresholds. IEEE Trans. Image Process. **22**(1), 31–42 (2013)
8. Derpanis, K.G., Wildes, R.P.: Dynamic texture recognition based on distributions of spacetime oriented structure. In: 2010 IEEE Conference on Computer Vision and Pattern Recognition (CVPR), pp. 191–198. IEEE (2010)
9. Zhang, J., Zhao, H., Liang, J.: Continuous rotation invariant local descriptors for texton dictionary-based texture classification. Comput. Vis. Image Underst. **117**(1), 56–75 (2013)
10. Law, M.W.K., Chung, A.C.S.: Three dimensional curvilinear structure detection using optimally oriented flux. In: Forsyth, D., Torr, P., Zisserman, A. (eds.) ECCV 2008. LNCS, vol. 5305, pp. 368–382. Springer, Heidelberg (2008). doi:10.1007/978-3-540-88693-8_27
11. Frangi, A.F., Niessen, W.J., Vincken, K.L., Viergever, M.A.: Multiscale vessel enhancement filtering. In: Wells, W.M., Colchester, A.C.F., Delp, S.L. (eds.) MICCAI 1998. LNCS, vol. 1496, pp. 130–137. Springer, Heidelberg (1998)
12. Breiman, L.: Random forests. Mach. Learn. **45**(1), 5–32 (2001)

Dual-Layer Groupwise Registration for Consistent Labeling of Longitudinal Brain Images

Minjeong Kim, Guorong Wu, Isrem Rekik, and Dinggang Shen[✉]

Department of Radiology and BRIC, University of North Carolina at Chapel Hill,
Chapel Hill, USA
{mjkim, dgshen}@med.unc.edu

Abstract. The growing collection of longitudinal images for brain disease diagnosis necessitates the development of advanced longitudinal registration and anatomical labeling methods that can respect temporal consistency between images. However, the characteristics of such longitudinal images and how they lodge into the image manifold are often neglected in existing labeling methods. Indeed, most of them independently align atlases to each target time-point image for propagating the pre-defined atlas labels to the subject domain. In this paper, we present a *dual-layer groupwise registration method* to consistently label anatomical regions of interest in brain images across different time-points using a multi-atlases-based labeling framework. Our framework can best enhance the labeling of longitudinal images through: **(1)** using the group mean of the longitudinal images of each subject (i.e., subject-mean) as a bridge between atlases and the longitudinal subject scans to align atlases to all time-point images jointly; and **(2)** using inter-atlas relationship in their nesting manifold to better register each atlas image to the subject-mean. These steps yield to a more consistent (from the joint alignment of atlases with all time-point images) and more accurate (from the manifold-guided registration between each atlases and the subject-mean image) registration, thereby eventually improving the consistency and accuracy for the subsequent labeling step. We have tested our dual-layer groupwise registration method to label two challenging longitudinal brain datasets (i.e., healthy infants and Alzheimer's disease subjects). Our experimental results have showed that our method achieves higher labeling accuracy while keeping the labeling consistency over time, when compared to the traditional registration scheme (without our proposed contributions). Moreover, the proposed framework can flexibly integrate with the existing label fusion methods, such as sparse-patch based methods, to improve the labeling accuracy of longitudinal datasets.

1 Introduction

Automatic and accurate region-of-interest (ROI) labeling has drawn significant attention in numerous medical image analysis studies, since it grounds the quantitative measurement of morphological structures related to brain disease or development across individuals or between groups. However, inter-subject anatomical variation in a

© Springer International Publishing AG 2016
L. Wang et al. (Eds.): MLMI 2016, LNCS 10019, pp. 69–76, 2016.
DOI: 10.1007/978-3-319-47157-0_9

population of brain images constitutes a key hurdle in achieving highly accurate ROI labeling. To partly overcome this difficulty, multi-atlas-based labeling approaches became more popular with the use of multiple atlases (with pre-defined labels) to propagate their labels to a target subject, then fusing them to obtain the final subject-specific labels. However, since the registration errors often occurs when registering multiple atlases to a subject image before the label fusion step, patch-based label fusion approaches have been proposed to reduce effects from these registration errors [1, 2]. These approaches can nicely incorporate neighboring information and also establish correspondences between a subject patch and atlas patches based on a patchwise similarity metric.

The potential registration errors may get more inflated when handling longitudinal brain data (and not only time-specific data). Hence, there is a need to develop advanced techniques to produce a longitudinally consistent registration and labeling that can accurately quantify subtle structural changes, which may be caused by brain development, aging or diseases. Notably, to devise a robust framework for consistent registration/labeling in the temporal domain, two key challenges must be overcome: (1) consecutive subject-specific registrations between different time-points would generate temporal registration errors (e.g., from brain atrophy or development across time), and (2) atlas-to-subject registration would engender spatial registration errors (from anatomical variations between subject and atlases). Therefore, to consistently label the ROIs in the longitudinal images, the atlas images with pre-labeled ROIs need to be warped in a temporally-constrained fashion to all time points of longitudinal images. However, the existing methods generally just register an atlas to each time-point image independently, or register different time-point images of the longitudinal scans to a pre-selected image at a certain time-point (used as a reference). This independence of registration may generate incoherent longitudinally registered images. Additionally, the existing methods only deployed pairwise registration to warp atlases to a target subject image. This strategy would also create a biased registration result due to the considerable anatomical difference between the atlases and the longitudinal subject images, which may cause inconsistent measurement of the small brain structure with longitudinal subtle changes (e.g., hippocampus).

To address these challenges, we propose a novel *dual-layer groupwise registration method,* which comprises two layers: (1) *Time-serial groupwise registration* to first register longitudinal images of the same subject. This estimates a subject-mean image as a common space to jointly align all different time-point images; and (2) *Manifold-guided registration* to label each time-point image by propagating the pre-defined ROIs from each of the multiple atlases, through the subject-mean image and with the help of neighboring atlases in the manifold. Then, subject-specific ROI labels, propagated from the aligned atlases, are fused using any label fusion method (e.g., sparse patch-based label fusion method [3]).

We tested our registration-labeling framework on two challenging longitudinal datasets from Alzheimer's disease (AD) patients and healthy infants, respectively. These two datasets present different challenges: AD subjects suffer from subtle but continuous anatomical changes, such as atrophy in hippocampal area, while structural brain images from infants show drastic changes both in shape and appearance especially in the first two years of postnatal development. Our dual-layer groupwise registration method showed a better labeling accuracy of the hippocampus in both datasets, compared to the traditional registration scheme, using the same multi-atlas-based label fusion method.

2 Method

Standard pairwise registration between the atlas to the target image is often used for labeling a single image with a single atlas. Intuitively, one could employ this standard pairwise registration in a serial fashion to label ROIs in a target longitudinal image sequence with multiple atlases. In other words, one can perform a series of pairwise registrations between N atlases $A = \{A_i | i = 1, \ldots, N\}$ and each of all T time-point subject images $I^t (t = 1, \ldots, T)$. Thus, the dense deformation field $F_t = \{f_t(x) | f_t(x) = x + u_{A_i \to I^t}(x), x \in \Omega_{A_i}\}$ for each pair of A_i and I^t can be estimated through this framework, where $u_{A_i \to I^t}(x)$ denotes the displacement of a point x in the atlas domain Ω_{A_i} to the image I^t in the longitudinal sequence.

However, as we pointed out before, this simple extension may generate both registration and labeling errors. To address this issue, we include the following two steps in our method for consistent labeling of a longitudinal image sequence: (1) the incorporation of a group mean of the target longitudinal images, called a subject-mean image I^M, as a bridge between atlases and the longitudinal images to align atlas images to all time-point images jointly; (2) the use of inter-atlas relationship between atlases in a manifold to better register each atlas image to the subject-mean. Thus, we can expect to achieve good temporal coherence between registered longitudinal images from the joint alignment of all time-point images with atlases (Step 1) as well as better spatial registration accuracy between the subject-mean image and atlases from the manifold guidance (Step 2).

Specifically, in the Step 1, we use a groupwise registration method to jointly register all time-point images I^t onto a common space, i.e., a subject-mean embedding space. In turn, this simultaneously generates the subject-mean image I^M and the intermediate deformation fields $F_{I^M \to I^t} = \{f_{I^M \to I^t}(x) | f_{I^M \to I^t}(x) = x + u_{I^M \to I^t}(x), x \in \Omega_{I^M}\}$ of all I^t towards the common space. In the Step 2, we propose a manifold-guided registration method to estimate the deformation fields from the best atlas images $B = \{B_i | i = 1, \ldots, P, P < N\}$ (i.e., $B \subset A$) to the subject-mean image I^M, denoted as $F_{B_i \to I^M} = \{f_{B_i \to I^M}(x) | B_i(x) = x + u_{B_i \to I^M}(x), x \in \Omega_{B_i}\}$. Finally, the deformation field F_t from B_i to each time-point image I^t in the longitudinal sequence is estimated by composing the deformation fields $F_{I^M \to I^t}$ and $F_{B_i \to I^M}$, i.e., $F_t = F_{I^M \to I^t} \circ F_{B_i \to I^M}$.

Figure 1 illustrates the overall idea of the proposed method, by comparison with the traditional scheme. The traditional registration scheme (Fig. 1(a)), independently aligns the atlases with each time-point image, which neglects the appealing properties of data distribution among atlases and the similarity of different time-point images of subject longitudinal sequence. In contrast, in our proposed framework (Fig. 1(b)), the registration between the atlases and different time-point images always goes through the subject-mean. Moreover, the manifold of atlases determines the deformation pathways from each atlas to the subject-mean by finding the best cost-efficient routes linking neighboring atlases in a graph hierarchy. Also, similarity of different time-point images is used in estimating subject-mean, and longitudinal consistency is further respected.

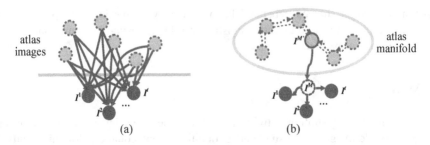

atlas images

atlas manifold

(a)   (b)

Fig. 1. Schematic illustration of the proposed registration framework (b) in comparison with the traditional registration framework (a).

2.1 Groupwise Time-Serial Image Registration

The goal of groupwise registration is to register all time-point images I^t to a common space by jointly estimating the deformation field $F_{I^M \to I^t}$ and the subject-mean image I^M. Specifically, we implement the groupwise registration method for longitudinal image sequence with implicit template [4]. First, all time-point images of the same subject are initially registered using groupwise affine registration, and then the initial subject-mean image can be built by averaging those affine-aligned images. Next, the consistent registration of longitudinal images to the subject-mean image and the updating of subject-mean image are performed by iterating the following two steps: **(1)** register each time-point image to the current subject-mean image by a pairwise registration algorithm; and **(2)** estimate the subject-mean image based on the current registration results of all time-point images. Specifically, at the $(k-1)^{th}$ iteration, each subject image I^t is deformed into I^t_{k-1} via its current estimated deformation field $F^{k-1}_{I^M \to I^t}$, where $I^t_{k-1}(x) = I_{k-1}(F^{k-1}_{I^M \to I^t}(x))$. Similarly, at the kth iteration, the mean image $I^{M_k}(x) = \frac{1}{T}\sum_{t=1}^{T} I^t_{k-1}(x)$ can be updated. Next, each time-point image I^t is registered to I^{M_k} using standard pairwise registration, thus obtaining its updated deformation field $F^k_{I^M \to I^t}$ for the $(k+1)^{th}$ iteration. In the end of groupwise registration, the subject-mean image I^M in the common space can be obtained, as well as the deformation field $F_{I_M \to I_t}$ of each time-point image I^t.

2.2 Manifold-Guided Registration of Atlases and Subject Image Sequence

We use a manifold-guided registration algorithm to rapidly and more accurately register all atlases to the subject-mean image I^M, with the help of other atlases by exploring their distribution on the atlas manifold. Specifically, the image graph is first built by computing the distance between all pairs of atlas images as weights of the graph edges that connect image nodes (atlases). Note that atlas images with high structural similarity are adjacently located in the graph; therefore, we use the built graph to progressively register each atlas to the subject-mean image by traversing the intermediate neighboring atlases one-by-one using the shortest path in the graph. In this way, the registration accuracy between each atlas and the subject-mean can be highly and incrementally improved by only estimating small deformations between similar atlases in the graph, thereby ascertaining a better propagation of the multi-atlas labels to the target different time-point images.

Specifically, we first use affinity propagation (AP) [5] to cluster all atlas images into several groups based on the distance matrix $D = [d_{ij}]_{N \times N}$, where each entry $d_{ij} = d(A_i, A_j)$ denotes the distance (i.e., image similarity) between the atlas $A_i(i = 1, \cdots, N)$ and the atlas $A_j(j = 1, \cdots, N)$. For each group, we build a graph to represent the interior image distribution by connecting only similar atlas images in the graph. Given a well-defined graph, we only calculate the deformation fields for the atlas images directly connected in the graph. This helps overcome the difficulty of directly registering atlas images with significant shape difference.

Given a target subject-mean image I^M, to which the atlases will be warped, we look for the most similar atlas image A_{i_0} among a group of atlases $A = \{A_i | i = 1, \ldots, N\}$ in the manifold. It is worth noting that the atlases in the same group of A_{i_0} are considered as the best atlases $B = \{B_i | i = 1, \ldots, P, P < N\}$. This can provide a straightforward solution on how to select atlases for the label fusion step, which highly influences the final labeling accuracy.

Next, we use deformable image registration to estimate the deformation F_{B_i, B_j} for the directly connected best atlases $B_i(i = 1, \cdots, P)$ and $B_j(j = 1, \cdots, P)$ in the graph. The goal of image registration is then to estimate the deformation field that warps B_i to the space of A_{i_0} using these directly connected atlases in the graph. In a traditional registration approach, the optimization of the deformation pathway could be very complex and prone to local minima, since the shape and appearance differences between A_{i_0} and B_i are typically large in the aging/developing brains. However, the graph structure built in the atlas manifold can provide an easier way to estimate the deformation pathway between B_i and A_{i_0} by concatenating intermediate deformations on the shortest route linking them. To locate the shortest route from an atlas image B_i to A_{i_0}, we apply Yen's algorithm, which explores multiple shortest paths between them. Finally, we can obtain the total deformation pathway $F_{A_{i_0} \to B_i}$ by sequentially composing the small deformations of all graph edges along the shortest route. Ultimately, we further refine the deformation between A_{i_0} and I^M using a pairwise registration method with reasonable performance [6]. These steps are applied to all pairs of those selected atlas images and the subject-mean. After we get the warped atlases in the subject-mean space, we use patch-based label fusion to determine the final labels for each voxel in the subject-mean image as described next.

2.3 Consistent ROI Labeling of Longitudinal Image Sequence

The limitation of patch-based label fusion methods [1, 2] stems from that the atlas patches with low patch similarity to the target patch can still contribute to label fusion, thus leading to possibly inaccurate labeling. Instead, sparse patch-based label fusion methods [3] have been applied to solve this issue. Specifically, the low-similar atlas patches are automatically excluded for label fusion, by employing a sparsity constraint to reconstruct each target patch only from a small number of atlas patches. Thus, the estimated sparse reconstruction coefficients (with zeros for many low-similar atlas patches) can be used for effective label fusion.

Using the deformation $F_t = F_{I^M \to I^t} \circ F_{B_i \to I^M}$, a set of P warped best atlas images $B' = \{B'_i | i = 1, \ldots, P\}$ and their corresponding label maps $L' = \{L'_i | i = 1, \ldots, P\}$ are obtained for propagating the labels from the warped atlases to each time-point image I^t. At each target point $x(x \in I^t)$ of each time-point image I^t, we can compute the patchwise similarities between all atlas patches within a certain search neighborhood $n(x)$, denoted as $\vec{\beta}_{i,y} \left(\vec{\beta}_{i,y} \subset B'_i, y \in n(x) \right)$, and the image patch $\vec{\alpha}_{I^t,x} (\vec{\alpha}_{I^t,x} \subset I^t)$ of I^t. Then, we can get the respective weighting vector $\vec{w} = \left[w_{i,y} \right]_{i=1,\ldots,P,y \in n(x)}$ to integrate the atlas labels for estimating a label for the target point x. We can further adopt the sparse representation to reconstruct the local patch at target point x of each time-point image I^t (represented by column vector $\vec{\alpha}_{I^t,x}$) from the adjacent atlas patches centered at nearby voxels y in all atlases, which are also represented by column vectors and organized into a matrix C. Therefore, the sparse representation can be formulated as $\hat{\vec{w}} = \arg \min_{\vec{w}} \left\| \vec{\alpha}_{I^t,x} - C\vec{w} \right\|^2 + \lambda \|\vec{w}_1\|$, s.t. $\vec{w} > 0$, where λ controls the strength of sparsity. With this estimated weight vector $\vec{w}$, we can also estimate a label for the target point x, as similarly done in the above.

3   Experimental Results

We evaluated our dual-layer registration framework in terms of both labeling consistency and labeling accuracy. Two longitudinal datasets, i.e., Alzheimer's disease (AD) patients from ADNI database and infant brain scans, were used in the following experiments. For AD dataset, 88 subjects with 3 time-point longitudinal scans, each with manual hippocampus labels, were first selected from ADNI database. 20 subjects among 88 subjects were used as the testing dataset (to-be-labeled) while the rest (i.e., 68 subjects) were considered as atlases. For infant dataset, we used 10 longitudinal infant brains with 5 time-points, acquired at birth to less than 2-years-old, with manual hippocampus labels delineated by an expert. Due to the small sample size, labeling was performed in a leave-one-out (LOO) fashion. To better take the advantage of manifold-guided registration by including more samples in the graph hierarchy, 20 infant subjects without hippocampus labels were also included in the construction of atlas manifold to provide more efficient routes between atlases and subject-mean image.

3.1   Evaluation of Longitudinal Labeling Consistency

We evaluated the consistency of longitudinal labeling by quantifying the trend of longitudinal hippocampus volumes, segmented using our proposed framework and the traditional registration scheme (i.e., pairwise registration between atlases and each time-point image in the longitudinal subject images) followed by sparse patch-based label fusion [3]. Figures 2 and 3 show the longitudinal hippocampal volumes measured by our framework (right panel) and the conventional method (left panel) averaged

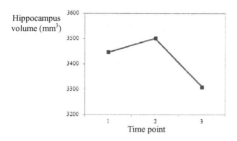
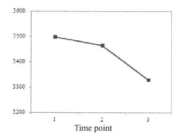

Fig. 2. Longitudinal hippocampal volumes segmented by our dual-layer registration framework (right) in comparison with those by the traditional registration scheme (left) for 20 AD subjects.

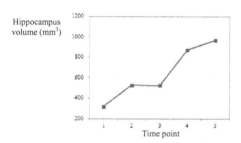
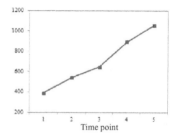

Fig. 3. Longitudinal hippocampal volumes segmented by our dual-layer registration framework (right) in comparison with those by the traditional registration scheme (left) for 10 infant subjects.

across 20 AD subjects and 10 infant subjects, respectively. One can see that the longitudinal hippocampal volume decreases more consistently due to disease progress (for AD subjects) or increases due to brain growth/development (for infant subjects), thus showing the effectiveness of consistent labeling enhanced by our dual-layer groupwise registration framework.

3.2   Evaluation of Longitudinal Labeling Accuracy

The overall hippocampus labeling accuracy of longitudinal brain sequences using our dual-layer registration method, followed by using several label fusion methods such as standard majority voting (MV), locally-weighted voting (LWV), non-local mean (NLM) [5] methods, and more advanced sparse patch-based label fusion (SPBL) [3], was evaluated in the comparison with the conventional registration framework. Table 1 compares the averaged Dice overlap ratios between manually-delineated hippocampus labels and the automatic labeling results by two methods, respectively. It shows that our dual-layer groupwise registration consistently helps achieve higher labeling accuracy for all four label fusion algorithms incorporated in our framework, compared to the traditional registration scheme, on both AD and infant datasets. This indicates that our proposed registration-labeling framework can integrate existing label fusion algorithms to immediately boost the final labeling accuracy.

Table 1. Quantitative comparisons between conventional method and our dual-layer groupwise registration framework for measuring longitudinal hippocampus in 20 AD subjects and 10 infant subjects. (unit: %).

	Conventional registration scheme				Our dual-layer registration framework			
	MV	LMV	NLM	SPBL	MV	LMV	NLM	SPBL
AD subjects	68.91	79.43	84.52	86.24	70.28	81.51	85.35	87.02
Infant subjects	60.24	62.56	58.13	62.98	62.52	63.70	59.98	65.07

4   Conclusion

We have proposed a dual-layer groupwise registration method for longitudinal brain labeling. Our method is anchored in two fundamental contributions. First, time-serial groupwise registration is applied to register longitudinal images of the same subject to estimate a subject-mean image as a common space to jointly align all different time-point images. Second, manifold-guided registration is proposed to label all subject time-point images by more accurately and rapidly propagating the pre-defined ROIs from each of the multiple atlases. Intensive evaluations were conducted using two compelling longitudinal AD and infant subjects that challenge our method with an opposing spectrum of image variability, from atrophy to drastic shape growth and dramatic appearance changes. Our experiments showed that our framework led to better labeling consistency and higher labeling accuracy of hippocampus for both datasets when compared to the traditional registration scheme. It is worth noting that the applications of our method are not limited to labeling hippocampus, but can be tested on various anatomical structures with time-serial scans. In future works, we will explore more high-order manifold neighborhoods for best atlas incremental selection and incorporate more advanced label fusion methods, e.g., group-sparsity based label fusion, in our dual-layer registration-labeling framework.

References

1. Coupé, P., et al.: Patch-based segmentation using expert priors: application to hippocampus and ventricle segmentation. NeuroImage **54**, 940–954 (2011)
2. Rousseau, F., et al.: A supervised patch-based approach for human brain labeling. IEEE Trans. Med. Imaging **30**, 1852–1862 (2011)
3. Zhang, D., Guo, Q., Wu, G., Shen, D.: Sparse patch-based label fusion for multi-atlas segmentation. In: Yap, P.-T., Liu, T., Shen, D., Westin, C.-F., Shen, L. (eds.) MBIA 2012. LNCS, vol. 7509, pp. 94–102. Springer, Heidelberg (2012)
4. Wu, G., et al.: Registration of longitudinal brain image sequences with implicit template and spatial–temporal heuristics. NeuroImage **59**, 404–421 (2012)
5. Frey, B.J., Dueck, D.: Clustering by passing messages between data points. Science **315**, 972–976 (2007)
6. Vercauteren, T., et al.: Diffeomorphic demons: efficient non-parametric image registration. NeuroImage **45**, S61–S72 (2009)

Joint Discriminative and Representative Feature Selection for Alzheimer's Disease Diagnosis

Xiaofeng Zhu[1], Heung-Il Suk[2], Kim-Han Thung[1], Yingying Zhu[1], Guorong Wu[1], and Dinggang Shen[1(✉)]

[1] Department of Radiology and BRIC,
University of North Carolina at Chapel Hill, Chapel Hill, USA
`dgshen@med.unc.edu`
[2] Department of Brain and Cognitive Engineering,
Korea University, Seongbuk-gu, Republic of Korea

Abstract. Neuroimaging data have been widely used to derive possible biomarkers for Alzheimer's Disease (AD) diagnosis. As only certain brain regions are related to AD progression, many feature selection methods have been proposed to identify informative features (*i.e.*, brain regions) to build an accurate prediction model. These methods mostly only focus on the feature-target relationship to select features which are discriminative to the targets (*e.g.*, diagnosis labels). However, since the brain regions are anatomically and functionally connected, there could be useful intrinsic relationships among features. In this paper, by utilizing both the feature-target and feature-feature relationships, we propose a novel sparse regression model to select informative features which are discriminative to the targets and also representative to the features. We argue that the features which are representative (*i.e.*, can be used to represent many other features) are important, as they signify strong "connection" with other ROIs, and could be related to the disease progression. We use our model to select features for both binary and multi-class classification tasks, and the experimental results on the Alzheimer's Disease Neuroimaging Initiative (ADNI) dataset show that the proposed method outperforms other comparison methods considered in this work.

1 Introduction

Magnetic Resonance Imaging (MRI) data have become one of the most commonly used neuroimaging data to obtain biomarkers for Alzheimer's Disease (AD), as they are widely available, non-invasive, affordable, and may show early signs of neurodegeneration in human brain [6,19]. As neuroimaging data are very high in dimension, most methods [4,17] prefer to use Region-Of-Interest (ROI)-based features instead of the original voxel values for analysis. However, not all the ROIs are related to disease progression, and thus a lot of feature selection methods have been proposed [4,15,20]. For example, Zhang and Shen [17] and

Electronic supplementary material The online version of this chapter (doi:10.1007/978-3-319-47157-0_10) contains supplementary material, which is available to authorized users.

© Springer International Publishing AG 2016
L. Wang et al. (Eds.): MLMI 2016, LNCS 10019, pp. 77–85, 2016.
DOI: 10.1007/978-3-319-47157-0_10

Wang *et al.* [15] used multi-task learning to select common features for classification and regression tasks, *i.e.,* features are jointly selected to discriminate both classification labels and clinical scores. These feature selection methods are task-oriented, as they exploit the feature-target relationship to select features which are discriminative to the targets. Feature-feature relationship, *e.g.,* correlations among features, however, is ignored in these methods.

The MRI ROI-based features are actually correlated or "connected" in some ways. This can be deduced based on the facts that the ROIs are anatomically and functionally connected [11,12,14]. Thus, we hypothesize that there exist intrinsic relationships among the features, *i.e.,* ROIs. We then devise a self-representation formulation to measure how well a feature can be used to represent other features. We argue that a more representative feature, *i.e.,* a feature which can be used to represent many other features, is more important and useful in AD study. In the context of brain connectivity, a more representative feature could also signify a strong "connection" between this feature and other features. Thus, a representation-oriented feature selection method, which selects representative features without considering the target information, can also be used for AD diagnosis.

In this study, we consider both the feature-target and feature-feature relationships to formulate a novel feature selection method. Our method combines the complementary advantages of both the task-oriented and the representation-oriented methods, to select features, which are both discriminative to the targets and representative to the other features. More specifically, our formulation consists of three components: (1) *task-oriented component*: to obtain a discriminative coefficient matrix, which denotes the discriminative power of the features to the targets in supervised learning; (2) *representation-oriented component*: to obtain a representative coefficient matrix, whose row denotes the representative power of a feature representing other features in unsupervised learning; (3) *joint sparsity constraint*: to remove features that are neither discriminative nor representative, by jointly penalizing the above discriminative and representative coefficient matrices via an $\ell_{2,1}$-norm regularization. We then use the selected features to conduct both binary and multi-class classification tasks for different stages of AD diagnosis.

The contributions of this paper are three-fold: (i) we utilize the self-representation characteristics of the MRI ROI-based data to extract the feature-feature relationship for conducting feature selection, while the previous methods [2,16] mostly used it to extract the sample-sample relationship for clustering purpose; (ii) we consider both the feature-target and feature-feature relationships in the formulation of a novel *joint* feature selection method, while most of the previous AD studies [18,20,21] utilized the feature-target relationship, thus ignoring intrinsic relationships among the features that could be also useful; and (iii) we simultaneously consider both binary and multi-class classification tasks, for a more practical clinical application, while most of the previous studies [15,17] focused on the binary classification for AD study.

2   Method

Let $\mathbf{X} \in \mathbb{R}^{n \times d}$ and $\mathbf{Y} \in \{0,1\}^{n \times c}$, denote the feature matrix and the target matrix of all MRI data, respectively, where n, d, and c denote the numbers of the samples (or subjects), the features, and the targets (*i.e.*, class labels), respectively. We use $\mathbf{x}^i$ and $\mathbf{x}_j$ to denote the i-th row (sample) and the j-th column (feature) of $\mathbf{X}$, respectively. The corresponding target vector for $\mathbf{x}^i$ is given as $\mathbf{y}^i = [y_{i1}, \ldots, y_{ij}, \ldots, y_{ic}] \in \{0,1\}^c$, where $y_{ij} = 1$ indicates that $\mathbf{x}^i$ is belonged to the j-th class, and vice versa.

2.1   Task-Oriented Supervised Feature Selection

In our case, a prediction task is defined as a problem using $\mathbf{X}$ to predict a single column (label) of $\mathbf{Y}$. If there are multiple columns of $\mathbf{Y}$, *e.g.*, in multi-class classification scenario, we will end up with a multi-task learning problem. In the task-oriented feature selection method, we aim to select features, which are useful in the prediction task(s), based on the feature-target relationship. The motivation of considering the feature-target relationship is that, the high-level representation $\mathbf{Y}$ is the abstraction of the low-level representation $\mathbf{X}$, thus they should have inherent relationships. In this paper, we assume that there exists a linear relationship between the feature matrix $\mathbf{X}$ and the target matrix $\mathbf{Y}$. By using a linear regression model, the feature-target relationship can be explained by using a coefficient matrix $\mathbf{W} \in \mathbb{R}^{d \times c}$, which maps $\mathbf{X}$ to $\mathbf{Y}$ to achieve a minimum prediction residual $\|\mathbf{Y} - \mathbf{XW}\|_F^2$, where $\mathbf{XW}$ is the prediction of $\mathbf{Y}$. As not all the features (*i.e.*, ROIs) are related to AD [15,17], we impose a sparsity constraint on $\mathbf{W}$ to select features that are discriminative to the targets. Then the resulting linear regression model with an added bias term and a sparsity constraint is given as

$$\min_{\mathbf{W},\mathbf{b}} \|\mathbf{Y} - \mathbf{XW} - \mathbf{eb}^T\|_F^2 + \lambda \|\mathbf{W}\|_{2,1}, \tag{1}$$

where $\mathbf{b} \in \mathbb{R}^{c \times 1}$ is a bias term, $\mathbf{e} \in \mathbb{R}^{n \times 1}$ denotes a vector with all ones, λ is a sparsity control parameter, $\| \cdot \|_F$ is the Frobenius norm, $\mathbf{b}^T$ is the transpose operator on $\mathbf{b}$, and $\| \cdot \|_{2,1}$ is the $\ell_{2,1}$-norm regularization, which is defined as $\|\mathbf{W}\|_{2,1} = \sum_i \sqrt{\sum_j w_{ij}^2}$. The least square loss function (*i.e.*, the first term in Eq. (1)) computes the sum of the prediction residuals, while the $\ell_{2,1}$-norm regularization (*i.e.*, the second term in Eq. (1)) helps in selecting common discriminative features for all the prediction tasks.

The use of the $\ell_{2,1}$-norm regularization in Eq. (1) is based on the assumption that, a feature that is important to represent a target could also be informative to other targets, and vice versa. Thus, such a feature should be jointly selected or un-selected in representing the targets. Specifically, each column of $\mathbf{W}$ denotes the coefficient vector for one task, while each row of $\mathbf{W}$ denotes the weight vector of a feature for all the prediction tasks. The $\ell_{2,1}$-norm regularization first groups features in each row of $\mathbf{W}$ with the ℓ_2-norm, and subsequently imposes row sparsity for the grouped features using the ℓ_1-norm. Thus, the $\ell_{2,1}$-norm regularization tends to cause all-zero value rows in $\mathbf{W}$. As each row of $\mathbf{W}$ corresponds to one feature in $\mathbf{X}$, this is equivalent to joint feature selection for all the targets, *i.e.*, selecting common brain regions that contribute to the clinical decision (*e.g.*, AD, progressive Mild Cognitive Impairment (pMCI), stable MCI (sMCI) and Normal Control (NC)).

2.2 Representation-Oriented Unsupervised Feature Selection

The previous AD studies have observed the following neurophysiological characteristics: (i) AD may affect multiple brain regions simultaneously, rather than just a single region [17]; and (ii) human brain is a complex system where the brain regions are functionally interacting with each other [10]. In this regards, we assume that there are dependencies among ROIs (*i.e.*, features), and thus devise a new regularizer to utilize this relational characteristic among ROIs for feature selection. Specifically, we define a linear regression model such that each feature $\mathbf{x}_i$ in $\mathbf{X}$ can be represented as a linear combination of other features:

$$\mathbf{x}_i \approx \sum_{j=1}^{d}(\mathbf{x}_j s_{ji}) + \mathbf{e}p_i = \mathbf{X}\mathbf{s}_i + \mathbf{e}p_i, \quad i = 1, \dots, d. \tag{2}$$

where s_{ij} is a weight between the i-th feature vector $\mathbf{x}_i$ and the j-th feature vector $\mathbf{x}_j$, and p_i is the bias term for the i-th feature. $\mathbf{s}_i = [s_{1i}, \cdots, s_{di}]^T$ is a weight vector, where each element indicates the contribution of the corresponding feature in representing $\mathbf{x}_i$. In matrix form, Eq. (2) is equivalent to $\mathbf{X} \approx \mathbf{X}\mathbf{S} - \mathbf{e}\mathbf{p}^T$, where $\mathbf{S} \in \mathbb{R}^{d \times d}$ is the coefficient matrix (with s_{ij} denotes its (i,j)-th element) and $\mathbf{p} = [p_1, \dots, p_j, \dots, p_d]^T \in \mathbb{R}^{d \times 1}$ is the bias vector. By regarding the representation of each feature as a task and devising a sparsity constraint across tasks with an $\ell_{2,1}$-norm regularization, we define a representation-oriented feature selection method as follows[1]:

$$\min_{\mathbf{S},\mathbf{p}} \|\mathbf{X} - \mathbf{X}\mathbf{S} - \mathbf{e}\mathbf{p}^T\|_F^2 + \alpha\|\mathbf{S}\|_{2,1}, \tag{3}$$

where α is a sparsity control parameter. The $\ell_{2,1}$-norm regularization $\|\mathbf{S}\|_{2,1}$ penalizes all coefficients in the same row of $\mathbf{S}$ together for joint selection of features in reconstructing the feature matrix $\mathbf{X}$.

The first term in Eq. (3) is a self-representation term, as $\mathbf{X}$ is approximated by a multiplication of a matrix to itself, *i.e.*, $\mathbf{X}\mathbf{S} + \mathbf{e}\mathbf{p}^T$ (we can ignore the bias term without lost of generality). Self-representation has been used in the literature to extract the sample-sample relationship [2,7], but, in our application,

---

[1] Note that since a vector $\mathbf{x}_i$ in the observation $\mathbf{X}$ can be used to represent itself, there always exists a feasible (trivial) solution. That is, its corresponding coefficient in $\mathbf{S}$ equals to one and all the other coefficients equal to zero. However, due to our assumption of dependencies among ROIs, *i.e.*, $rank(\mathbf{X}) < \min(n, d)$, where $rank(\mathbf{X})$ indicates the rank of the matrix $\mathbf{X}$, there also exist non-trial solutions in the space of $\mathbf{I} - null(\mathbf{X})$ [7], where $null(\mathbf{X})$ stands for the null space of $\mathbf{X}$.

we use it to extract the feature-feature relationship, as each element of $\mathbf{S}$ can be regarded as a proximity measure between two features. Specifically, each column of $\mathbf{S}$ indicates how other features are used to represent a feature in $\mathbf{X}$, while each row of $\mathbf{S}$ indicates how useful of a feature in representing other features. Moreover, the ℓ_2-norm value of each row of $\mathbf{S}$ indicates the representativeness of a feature, *i.e.*, how much contribution is the feature in representing others. In this study, we argue that a more representative feature (ROI) is more desirable, as it could be the main ROI that affects the disease progression, thus justifying the use of $\ell_{2,1}$-norm in the second term of Eq. (3).

2.3 Proposed Objective Function

We propose to combine the task-oriented feature selection method in Eq. (1) and the representation-oriented feature selection method in Eq. (3) into a unified framework, to take advantages of these two feature selection methods, *i.e.*, complementary relationships of the feature-target and feature-feature relationships. The final objective function is given as follows:

$$\min_{\mathbf{W},\mathbf{b},\mathbf{S},\mathbf{p}} \|\mathbf{Y} - \mathbf{X}\mathbf{W} - \mathbf{e}\mathbf{b}^T\|_F^2 + \beta\|\mathbf{X} - \mathbf{X}\mathbf{S} - \mathbf{e}\mathbf{p}^T\|_F^2 + \lambda\|[\mathbf{W},\mathbf{S}]\|_{2,1} \quad (4)$$

where $\mathbf{A} = [\mathbf{W},\mathbf{S}] \in \mathbb{R}^{d\times(c+d)}$ is defined as a joint analyzer, *i.e.*, a horizontal concatenation of $\mathbf{W}$ and $\mathbf{S}$. Each row of $\mathbf{A}$ reflects the importance of a feature in jointly predicting the targets and representing other features.

We illustrate our formulation in Fig. 1. In brief, our formulation iteratively learns the coefficient matrices from both the task-oriented (the first term in Eq. (4)) and representation-oriented (the second term in Eq. (4)) feature selection methods until Eq. (4) achieves its optimal solution. The $\ell_{2,1}$-norm regularization in the third term of Eq. (4) encourages joint row sparsity in $\mathbf{A}$, *i.e.*, it encourages to have rows of all-zero values in $\mathbf{A}$. Since each row of $\mathbf{A}$ is corresponding to a

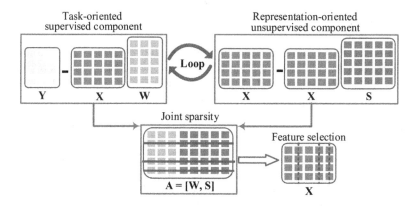

Fig. 1. The framework of the proposed method, where the solid red lines and the dot red lines, respectively, imply removing the rows of $\mathbf{A}$ and the columns (*i.e.*, features) of $\mathbf{X}$. (Color figure online)

feature index in $\mathbf{X}$, an all-zero value row indicates to unselect the corresponding feature in $\mathbf{X}$. Since $\mathbf{W}$ and $\mathbf{S}$ give us the discriminative and representative information about the features, respectively, the selected features are discriminative and representative. Given the selected features, we use them to train a support vector machine (SVM) as our classifier.

3 Experimental Results

We conducted experiments using the ADNI dataset ('www.adni-info.org') to compare the proposed method with the comparison methods, including "Original", Fisher Score (FS) [1], Laplacian Score (LS) [5], SELF-representation (SELF) [18], Multi-Modal Multi-Task (M3T) [17], and Sparse Joint Classification and Regression (SJCR) [15]. "Original" method uses all the original features for classification, without any feature selection. Both FS and LS are the classic supervised (task-oriented) feature selection methods in machine learning. SELF is our unsupervised representation-oriented feature selection method, with the objective function given in Eq. (3). M3T and SJCR are the most recent task-oriented methods for AD diagnosis.

In our experiments, we used the baseline MRI data including 226 NC, 186 AD, and 393 MCI subjects. MCI subjects were clinically subdivided into 118 pMCI and 124 sMCI by checking which subjects have converted to AD within 24 months. We preprocessed MRI images by sequentially conducting spatial distortion correction, skull-stripping, and cerebellum removal, and then segmented MRI images into gray matter, white matter, and cerebrospinal fluid. We further parcellated MRI images into 93 ROIs based on a Jacob template, followed by computing the gray matter tissue volumes of the ROIs as features. With this, we obtained 93 gray matter volumes from one MRI image.

We considered two binary classification tasks (*i.e.*, AD vs. NC and pMCI vs. sMCI) and two multi-class classification tasks (*i.e.*, AD vs. NC vs. MCI (3-Class) and AD vs. NC vs. pMCI vs. sMCI (4-Class). The performance metrics used are classification ACCuracy (ACC), SENsitivity (SEN), SPEcificity (SPE), and Area Under Curve (AUC) for binary classification, while we only used ACC for multi-class classification.

We used 10-fold cross-validation to test all the methods, and employed a nested 5-fold cross-validation for model selection, where the parameter values were chosen from the ranges of $\{10^{-5}, 10^{-3} \ldots, 10^{5}\}$ for all methods. We repeated the whole process 10 times and report the average results in this paper.

3.1 Classification Results

We summarize the results of all the methods in Table 1, with the following observations: (i) In the binary classification tasks, the proposed method outperforms all the comparison methods, with the improvement of average classification accuracies over other methods as 8.50 % (vs. Original), 3.80 % (vs. FS), 4.55 % (vs. LS), 4.99 % (vs. SELF), 3.30 % (vs. SJCR), and 3.75 % (vs. M3T), respectively. Based on these results, we confirm the superiority of our proposed method, which considers both the feature-target and feature-feature relationships, and selects

Table 1. Classification performance for all the methods.

Methods	AD vs. NC				pMCI vs. sMCI				3-Class	4-Class
	ACC	SEN	SPE	AUC	ACC	SEN	SPE	AUC	ACC	ACC
Original	0.781*	0.856*	0.725*	0.799*	0.645*	0.623*	0.601*	0.700*	0.494*	0.482*
FS	0.854*	0.862*	0.775*	0.852*	0.686*	0.651*	0.647*	0.732*	0.573*	0.513*
LS	0.852*	0.873*	0.758*	0.860*	0.673*	0.648*	0.638*	0.738*	0.579*	0.527*
SELF	0.844*	0.872*	0.782*	0.818*	0.673*	0.670*	0.655*	0.734*	0.593*	0.536*
M3T	0.875*	0.871*	0.788*	0.897*	0.675*	0.678*	0.697*	0.775*	0.607*	0.553*
SJCR	0.861*	0.853*	0.762*	0.883*	0.680*	0.664*	0.668*	0.766*	0.603*	0.540*
Proposed	**0.903**	**0.915**	**0.819**	**0.912**	**0.713**	**0.681**	**0.755**	**0.781**	**0.639**	**0.593**

$\star$ (or $*$): Statistically significant results with $p < 0.05$ (or $p < 0.001$) between our method and all other comparison methods using paired-sample t-tests.

the discriminative and representative features jointly. (ii) In the multi-class classification tasks, our method also outperforms all the comparison methods. For example, in the 3-class classification, our proposed method achieves an average classification accuracy of 63.9%, an improvement of 14.5% (vs. Original), 6.6% (vs. FS), 6.0% (vs. LS), 4.6% (vs. SELF), 3.2% (vs. M3T), and 3.6% (vs. SJCR), respectively. In the 4-class classification, our proposed method achieves an average classification accuracy of 59.3%, an improvement of 11.1% (vs. Original), 8.0% (vs. FS), 6.6% (vs. LS), 5.7% (vs. SELF), 4.0% (vs. M3T), and 5.3% (vs. SJCR), respectively. (iii) We found that the representation-oriented feature selection method (*i.e.*, SELF) alone performs relatively poor, compared with the task-oriented feature selection methods (*i.e.*, FS, LF, M3T, and JCSR). This is probably due to its unsupervised learning, *i.e.*, without using target information. However, when it is used in conjunction with a task-oriented method, as in our proposed method, it helps enhance classification accuracies. This confirms our assumption that complementary information between the feature-target and the feature-feature relationships is useful for AD diagnosis.

3.2 Most Discriminative Brain Regions

Figure 2 shows the frequency map of the proposed feature selection method, *i.e.*, how frequently a feature is selected in 100 experiments, for all the classification tasks. From the figure, we observe that: (i) Our method, on average, selected 58.0 (AD vs. NC), 53.0 (pMCI vs. sMCI), 50.6 (3-Class), and 35.3 (4-Class) numbers of features, out of 93 features (as known as ROIs), respectively. (ii) The commonly top selected regions in all four different classification tasks are uncus right (22), hippocampal formation right (30), uncus left (46), middle temporal gyrus left (48), hippocampal formation left (69), amygdala left (76), middle temporal gyrus right (80), and amygdala right (83), where the number in the parentheses represents an index of the respective ROI. These regions are consistent with the regions selected in the previous literature that worked on binary classification [17]. In addition, these regions also have been reported to be closely related to AD and its prodromal stage (*i.e.*, MCI) in clinical diagnosis [3,8]. In this regard, these regions could be used as the potential biomarkers

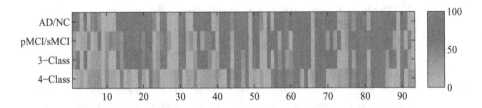

Fig. 2. The frequency map (*i.e.,* how frequent a feature (one of 93 ROIs) is selected in 100 experiments) of the proposed feature selection method for four different types of classification tasks. The horizontal axis indicates the indices of ROIs, while their full names can be found in the Supplementary Material.

for AD or MCI diagnosis. It is worth noting that the comparison methods also selected most of the above ROIs, but with a lesser frequency and consistency than our method.

4   Conclusion

In this paper, we proposed a novel feature selection method to consider both the feature-target relationship and the feature-feature relationship, by combining a task-oriented supervised method and a representation-oriented unsupervised method into a linear regression framework. Our proposed method selected features, which are discriminative to the targets and also representative to the other features. Our experimental results on the ADNI MRI data validated the effectiveness of our proposed method in both binary classification and multi-class classification tasks. In the future work, we will extend our proposed framework to the dataset with incomplete information [9,13,22].

Acknowledgements. This work was supported in part by NIH grants (EB006733, EB008374, EB009634, MH100217, AG041721, AG042599). Heung-Il Suk was supported in part by Institute for Information & communications Technology Promotion (IITP) grant funded by the Korea government (MSIP) (No.B0101-16-0307, Basic Software Research in Human-level Lifelong Machine Learning (Machine Learning Center)). Xiaofeng Zhu was supported in part by the National Natural Science Foundation of China under grants 61573270 and 61263035.

References

1. Duda, R.O., Hart, P.E., Stork, D.G.: Pattern Classification. Wiley, Hoboken (2012)
2. Elhamifar, E., Vidal, R.: Sparse subspace clustering: algorithm, theory, and applications. IEEE Trans. Pattern Anal. Mach. Intell. **35**(11), 2765–2781 (2013)
3. Fox, N.C., Schott, J.M.: Imaging cerebral atrophy: normal ageing to Alzheimer's disease. Lancet **363**(9406), 392–394 (2004)
4. Guerrero, R., Ledig, C., Rueckert, D.: Manifold alignment and transfer learning for classification of Alzheimer's disease. In: Wu, G., Zhang, D., Zhou, L. (eds.) MLMI 2014. LNCS, vol. 8679, pp. 77–84. Springer, Heidelberg (2014)

5. He, X., Cai, D., Niyogi, P.: Laplacian score for feature selection. In: NIPS, pp. 507–514 (2005)
6. Huang, L., Jin, Y., Gao, Y., Thung, K., Shen, D., Initiative, A.D.N., et al.: Longitudinal clinical score prediction in alzheimers disease with soft-split sparse regression based random forest. Neurobiol. Aging **46**, 180–191 (2016)
7. Liu, G., Lin, Z., Yan, S., Sun, J., Yu, Y., Ma, Y.: Robust recovery of subspace structures by low-rank representation. IEEE Trans. Pattern Anal. Mach. Intell. **35**(1), 171–184 (2013)
8. Misra, C., Fan, Y., Davatzikos, C.: Baseline and longitudinal patterns of brain atrophy in MCI patients, and their use in prediction of short-term conversion to AD: results from ADNI. NeuroImage **44**(4), 1415–1422 (2009)
9. Qin, Y., Zhang, S., Zhu, X., Zhang, J., Zhang, C.: Semi-parametric optimization for missing data imputation. Appl. Intell. **27**(1), 79–88 (2007)
10. Sato, J.R., Hoexter, M.Q., Fujita, A., Rohde, L.A.: Evaluation of pattern recognition and feature extraction methods in ADHD prediction. Front. Syst. Neurosci. **6**, 68 (2012)
11. Suk, H., Wee, C., Lee, S., Shen, D.: Supervised discriminative group sparse representation for mild cognitive impairment diagnosis. Neuroinformatics **13**(3), 277–295 (2015)
12. Suk, H., Wee, C., Lee, S., Shen, D.: State-space model with deep learning for functional dynamics estimation in resting-state fMRI. NeuroImage **129**, 292–307 (2016)
13. Thung, K., Wee, C., Yap, P., Shen, D.: Neurodegenerative disease diagnosis using incomplete multi-modality data via matrix shrinkage and completion. NeuroImage **91**, 386–400 (2014)
14. Thung, K., Wee, C., Yap, P., Shen, D.: Identification of progressive mild cognitive impairment patients using incomplete longitudinal MRI scans. Brain Struct. Funct. 1–17 (2015)
15. Wang, H., Nie, F., Huang, H., Risacher, S., Saykin, A.J., Shen, L.: Identifying AD-sensitive and cognition-relevant imaging biomarkers via joint classification and regression. In: Fichtinger, G., Martel, A., Peters, T. (eds.) MICCAI 2011, Part III. LNCS, vol. 6893, pp. 115–123. Springer, Heidelberg (2011)
16. Zhang, C., Qin, Y., Zhu, X., Zhang, J., Zhang, S.: Clustering-based missing value imputation for data preprocessing. In: INDIN, pp. 1081–1086 (2006)
17. Zhang, D., Shen, D.: Multi-modal multi-task learning for joint prediction of multiple regression and classification variables in Alzheimer's disease. NeuroImage **59**(2), 895–907 (2012)
18. Zhu, P., Zuo, W., Zhang, L., Hu, Q., Shiu, S.C.K.: Unsupervised feature selection by regularized self-representation. Pattern Recogn. **48**(2), 438–446 (2015)
19. Zhu, X., Suk, H., Lee, S., Shen, D.: Canonical feature selection for joint regression and multi-class identification in Alzheimers disease diagnosis. Brain Imaging Behav. 1–11 (2015)
20. Zhu, X., Suk, H.-I., Shen, D.: Multi-modality canonical feature selection for Alzheimer's disease diagnosis. In: Golland, P., Hata, N., Barillot, C., Hornegger, J., Howe, R. (eds.) MICCAI 2014, Part II. LNCS, vol. 8674, pp. 162–169. Springer, Heidelberg (2014)
21. Zhu, X., Suk, H., Wang, L., Lee, S.W., Shen, D., Alzheimer's Disease Neuroimaging Initiative, et al.: A novel relational regularization feature selection method for joint regression and classification in ad diagnosis. Med. Image Anal. (2015)
22. Zhu, X., Zhang, S., Jin, Z., Zhang, Z., Xu, Z.: Missing value estimation for mixed-attribute data sets. IEEE Trans. Knowl. Data Eng. **23**(1), 110–121 (2011)

Patch-Based Hippocampus Segmentation Using a Local Subspace Learning Method

Yan Wang[1], Xi Wu[2(✉)], Guangkai Ma[3], Zongqing Ma[1], Ying Fu[2], and Jiliu Zhou[1,2]

[1] College of Computer Science, Sichuan University, Chengdu, China
[2] Department of Computer Science,
Chengdu University of Information Technology, Chengdu, China
wuxi@cuit.edu.cn
[3] Space Control and Inertial Technology Research Center,
Harbin Institute of Technology, Harbin, China

Abstract. Patch-based segmentation methods utilizing multiple atlases have been widely studied for alleviating some misalignments when registering atlases to the target image. However, weights assigned to the fused labels are typically computed based on predefined features (e.g. simple patch intensities), thus being not necessarily optimal. Due to lack of discriminating features for different regions of an anatomical structure, the original feature space defined by image intensities may limit the segmentation accuracy. To address these problems, we propose a novel local subspace learning based patch-wise label propagation method to estimate a voxel-wise segmentation of the target image. Specifically, multi-scale patch intensities and texture features are first extracted from the image patch in order to acquire the abundant appearance information. Then, margin fisher analysis (MFA) is applied to neighboring samples of each voxel to be segmented from the aligned atlases, in order to extract discriminant features. This process can enhance discrimination of features for different local regions in the anatomical structure. Finally, based on extracted discriminant features, the k-nearest neighbor (kNN) classifier is used to determine the final label for the target voxel. Moreover, for the patch-wise label propagation, we first translate label patches into several discrete class labels by using the k-means clustering method, and then apply MFA to ensure that samples with similar label patches achieve a higher similarity and those with dissimilar label patches achieve a lower similarity. To demonstrate segmentation performance, we comprehensively evaluated the proposed method on the ADNI dataset for hippocampus segmentation. Experimental results show that the proposed method outperforms several conventional multi-atlas based segmentation methods.

1 Introduction

Several neuroscience studies have shown that the hippocampus structure plays a crucial role in human memory and orientation [1, 2]. Hippocampus dysfunction involves a variety of diseases, such as Alzheimer's diseases, schizophrenia, dementia, and epilepsy. As a result, accurate segmentation of the hippocampus structure is very necessary for further studies. However, due to its small size, high variability, low contrast,

© Springer International Publishing AG 2016
L. Wang et al. (Eds.): MLMI 2016, LNCS 10019, pp. 86–94, 2016.
DOI: 10.1007/978-3-319-47157-0_11

and discontinuous boundaries in MR images, it is therefore a challenging task to develop accurate and reliable techniques for hippocampus segmentation.

Many segmentation methods have proposed recently. Among these methods, atlas-based methods have attracted great interest [3, 4]. This technique first employs deformable image registration as an important step to construct correspondences between pre-labeled atlas images and the target image (under segmentation). Then, using the acquired deformation field, labels in the atlas are propagated to the target image space. Obviously, anatomical differences between target and atlas images affect the image registration accuracy and greatly influence the final segmentation performance.

To alleviate the impact of anatomical variability in atlas-based segmentation, multi-atlas based methods have been extensively studied in recent years [5, 6]. By fusing the propagated labels of multiple atlases in a target image space, multi-atlas based methods can obtain a more robust and accurate segmentation result. Specifically, in a typical multi-atlas based segmentation approach, an additional label fusion model is utilized to combine the all propagated atlas labels to generate a segmentation result for the target image. The performance of multi-atlas based segmentation methods relies on both the registration accuracy and the effectiveness of the label fusion strategy. Therefore, in addition to optimizing the registration, many researchers focus on improving segmentation performance by utilizing more effective label fusion methods. Particularly, patch-based label propagation methods have been developed recently, and are regarded as an important direction for multi-atlas based segmentation. It has been demonstrated that patch-based label propagation methods are robust in several segmentation studies [5]. These methods have been proposed based on a basic assumption, that is, if two image patches are similar in appearance, they should have the same anatomical label. However, the definition of patch-based similarity is often handcrafted using predefined features such as image intensity, which may not be sufficiently effective for different sub-regions of hippocampus segmentation.

In this paper, we present a novel local subspace learning based patch-wise label propagation method. Here, patch-wise refers to the process in which each voxel in an atlas is assigned with one label patch, instead of a single label, for label propagation. First, we linearly register each atlas to the target image. Then, for each target voxel to be segmented, we generate a candidate training set from the voxels of aligned atlases within a spatial neighborhood. For each sampled voxel in atlases, its feature representation is extracted from the image patch with abundant texture information and multi-scale intensity information. Meanwhile, to preserve local anatomical structure information in the segmentation, we utilize label patch, instead of label of the voxel as the structured class label. To perform supervised learning based on the training set, a k-means clustering algorithm is employed to divide structured class labels into two subclasses with unique subclass labels. Then, according to assigned subclass labels of training samples, a local discriminant subspace is learned based on margin fisher analysis (MFA) strategy [8]. Afterwards, all training samples are projected into the learned subspace. When testing the label of the target voxel to be segmented, we adopt the k-nearest neighbor (kNN) classifier in the learned subspace to propagate label patches of training samples to the target voxel. Validated on ADNI dataset, our proposed method outperforms other state-of-the-art methods.

2 Method

2.1 Multi-atlas Based Segmentation Method

Given a target image I to be segmented and N atlases $\tilde{A} = \{(\tilde{I}_i, \tilde{L}_i) | i = 1, 2, \ldots N\}$, where $\tilde{I}_i$ represents an atlas image and $\tilde{L}_i$ is it's corresponding segmentation label with a value of $+1$ indicating the hippocampus region and -1 indicating non-hippocampus regions. In the multi-atlas based method, each atlas image is first spatially registered to the target image, thereby estimating the warping function. Then, the associated atlas labels are further propagated to the target image space based on the acquired warping function. Finally, all propagated atlas labels are fused for generating a segmentation result for the target image using a specific label fusion strategy.

Specifically, for the target voxel x, the candidate training set consists of the image patches $\{P_y^i | y \in V_x, i = 1, \ldots, N\}$ associated with the corresponding label patches $\{S_y^i | y \in V_x, i = 1, \ldots, N\}$ from aligned atlas images and the corresponding label maps. In this case, P_y^i is the image patch centered at the voxel y on the i-th atlas image, S_y^i is the corresponding label patch centered at the voxel y on the label maps of the i-th atlas, and V_x is the spatial neighborhood of the voxel x. Let Ω denote the voxel set of the label patch and a_c be the center location. We differentiate between two methods of label propagation: (1) voxel-wise (VW) label propagation which only utilizes the label at the center location of the label patch $S_y^i(a_c)$ and (2) patch-wise (PW) label propagation [7] which utilizes the entire label patch S_y^i. For voxel-wise label propagation, the label estimation of the target voxel x is obtained as follows:

$$\hat{L}^{VW}(x) = \frac{\sum_{i=1}^{N} \sum_{y \in V_x} w\left(P_x, P_y^i\right) S_y^i(a_c)}{\sum_i^N \sum_{y \in V_x} w\left(P_x, P_y^i\right)}, \tag{1}$$

where $w\left(P_x, P_y^i\right) = \exp(-\frac{\|P_x - P_y^i\|_2^2}{\sigma_x})$ is the weight assigned to the label $S_y^i(a_c)$. For the patch-wise label propagation, the estimation of the label patch centered at the target voxel x is first obtained as follows:

$$\hat{S}_x^{PW}(a) = \frac{\sum_{i=1}^{N} \sum_{y \in V_x} w\left(P_x, P_y^i\right) S_y^i(a)}{\sum_i^N \sum_{y \in V_x} w\left(P_x, P_y^i\right)}, a \in \Omega. \tag{2}$$

When testing the neighbor voxels of the voxel x, their corresponding label patches are also estimated, which can load the overlapped estimations for the voxel x from the estimated label patches of its neighbor voxels. Therefore, we adopt an averaging method to fuse the overlapped estimations and use it as the final label estimation $\hat{L}(x)$.

2.2   Local Subspace Learning Based Patch-Wise Label Propagation Method

In this section, we present our proposed method. First, we extract abundant texture information and multi-scale intensity information from the image patch as the feature representation for each voxel. Then, to enhance feature discrimination, margin fisher analysis (MFA) is employed to ensure that samples with the same label have feature a higher similarity while samples with different labels include a lower similarity. For simplicity, we first describe our method using voxel-wise label propagation and further extend it to patch-wise label propagation. Figure 1 schematically illustrates the overview of this local subspace learning based label propagation method that consists of a training stage and a testing stage.

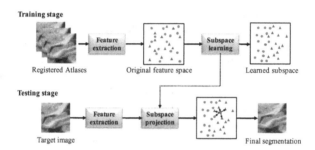

Fig. 1. Schematic illustration of the local subspace learning based label propagation method using voxel-wise label propagation.

Similar to typical multi-atlas based segmentation methods, we first linearly register each atlas to the target image. In the training stage, we generate the candidate training set for each target voxel to be segmented in the target image, using voxels of registered atlases within a spatial neighborhood of the target voxel. Then, for each training sample, a set of features is extracted for capturing effective information from the hippocampus using abundant texture descriptors and multi-scale patch intensities. Moreover, its associated class label is determined by the label of the voxel on the label map. In the subspace learning submodule, we learn a local discriminant subspace from the candidate training samples by using MFA. Afterwards, all the training samples are projected into the learned subspace.

In the testing stage, a kNN classifier is employed in the learned subspace to estimate the label of the target voxel. Specifically, the feature representation of the target voxel is first extracted from its surroundings in the target image and then projected into the learned subspace. Finally, the target voxel is compared with each training sample in the learned subspace, and the final label of the target voxel is determined by the most common label of the k-nearest neighbor samples. Next, we present details of the proposed segmentation method.

Generation of a Candidate Training Set: Given one target voxel x of the target image, voxels in its neighborhood $V(x)$ (with the size $\omega \times \omega \times \omega$) of all atlases are used to generate the training samples. This produces $N \times \omega \times \omega \times \omega$ candidate training samples $\{(\vec{f}_{i,j}, l_{i,j}) | i = 1, 2, \ldots N, j \in V(x)\}$, where $\vec{f}_{i,j}$ is a feature vector extracted from voxel j of the i th atlas, and $l_{i,j} \in \{+1, -1\}$ is the segmentation label of each candidate training sample. In order to balance the positive and negative samples for subspace learning, we respectively extract the same number of training samples from the hippocampus and non-hippocampus regions. Specifically, for the positive training samples, we select the q_1 most similar samples with the target image patch and randomly select another q_2 samples from the remaining training samples in the hippocampus region. In a similar manner, $q_1 + q_2$ negative samples are selected from the non-hippocampus regions, in which q_1 are the most similar with the target image patch and q_2 are randomly selected.

Feature Extraction: Abundant texture features and multi-scale intensity features are extracted. Specifically, the texture features consist of outputs from the first-order difference filters (FODs), second-order difference filters (SODs), 3D Hyperplan filters, 3D Sobel filters, Laplacian filters and range difference filters. For multi-scale intensity features, we use different Gaussian filters to replace the original intensity values with convolved intensity values. Here, a multi-scale strategy is proposed, which encodes both local and semi-local image information to characterize an image patch [9]. Specifically, the entire image patch is first divided into several non-overlapping scales, propagating from the center voxel to the boundaries of the patch. Considering the final purpose of the segmentation procedure is to determine the label of the center voxel, we use a fine scale to capture the center information of the image patch, and increasingly larger scales to capture coarse scale information as the distance to the patch center increases. Some other feature extraction method can also be used here [10, 11].

MFA-Based Subspace Learning: For simplicity, we use $U = [u_1, u_2, \ldots, u_M], u_i \in \mathbb{R}^d$ to denote training samples together with the corresponding class labels $\{y_1, y_2, \ldots, y_M\}, y_i \in \{+1, -1\}$. Here, M is the number of training samples, and d is the feature dimension. Margin fisher analysis (MFA) [8] aims to learn a subspace in which the intra-class manifold is compacted (i.e., intra-class compactness), while the manifold margin between different classes is enlarged based on the margin criteria (i.e., inter-class separability). Specifically, two undirected graphs, the intrinsic graph $G^I = \{U, S^I\}$ and the penalty graph $G^I = \{U, S^P\}$ are constructed according to graph embedding theory to respectively characterize the intra-class manifold structure and the manifold margin of different classes. In this case, U is the training samples set, and $S^I, S^P \in \mathbb{R}^{M \times M}$ are the corresponding similarity matrices. To characterize intra-class compactness, the similarity matrix S^I is defined as follows:

$$S_{ij}^I = \begin{cases} 1, & \text{if } i \in N_{k_1}^+(j) \text{ or } j \in N_{k_1}^+(i) \\ 0, & \text{else} \end{cases} \tag{3}$$

where $N_{k_1}^+(j)$ indicates the index set of the k_1 nearest neighbors of u_j in the same class. On the other hand, MFA defines the similarity matrix S^P to characterize interclass separability with the margin criteria, as follows:

$$S_{ij}^P = \begin{cases} 1, & \text{if } (i,j) \in P_{k_2}(y_i) \text{ or } (i,j) \in P_{k_2}(y_j) \\ 0, & \text{else} \end{cases} \tag{4}$$

where $P_{k_2}(y)$ is a set of data pairs that are the k_2 nearest pairs among the set $\{(i,j), y_i = y, y_j \neq y\}$. The adjacency relationships of the intrinsic and penalty graphs for MFA are illustrated in Fig. 2.

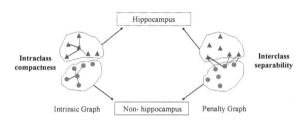

Fig. 2. Adjacency relationships of intrinsic and penalty graphs for MFA.

Then, the corresponding diagonal matrix D and the Laplacian matrix L of the intrinsic graph G^I are defined as

$$L = D - S, \quad D_{ii} = \sum_{j \neq i} S_{ij} \; \forall i. \tag{5}$$

The Lapaican matrix L^P of the penalty graph G^P can be defined similarly to Eq. (14). Finally, according to the graph embedding framework, the subspace projection matrix $\Phi_{\text{MFA}} \in \mathbb{R}^{d \times p}$, where p is the dimension of the subspace, can be computed by solving the objective function

$$\Phi_{\text{MFA}}^* = \arg\max_{\Phi_{\text{MFA}}} \frac{Tr\left(\Phi_{\text{MFA}}^T ULU^T \Phi_{\text{MFA}}\right)}{Tr\left(\Phi_{\text{MFA}}^T UL^P U^T \Phi_{\text{MFA}}\right)} \tag{6}$$

where $Tr(\cdot)$ is the trace operator of the matrix. Specifically, the projection matrix Φ_{MFA} consists of the eigenvectors corresponding to the largest eigenvalues of matrix $\left(\Phi_{\text{MFA}}^T ULU^T \Phi_{\text{MFA}}\right)^{-1} \left(\Phi_{\text{MFA}}^T UL^P U^T \Phi_{\text{MFA}}\right)$. After obtaining the projection function Φ_{MFA}, each feature representation u_i is projected into the learned space as follows:

$$w_i = \Phi_{\text{MFA}}^T \cdot u_i \tag{7}$$

Patch-Wise Label Propagation: In order to preserve local anatomical structure information in the segmentation, we extend our method to patch-wise label propagation. For patch-wise label propagation, each voxel is assigned with one label patch. Specifically, we extend the class label $y_i \in \mathbb{R}(i = 1, \ldots, M)$ of each voxel to the structured class label patch $Y_i \in \mathbb{R}^{t \times t \times t}$ corresponding to the label patch centered at the voxel, where $t \times t \times t$ is the size of the label patch. However, for the training set U together with the corresponding structured class label set $\{Y_1, \ldots, Y_M\}$, MFA cannot be directly used to learn the subspace. In order to perform MFA similar to that in the original class label space, we adopt k-means cluster method to $\{Y_1, \ldots, Y_M\}$, and then obtain the corresponding subclass labels $\{y_1', \ldots, y_M'\}, y_i' \in \{+1, -1\}$ in the unsupervised manner. Then, we replace $\{Y_1, \ldots, Y_M\}$ by $\{y_1', \ldots, y_M'\}$ and combine them with U to learn the subspace using MFA. In this case, samples with similar label patches are compacted and samples with dissimilar label patches are separated.

3   Experiments

Dataset: ADNI[1] dataset was used to evaluate the proposed method for hippocampus segmentation and compare it with other state-of-the-art segmentation methods. The ADNI dataset contains the segmentations of the left and right hippocampus of brain MRIs, which have been manually labeled by expert. The size of each MR image is $256 \times 256 \times 256$, and the voxel size is $1 \times 1 \times 1$ mm^3. We randomly selected 64 subjects to evaluate both performances of our method and the comparison methods. The selected subset of ADNI includes 16 normal control (NC), 32 MCI (Mild Cognitive Impairment) subjects, and 16 Alzheimer Disease (AD) subjects.

Validation Methodology: We use leave-one-out cross-validation to evaluate the performance of the proposed method, as well as two conventional multi-atlas based segmentation methods which are non-local patch-based label propagation (NPL) [5] and sparse patch-based label propagation (SPL) [6]. In this experiment, we calculated dice similarity coefficient (DSC), jaccard similarity coefficient (JSC), precision index (PI), recall index (RI). All these measures lie between 0 and 1 where the larger the value the more accurate/better. Additionally, hausdorff distance (HD) was also calculated whose lower value represents better segmentation performance.

Parameters: In the training stage, for the candidate training set, we set the search neighborhood V_x as $7 \times 7 \times 7$ and the number of training samples as 500. In the MFA, values for k_1 and k_2 are respectively set as 10 and 40, and the dimension p of learned subspace is set as 150. We set the intensity image patch size as $11 \times 11 \times 11$ for the feature extraction and the label patch size as $7 \times 7 \times 7$ for the label propagation. In the testing stage, we set the number k of nearest neighbors in the kNN classifier as 5.

Results: The mean and standard deviation values for the segmentation performance achieved using NLP, SLP, and our method are reported in Table 1. As shown in the table, our method obtains the best segmentation performance, followed by the SPL and NPL. Among the compared methods, NLP achieved the worst performance due to the lack of discriminating features and highly-correlated candidate patches which repeatedly produced the labeling errors. In terms of average performance for DSC, JSC, PI, RI, and HD, our method obtains statistically significant improvements (p-value <0.001)

---

[1] http://www.adni-info.org/.

Table 1. The mean and standard deviation of DSC, JSC, PI, RI and HD (mm) of left and right hippocampus, produced by NLP, SPL and Our method respectively. Values in the left and right of '/' respectively denote the segmentation accuracy of the left and right hippocampus.

	DSC	JSC	PI	RI	HD
NLP	0.848/0.865	0.752/0.764	0.878/0.883	0.857/0.864	2.341/2.139
	(0.071/0.031)	(0.074/0.050)	(0.087/0.059)	(0.045/0.039)	(0.532/0.536)
SPL	0.868/0.880	0.763/0.778	0.887/0.878	0.866/0.875	1.999/1.796
	(0.057/0.033)	(0.073/0.050)	(0.067/0.044)	(0.037/0.039)	(0.445/0.388)
Our method	0.879/0.889	0.773/0.789	0.903/0.914	0.879/0.889	1.857/1.753
	(0.047/0.030)	(0.064/0.045)	(0.066/0.043)	(0.033/0.039)	(0.369/0.348)

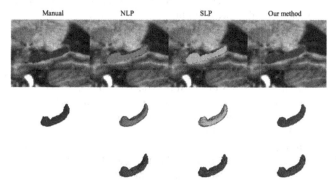

Fig. 3. Hippocampal segmentation results obtained by different methods. The first row shows segmentation results produced by different methods, the second row demonstrates their corresponding surface rendering results, and the third row shows differences between results of manual and automatic segmentation methods (red: manual segmentation results, green: automated segmentation results, blue: overlap between them). (Color figure online)

compared with NLP and SPL. Figure 3 shows segmentation results for a subject randomly chosen from the dataset. It is evident that, compared to the NLP and SLP, the segmentation produced by our method is closer to the manual segmentation. All experimental results indicated that the proposed method performed consistently better than other segmentation methods.

4   Conclusion

In this paper, we propose a novel local subspace learning based patch-wise label propagation method for hippocampus segmentation. Specifically, instead of using simple patch intensities to compute the similarity, multi-scale patch intensities and abundant texture features are extracted from image patches. In order to enhance feature discrimination, MFA is then utilized to extract the most discriminant features for each voxel to be segmented. Then, based on the extracted features, kNN classifier is used to determine the final label for the voxel. Furthermore, to take advantage of anatomical structure information in the segmentation, we extend MFA to the patch-wise label propagation. Experimental results demonstrate the superior performance of our method, as compared with traditional multi-atlas based segmentation methods.

References

1. Devanand, D.P., Pradhaban, G., Liu, X., Khandji, A., De, S.S., Segal, S., et al.: Hippocampal and entorhinal atrophy in mild cognitive impairment: prediction of Alzheimer disease. Retour Au Numéro **68**(11), 828–836 (2007)
2. Zarei, M., Beckmann, C.F., Binnewijzend, M.A.A., Schoonheim, M.M., Oghabian, M.A., Sanz-Arigita, E.J., et al.: Functional segmentation of the hippocampus in the healthy human brain and in Alzheimer's disease. NeuroImage **66c**, 28–35 (2013)
3. Wachinger, C., Sharp, G.C., Golland, P.: Contour-driven regression for label inference in atlas-based segmentation. In: Mori, K., Sakuma, I., Sato, Y., Barillot, C., Navab, N. (eds.) MICCAI 2013, Part III. LNCS, vol. 8151, pp. 211–218. Springer, Heidelberg (2013)
4. Pluim, J.P.W: Evaluating and improving label fusion in atlas-based segmentation using the surface distance. In: Proceedings of the SPIE, vol. 7962, no. 3, pp. 215–230 (2011)
5. Coupé, P., Manjón, J.V., Fonov, V., Pruessner, J., Robles, M., Collins, D.L.: Patch-based segmentation using expert priors: application to hippocampus and ventricle segmentation. NeuroImage **54**(2), 940–954 (2011)
6. Rousseau, F., Habas, P.A., Studholme, C.: A supervised patch-based approach for human brain labeling. IEEE Trans. Med. Imaging **30**(10), 1852–1862 (2011)
7. Yan, S., Xu, D., Zhang, B., Zhang, H.J., Yang, Q., Lin, S.: Graph embedding and extensions: a general framework for dimensionality reduction. IEEE Trans. Pattern Anal. Mach. Intell. **29**(1), 40–51 (2007)
8. Wu, G., Kim, M., Sanroma, G., Qian, W., Munsell, B.C., Shen, D.: Hierarchical multi-atlas label fusion with multi-scale feature representation and label-specific patch partition. NeuroImage **106**, 34–46 (2015)
9. Zhang, J., Liang, J., Zhao, H.: Local energy pattern for texture classification using self-adaptive quantization thresholds. IEEE Trans. Image Process. **22**(1), 31–42 (2013)
10. Zhang, J., Zhao, H., Liang, J.: Continuous rotation invariant local descriptors for texton dictionary-based texture classification. Comput. Vis. Image Underst. **117**(1), 56–75 (2013)

Improving Single-Modal Neuroimaging Based Diagnosis of Brain Disorders via Boosted Privileged Information Learning Framework

Xiao Zheng[1], Jun Shi[1(✉)], Shihui Ying[2], Qi Zhang[1], and Yan Li[3]

[1] School of Communication and Information Engineering,
Shanghai University, Shanghai, China
junshi@staff.shu.edu.cn
[2] Department of Mathematics, School of Science,
Shanghai University, Shanghai, China
[3] College of Computer Science and Software Engineering,
Shenzhen University, Shenzhen, China

Abstract. In clinical practice, it is more prevalent to use only a single-modal neuroimaging for diagnosis of brain disorders, such as structural magnetic resonance imaging. A neuroimaging dataset generally suffers from the small-sample-size problem, which makes it difficult to train a robust and effective classifier. The learning using privileged information (LUPI) is a newly proposed paradigm, in which the privileged information is available only at the training phase to provide additional information about training samples, but unavailable in the testing phase. LUPI can effectively help construct a better predictive rule to promote classification performance. In this paper, we propose to apply LUPI for the single-modal neuroimaging based diagnosis of brain diseases along with multi-modal training data. Moreover, a boosted LUPI framework is developed, which performs LUPI-based random subspace learning and then ensembles all the LUPI classifiers with the multiple kernel boosting (MKB) algorithm. The experimental results on two neuroimaging datasets show that LUPI-based algorithms are superior to the traditional classifier models for single-modal neuroimaging based diagnosis of brain disorders, and the proposed boosted LUPI framework achieves best performance.

1 Introduction

In recent years, the multi-modal neuroimaging based computer-aided diagnosis for brain disorders has attracted considerable attention. However, it is more prevalent to use only a single-modality for diagnosis in clinical practice. For example, although combination of structural magnetic resonance imaging (sMRI) and positron emission tomography (PET) biomarkers can improve the diagnosis accuracy of Alzheimer's disease (AD) [1], PET scanner is extremely expensive resulting in limited supply. Therefore, sMRI is still the most commonly used neruoimaging technique for brain due to its advantages on easy operation and visualization of anatomical structures.

A neuroimaging dataset generally has small labeled samples and may suffer from the small-sample-size problem [2]. Therefore, it is still a challenging task to train a robust

L. Wang et al. (Eds.): MLMI 2016, LNCS 10019, pp. 95–103, 2016.
DOI: 10.1007/978-3-319-47157-0_12

and accurate classifier from small single-modal neuroimaging dataset. To address this issue, many efforts have been devoted, such as the semi-supervised learning and even transfer learning. For example, Filipovych et al. proposed a semi-supervised learning based algorithm for AD classification with MRI images, in which the data of mild cognitive impairment (MCI) patients are considered as unlabeled samples [3]; Cheng et al. proposed a transfer learning based algorithm to predict the conversion of MCI to AD with MRI and PET images, which used the data from AD patients and normal controls (NC) as the auxiliary domains to enlarge training dataset [4].

Recently, Vapnik and Vashist propose a new learning paradigm, namely learning using privileged information (LUPI), in which the privileged information is available only at the training phase to provide additional information about training samples, but unavailable in the testing phase [5]. This privileged information can effectively help construct a better predictive rule to promote classification performance [5]. Since there are already some multi-modal neuroimaging datasets, LUPI has the potential to train a more robust and effective predictive model for the single-modal neuroimaging based diagnosis with additional modalities. It should be noted that an unprivileged and privileged sample pair has the same label, because they come from the same subject. This is one of the main difference between LUPI and transfer learning.

The commonly used LUPI classifier is an extension of support vector machine (SVM), known as SVM+ [5], which uses both unprivileged and privileged samples to construct an optimal hyperplane. To improve the performance of SVM+, many efforts have been devoted to mainly use more effective optimization solutions for SVM+ [6].

It is worth noting that features extracted from neuroimaging data may have high feature dimensionalities. Therefore, it is suitable to adopt a random subspace (RS) ensemble algorithm for these high-dimensional features, because RS ensemble is less sensitive to noise and redundant features, and outperforms single classifiers for neuroimaging data classification [7].

In this paper, we propose a novel boosted-LUPI-based classification framework for the single-modal neuroimaging based diagnosis of brain diseases along with privileged information. Specifically, the high-dimensional features of one modality are randomly split into several subspaces, and each feature subspace is then used to train an SVM+ classifier together with the features from another modality. A multiple kernel boosting (MKB) based boosted-SVM+ (SVM+-MKB) algorithm is then developed to ensemble all the SVM+ classifiers trained with different subspace features, which can promote the predictive performance.

2   Boosted-LUPI-Based Classification Framework

As shown in Fig. 1, the proposed boosted-LUPI-based classification framework consists of three components: random subspace feature sampling, LUPI and MKB learning. In the training stage, the higher-dimensionality features in one modality data (unprivileged data or privileged data) are randomly split into k subspaces, which form k groups of input features together with the features from another modality data. Each feature group is then fed to a SVM+ to train toally k classifiers. All the classifiers are finally boosted by MKB to build a strong classifier. In the testing phase, only the unprivileged data are fed to the trained strong predictive model.

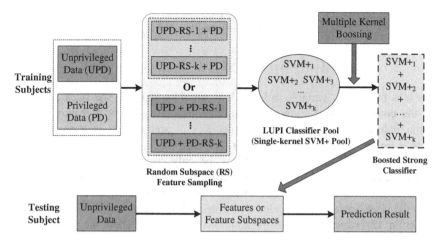

Fig. 1. Flowchart of the boosted LUPI classification framework

In this work, the multiple LUPI classifiers are boosted to a strong classifier by the MKB algorithm, which has shown its advantages of simplicity and effectiveness [8]. However, other boosting methods also can be used instead of MKB in this boosted-LUPI-based classification framework.

2.1 Random Subspace Feature Sampling

Let $\{(x_i, x_i', y_i)\}_{i=1}^n$ be n training samples, where x_i is a d-dimensional unprivileged sample in space X, x_i' is a d'-dimensional privileged sample belonging to space X$'$, which is different from the space X, and y_i is the corresponding label value.

Since in LUPI, there are two data space, namely X and X$'$, we generally select the data with higher feature dimensionality for random subspace feature sampling, while keep another data unaltered. For example, if the feature dimensionality d' of privileged data x_i' is larger than that of unprivileged data x_i, we then randomly split the d'-dimensional features into k subsets. It is worth noting that the privileged and un privileged data could be split into k subsets, respectively, in case they both have very high feature dimensionalities.

Each feature subset together with another dataset will then be fed to SVM+ to train k classifiers in total. Notably, the privileged information is only provided at the training stage, while during the testing phase, only the test data in space X will be input to all the k SVM+ classifiers for prediction.

2.2 Privileged Information Learning

The SVM-based LUPI paradigm is described as follows [5]. A standard soft-margin SVM classifier should solve the following optimization problem:

$$\min_{w,b,\xi} \phi(\mathbf{w}, b, \xi) = \frac{1}{2} \|\mathbf{w}\|^2 + C \sum_{i=1}^{N} \xi_i \tag{1}$$

$$\text{s.t.} \quad y_i\left((\mathbf{w}^T \phi(x)) + b\right) \geq 1 - \xi_i, \quad \xi_i \geq 0, i = 1, \ldots n$$

where $\mathbf{w}$ is the weight variable, b is the bias variable, and ξ_i is the slack variable to relax the constraints and allow some misclassification. $\phi(x)$ is a feature mapping function induced by the associated kernel $K(\cdot, \cdot)$, and $C > 0$ is a regularization parameter for the tradeoff of margin error.

In the standard SVM, nonnegativity is the only constraint on ξ_i. In LUPI, the privileged information can be used to introduce additional constraints on the slack variables (errors) for training samples, which leads to the main idea of SVM+. That is to say, the slack variable is modeled and restricted by the so-called 'correcting functions' in Eq. (2), which represents the additional information about the data in SVM+.

$$\xi_i'\left(x_i'\right) = \varphi\left(x_i', \mathbf{w}'\right) = \mathbf{w}'^T \phi'\left(x_i'\right) + b' \tag{2}$$

When using the correcting function to replace the slack variable $\xi_i \geq 0$ in the hinge loss in the original SVM, we then get the following primal problem:

$$\min_{w,b,\xi} \phi\left(\mathbf{w}, b, \xi'\right) = \frac{1}{2}\left(\|\mathbf{w}\|^2 + \gamma \|\mathbf{w}'\|^2\right) + C \sum_{i=1}^{N} \xi_i' \tag{3}$$

$$\text{s.t.} \quad y_i\left((\mathbf{w}^T \phi(x)) + b\right) \geq 1 - \xi_i', \quad \xi_i' \geq 0, i = 1, \ldots n$$

The optimization problem of Eq. (3) then can be solved by constructing the Lagrangian

$$\begin{aligned} L\left(\mathbf{w}, b, \mathbf{w}', b', \alpha, \beta\right) &= \frac{1}{2}\left(\|\mathbf{w}\|^2 + \gamma \|\mathbf{w}'\|^2\right) + C \sum_{i=1}^{N} [\mathbf{w}'^T \phi'\left(x_i'\right) + b'] \\ &- \sum_{i=1}^{N} \alpha_i \left[y_i\left((\mathbf{w}^T \phi(x)) + b\right) - 1 + \left(\mathbf{w}'^T \phi'\left(x_i'\right) + b'\right)\right] \\ &- \sum_{i=1}^{N} \beta_i \left(\mathbf{w}'^T \phi'\left(x_i'\right) + b'\right) \end{aligned} \tag{4}$$

where $\alpha_i \geq 0$ and $\beta_i \geq 0$.

Let the decision function and the corresponding correcting function be the forms:

$$f(x, \alpha) = \sum_{i=1}^{N} \alpha_i y_i K(x_i, x) + b \tag{5}$$

and

$$f'\left(x', \beta\right) = \frac{1}{\gamma} \sum_{i=1}^{N} (\alpha_i + \beta_i - C) K'\left(x_i', x'\right) + b' \tag{6}$$

where K and K' are the kernel functions. By applying KKT conditions, the corresponding dual problem only depends on α and β as follows:

$$
\max\nolimits_{\alpha,\beta} \sum\nolimits_{i=1}^{N} \alpha_i - \sum\nolimits_{i=1}^{N} \sum\nolimits_{j=1}^{N} \alpha_i \alpha_j y_i y_j K\left(x_i, x_j\right) -
$$
$$
\frac{1}{2\gamma} \sum\nolimits_{i=1}^{N} \sum\nolimits_{j=1}^{N} (\alpha_i + \beta_i - C)(\alpha_j + \beta_j - C) K'\left(x_i', x_j'\right) \tag{7}
$$

$$
\text{s.t.} \ \sum\nolimits_{i=1}^{N} (\alpha_i + \beta_i - C) = 0, \ \ \sum\nolimits_{i=1}^{N} y_i \alpha_i = 0, \ \ \alpha_i \geq 0, \ \ \beta_i \geq 0
$$

Equation (7) is a standard quadratic programming problem, which can be solved by several conventional methods. Once the optimal α and β are obtained, the new test sample x can be predicted by Eq. (5).

2.3 Multiple Kernel Boosting Learning

As shown in Fig. 1, a pool of SVM+ classifiers are generated, when we apply SVM+ to each group of subspace features and unaltered features. In order to effectively ensemble these classifiers, we treat all SVM+ classifiers as weak classifiers and then learn a strong classifier using the boosting method.

In this work, we develop a boosted SVM+ with a similar way to the multiple kernel boosting (MKB) method [8], which combines several SVMs of different kernels.

In multiple kernel learning (MKL), let $\{K_l\}_1^M$ be the kernel set, the combination of multiple kernels can be defined as

$$
K(x, x_i) = \sum\nolimits_{l=1}^{M} \eta_l K_l(x, x_i), \quad \text{s.t. } \eta_l \geq 0 \text{ and } \sum\nolimits_{l=1}^{M} \eta_l = 1 \tag{8}
$$

where η_l is the kernel weight. Then, the decision function is given by

$$
Y(x) = \sum\nolimits_{i=1}^{N} \eta_l \sum\nolimits_{l}^{M} \mu_i y_i K_l(x, x_i) + \tilde{b} = \sum\nolimits_{l}^{M} \eta_l (\mu^{\mathrm{T}} \mathbf{K}_l(x) + \tilde{b}_l) \tag{9}
$$

where μ_i is the Lagrange multiplier, $\mu = [\mu_1 y_1, \mu_2 y_2 \ldots \mu_N y_N]^{\mathrm{T}}$, and $\tilde{b} = \sum\nolimits_{l=1}^{M} \tilde{b}_l$.

Since there are multiple SVM+ classifiers obtained from different subspace features, we can convert the standard MKL formulation to a linear combination of the real outputs of multiple single-kernel SVM+ classifiers based on Eqs. (5) and (9).

The key problem now becomes how to optimize the weights η_j, which is propsed to be computed by the classical Adaboost method here. By combining Eqs. (5) and (9) can be rewritten as

$$
Y(x) = \sum\nolimits_{j=1}^{J} \eta_j f_j(x) \tag{10}
$$

where J denotes the number of iterations in the boosting process. Equation (9) means that each SVM+ is considered as a weak classifier, and the final strong classifier $Y(x)$ is the weighted combination of all the weak classifiers.

The weighted classification error of a single SVM+ classifier at the j-th iteration is defined as

$$\varepsilon_j = \frac{\sum_{i=1}^{N} \omega(i)|f_j(x_i)|(\text{sign}(-y_i f_j(x_i)) + 1)/2}{\sum_{i=1}^{N} \omega(i)|f_j(x_i)|} \tag{11}$$

where $\omega(i)$ is the weight of the training samples.

After J iterations, all the η_j and $f_j(x_i)$ are calculated and the final boosted classifier is achieved.

3 Experiment and Results

Two neuroimaging datasets, namely the MLSP schizophrenia MRI dataset (www. kaggle.com/c/mlsp-2014-mri/) [9] and Alzheimer's Disease Neuroimaging Initiative (ADNI) database [10], are used in this work.

The proposed SVM+-MKB algorithm is compared with the following algorithms: (1) the standard SVM classifier with only the unprivileged sMRI data; (2) the kernel canonical correlation analysis (KCCA), a commonly used two-view learning algorithm, which is performed to jointly train two data representation models for both modality data, and only the model of unprivileged data is used to generate new feature representation for a standard SVM classifier during the testing phase; (3) the heterogeneous feature augmentation (HFA) based transfer learning algorithm with SVM classifier [11], which uses the privileged information in SVM+ as the source domain and unprivileged data as the target domain; (4) SVM+; (5) the voting-based SVM+, which ensembles the classifiers in the SVM+ pool by majority-voting method.

3.1   Experiment on MLSP Schizophrenia Dataset

The first experiment is conducted on the MLSP schizophrenia dataset with sMRI and fMRI images as multi-modal neuroimaging data [9]. Only the training set data are used in this work, which include 40 schizophrenia patients and 46 NC. Totally 32 features are extracted from gray matter density with the source-based morphometry from sMRI data, and 378-dimensional functional network connectivity (FNC) features are extracted from fMRI data in MLSP schizophrenia challenge [9]. For details about the multi-modal feature extraction, please refer to [9].

In this experiment, sMRI is selected as the unprivileged data for the single-modal diagnosis tool and fMRI as the privileged information. Moreover, the 378-dimensional features of fMRI are randomly split into 10 subsets for boosting. The 5-fold cross-validation strategy is performed, and this process is repeated for 5 times independently so as to avoid the bias introduced by randomly partitioning dataset in the cross-validation.

Table 1 shows the classification results of different algorithms. It is observed that all the three SVM+-based algorithms outperform SVM and KCCA algorithms, which indicates the effectiveness of LUPI for single-modal neuroimaging based diagnosis.

Table 1. Classification results of different algorithms on schizophrenia dataset (unit: %)

	Accuracy	Sensitivity	Specificity
SVM	68.38 ± 3.21	58.50 ± 4.54	76.93 ± 4.36
KCCA	58.22 ± 3.25	51.50 ± 4.18	64.09 ± 4.97
HFA	72.16 ± 2.06	68.00 ± 1.12	75.78 ± 3.42
SVM+	72.55 ± 3.77	67.50 ± 3.06	76.89 ± 5.42
SVM+-Voting	73.03 ± 3.86	68.00 ± 3.26	77.38 ± 4.93
SVM+-MKB	**75.10 ± 3.24**	**69.50 ± 2.10**	**79.91 ± 4.88**

SVM+ is slightly better than HFA-based transfer learning algorithm on classification accuracy and specificity. Notably, the proposed SVM+-MKB algorithm has the best performance with the mean classification accuracy, sensitivity and specificity of 75.10 ± 3.24 %, 69.50 ± 2.10 % and 79.91 ± 4.88 %, respectively, which achieves at least 2.55 %, 1.50 % and 2.53 % improvements, compared with all other algorithms.

3.2 Experiment on ADNI Dataset

Since diagnosis of MCI is more difficult than diagnosis of AD, in the second experiment on ADNI dataset, we used the sMRI images from 99 MCI patients and 52 NCs for classification, together with their corresponding cerebrospinal fluid (CSF) data Each MR image is partitioned into 93 brain ROIs, and the volumes of gray matter tissue are then calculated for each ROI as features [1]. CSF $A\beta_{42}$, t-tau and p-tau are used as the CSF features [1]. CSF data are used as privileged information, while 93 MRI features are randomly split into five subsets. The 10-fold cross-validation strategy is performed, which is repeated for 10 times independently.

Table 2 gives the classification results of different algorithms. As can been seem that all the SVM+-based algorithms are still superior to SVM and KCCA algorithms, and boosted SVM+ again acheves best performance with the mean accuracy 75.76 ± 1.44 %, sensitivity 86.39 ± 2.79 % and specificity 55.47 ± 4.97 %, improving at least 2.99 %, 1.07 % and 4.84 %, respectively, compared with all other algorithms.

Table 2. Classification results of different algorithms on ADNI dataset (unit: %)

	Accuracy	Sensitivity	Specificity
SVM	71.56 ± 2.37	84.24 ± 2.79	47.37 ± 3.88
KCCA	65.08 ± 2.91	81.71 ± 3.79	33.77 ± 6.20
HFA	72.75 ± 1.56	82.54 ± 2.19	52.93 ± 5.06
SVM+	72.77 ± 1.56	84.57 ± 1.62	50.63 ± 2.23
SVM+-Voting	72.60 ± 2.08	85.32 ± 2.77	48.70 ± 4.79
SVM+-MKB	**75.76 ± 1.44**	**86.39 ± 2.79**	**55.47 ± 4.97**

4 Conclusion

Summary, we propose a boosted LUPI framework to train a more effective classifier model for single-modal neuroimaging based diagnosis of brain disorders along with multi-modal training data. The results on two datasets indicate that the LUPI-based algorithms is superior to the traditional classifier model using sMRI as the single-modelity, because the privileged data provides additional information for helping train a more discriminating hyperplane in SVM classifier. Moreover, the proposed boosted SVM+ outperforms all compared algorithms, including the commonly used HFA-based transfer learning algorithm. It suggests that our boosted LUPI framework has the potential in single-modal neuroimaging based diagnosis of brain disorders.

In future work, more boosting learning algorithms should be studied for the ensemble of SVM+ pool to further improve the performance of boosted SVM+. Other MKL algorithms should also be investigated, which can directly optimize the combination of multiple kernels in SVM+ without Adaboost. Moreover, we will focus on the semi-supervised LUPI to involve more unlabeled neuroimaging data for superior performance.

Acknowledgments. This work is supported by the National Natural Science Foundation of China (61471231, 61401267, 11471208, 61201042, 61471245, U1201256), the Projects of Guangdong R/D Foundation and the New Technology R/D projects of Shenzhen City.

References

1. Zhang, D.Q., Wang, Y.P., Zhou, L.P., Yuan, H., Shen, D.G.: ADNI: multimodal classification of Alzheimer's disease and mild cognitive impairment. NeuroImage **55**(3), 856–867 (2011)
2. Mwangi, B., Tian, T.S., Soares, J.C.: A review of feature reduction techniques in neuroimaging. Neuroinformatics **12**(2), 229–244 (2014)
3. Filipovych, R., Davatzikos, C.: Semi-supervised pattern classification of medical images: application to mild cognitive impairment (MCI). NeuroImage **55**(3), 1109–1119 (2011)
4. Cheng, B., Liu, M.X., Zhang, D.Q., Munsell, B.C., Shen, D.G.: ADNI: domain transfer learning for MCI conversion prediction. IEEE Trans. Biomed. Eng. **62**(7), 1805–1817 (2015)
5. Vapnik, V., Vashist, A.: A new learning paradigm: learning using privileged information. Neural Netw. **22**, 544–557 (2009)
6. Pechyony, D., Izmailov, R., Vashist, A., Vapnik, V.: SMO-style algorithms for learning using privileged information. In: DMIN, pp. 235–241 (2010)
7. Kuncheva, L.I., Rodríguez, J.J., Plumpton, C.O., Linden, D.E.J., Johnston, S.J.: Random subspace ensembles for fMRI classification. IEEE Trans. Med. Imaging **29**(2), 531–542 (2010)
8. Yang, F., Lu, H.C., Yang, M.H.: Robust visual tracking via multiple kernel boosting with affinity constraints. IEEE Trans. Circuits Syst. Video Technol. **24**(2), 242–254 (2014)
9. Silva, R.F., Castro, E., Gupta, C.N., Cetin, M., Arbabshirani, M., Potluru, V.K., Plis, S.M., Calhoun, V.D.: The tenth annual MLSP competition schizophrenia classification challenge. In: MLSP, pp. 1–6 (2014)

10. Jack, C.R., Bernstein, M.A., Fox, N.C., et al.: The Alzheimer's disease neuroimaging initiative (ADNI): MRI methods. J. Magn. Reson. Imaging **27**, 685–691 (2008)
11. Li, W., Duan, L.X., Xu, D., Tsang, I.W.: Learning with augmented features for supervised and semi-supervised heterogeneous domain adaptation. IEEE Trans. Pattern Anal. Mach. Intell. **36**(6), 1134–1148 (2014)

A Semi-supervised Large Margin Algorithm for White Matter Hyperintensity Segmentation

Chen Qin[1]([✉]), Ricardo Guerrero Moreno[1], Christopher Bowles[1],
Christian Ledig[1], Philip Scheltens[2], Frederik Barkhof[2],
Hanneke Rhodius-Meester[2], Betty Tijms[2], Afina W. Lemstra[2],
Wiesje M. van der Flier[2], Ben Glocker[1], and Daniel Rueckert[1]

[1] Department of Computing, Imperial College London, London, UK
c.qin15@imperial.ac.uk
[2] Department of Neurology, VU University Medical Center,
Amsterdam, The Netherlands

Abstract. Precise detection and quantification of white matter hyperintensities (WMH) is of great interest in studies of neurodegenerative diseases (NDs). In this work, we propose a novel semi-supervised large margin algorithm for the segmentation of WMH. The proposed algorithm optimizes a kernel based max-margin objective function which aims to maximize the margin averaged over inliers and outliers while exploiting a limited amount of available labelled data. We show that the learning problem can be formulated as a joint framework learning a classifier and a label assignment simultaneously, which can be solved efficiently by an iterative algorithm. We evaluate our method on a database of 280 brain Magnetic Resonance (MR) images from subjects that either suffered from subjective memory complaints or were diagnosed with NDs. The segmented WMH volumes correlate well with the standard clinical measurement (Fazekas score), and both the qualitative visualization results and quantitative correlation scores of the proposed algorithm outperform other well known methods for WMH segmentation.

1 Introduction

White matter hyperintensities (WMH) are areas of the brain in cerebral white matter (WM) that appear bright on T2-weighted fluid attenuated inversion recovery (FLAIR) magnetic resonance (MR) images due to localized, pathological changes in tissue composition [12]. WMH are commonly observed in elderly subjects and subjects with neurodegenerative diseases (NDs), such as vascular dementia (VaD), Alzheimer's disease (AD) and dementia with Lewy Bodies (DLB). Current research [2,5] indicates that the WMH volume in subjects with dementia is significantly higher than that of a normal aging population, and the presence, severity and distribution of WMH also vary between different disorders. Clinically, the amount of WMH is usually characterized by the Fazekas score [3], which is useful in the assessment of subjects with possible dementia. However, such visual rating scales show poor sensitivity to clinical group differences and

© Springer International Publishing AG 2016
L. Wang et al. (Eds.): MLMI 2016, LNCS 10019, pp. 104–112, 2016.
DOI: 10.1007/978-3-319-47157-0_13

may also incur high intra- and inter-rater variability [2]. Thus, more reliable and precise methods for quantifying and analyzing WMH are still desirable.

Recently, several techniques that seek to automatically and precisely segment and quantify WMH have been put forward [2]. In the supervised setting, machine learning methods such as k-nearest neighbor (kNN) [1], support vector machines (SVM) [7] and random forests [5] have been applied to the problem of WMH segmentation. These approaches learn the characteristic features of lesions from training samples that have been manually segmented by an expert. Such supervised methods can achieve good performance, however, they rely on the manual segmentation which is costly, time consuming and inevitably contains some mislabelled training data. In contrast, unsupervised segmentation methods do not require labelled training data. Most approaches employ clustering techniques to group similar voxels, such as fuzzy C-means clustering [4] and EM-based algorithms [6]. A different type of approach considers lesions as outliers to normal tissues [11,14]. Recently, a lesion growth algorithm [10] has been developed, which constructs a conservative lesion belief map with a pre-chosen threshold (τ), followed by the initial map being grown along voxels that appear hyperintense in the FLAIR image. However, such unsupervised approaches can not always produce satisfactory results in subjects with NDs, since WMH in those subjects are often small and irregular, and also heterogeneous within and across subjects [5].

In this work, we propose a semi-supervised large margin approach for WMH segmentation, which identifies WMH as outliers, i.e., patterns deviating from normal data. Specifically, our method optimizes a kernel based max-margin objective function formulated by both the limited labelled information and a large amount of unlabelled data. We show that the framework jointly learns a large margin classifier and a label assignment, which is solved by updating the classifier and the label indicator alternatingly. The main idea of the proposed approach is to tackle the uncertainty of unlabelled input data with the help of a small proportion of labelled ones, and to discover outliers by training a large margin classifier which maximizes the average margins of judged inliers and outliers. Instead of assuming that data is generated from a particular distribution as most of other outlier detection methods do [11,14], which may not hold true for WMH segmentation, our method assumes that neighboring samples tend to have consistent classifications that are guided by available labelled data. Quantitative and qualitative results indicate that the proposed method outperforms the current well known methods on a large database of subjects with NDs.

2   Unsupervised One-Class Learning

Let $\mathcal{X} = \left\{\mathbf{x}_i \in \mathbf{R}^d\right\}_{i=1}^n$ denote a set of n unlabelled input samples, and y_i represent the corresponding soft label that assigns normal samples a positive value (c^+) while a negative value (c^-) for outliers. Additionally, let $\mathcal{H}$ be a reproducing kernel Hilbert space (RKHS) of the function: $f(\mathbf{x}) = \sum_{i=1}^n \kappa(\mathbf{x}, \mathbf{x}_i)\alpha_i$, with associated kernel κ as the functional base and the expansion coefficient α. The unsupervised one-class learning (UOCL) proposed by Liu et al. [9] is an unsupervised algorithm that uses a self-guided labelling procedure to discover potential outliers in the data. This method aims to separate the positive samples from outliers by training a large margin classifier, which is obtained from minimizing the following objective function:

$$\min_{f\in\mathcal{H},\{y_i\}} \sum_{i=1}^{n} \left(f(\mathbf{x}_i)-y_i\right)^2 + \gamma_1 \|f\|_{\mathcal{M}}^2 - \frac{2\gamma_2}{n_+} \sum_{i,y_i>0} f(\mathbf{x}_i) \tag{1}$$
$$s.t. \quad y_i \in \{c^+, c^-\}, \ \forall i \in [1:n], \ 0 < n_+ = |\{i|y_i>0\}| < n.$$

Here, the first term in function (1) uses the squared loss to make the classification function consistent with the label assignment. The second term is a manifold regularizer, which endows f with the smoothness along the intrinsic manifold structure $\mathcal{M}$ underlying the data. Here $\|f\|_{\mathcal{M}}^2$ can be formulated as $\mathbf{f}^{\mathrm{T}}\mathbf{L}\mathbf{f}$, in which $\mathbf{f} = \left[f(\mathbf{x}_1), \cdots, f(\mathbf{x}_n)\right]^{\mathrm{T}}$, and $\mathbf{L}$ is the graph Laplacian matrix. The last term represents the margin averaged over the judged positive samples, which aims to push the majority of the inliers as far away as possible from the decision boundary $f(\mathbf{x}) = 0$. The importance of all three terms are balanced by the trade-off parameters γ_1 and γ_2. For more details, please refer to [9].

This minimization problem is solved by an alternating optimization scheme, with the continuous function f and discrete label assignment y_i being optimized iteratively. The method has been shown to be robust to high outlier proportion, which is a highly desirable trait in WMH segmentation of subjects with NDs.

3   Semi-supervised Large Margin Algorithm

When it comes to the WMH segmentation, the classification results of UOCL are not always satisfactory. Since outliers originate from low-density samples and are later separated from high-density regions without guidance from labelled information, the UOCL method can produce many false positives when segmenting WMH, such as identifying edges and partial volume as outliers. To address this problem, we extend the UOCL method to a semi-supervised large margin algorithm (SSLM). A limited amount of labelled data is introduced to provide some guidance for unlabelled samples, with the aim of improving its performance over unsupervised methods as well as reducing the need of expensive labelled data required in fully supervised learning.

3.1   Learning Model

Following the notations defined in Sect. 2, we define L as a labelled data set and U as the unlabelled data set, which, in WMH segmentation case, represent sets of voxels with known and unknown labels respectively. The objective function of our proposed model is formulated as:

$$\min_{f \in \mathcal{H}, \{y_i\}} \sum_{\mathbf{x}_i \in U} (f(\mathbf{x}_i) - y_i)^2 + \lambda \sum_{\mathbf{x}_j \in L} (f(\mathbf{x}_j) - y_j)^2 + \gamma_1 \|f\|_{\mathcal{M}}^2$$

$$- \frac{2\gamma_2}{n_+} \sum_{k, y_k > 0} f(\mathbf{x}_k) + \frac{2\gamma_3}{n_-} \sum_{k, y_k < 0} f(\mathbf{x}_k), \qquad (2)$$

$$s.t. \quad y_i \in \{c^+, c^-\}, \ n_+ = |\{i|y_i > 0\}|, \ n_- = |\{i|y_i < 0\}|,$$

where $\mathbf{x}_k \in L \cup U$, $\lambda, \gamma_1, \gamma_2$ and γ_3 are trade-off parameters controlling the model, and n_+ and n_- are numbers of positive and negative samples respectively during the learning. In this model, we introduce a new term $\sum_{\mathbf{x}_j \in L} (f(\mathbf{x}_j) - y_j)^2$ that represents squared loss for labelled data. This enables the classification to be informed by the available labels, thereby allowing it to better discriminate between inliers and outliers. Additionally, motivated by [13], we also introduce a new term $\sum_{k, y_k < 0} f(\mathbf{x}_k)/n_-$ into the objective function (2), which aims to maximize the average margin between the judged outliers and the decision boundary. The last two terms in objective function (2) work together to push the positive samples and outliers far away from the decision boundary, thus enabling these two groups of data to be far away from each other.

For a more concise notation, we further define the vectorial kernel mapping $\mathbf{k}(\mathbf{x}) = [\kappa(\mathbf{x}_i, \mathbf{x}), \cdots, \kappa(\mathbf{x}_n, \mathbf{x})]^{\mathrm{T}}$, and the kernel matrix $\mathbf{K} = [\kappa(\mathbf{x}_i, \mathbf{x}_j)]_{1 \le i, j \le n}$, so the target function can be expressed as $f(\mathbf{x}) = \alpha^{\mathrm{T}} \mathbf{k}(\mathbf{x})$ and $\mathbf{f} = \mathbf{K}\alpha$, in which $\alpha = [\alpha_1, \cdots, \alpha_n]^{\mathrm{T}} \in R^n$. Then the objective function can be rewritten as

$$\min_{\alpha, \mathbf{y}} \alpha^{\mathrm{T}} \mathbf{K} (\mathbf{\Lambda} + \gamma_1 \mathbf{L}) \mathbf{K} \alpha - 2\alpha^{\mathrm{T}} \mathbf{K} \mathbf{\Lambda} \mathbf{y} + \mathbf{y}^{\mathrm{T}} \mathbf{\Lambda} \mathbf{y} - 2\alpha^{\mathrm{T}} \mathbf{K} \tilde{\mathbf{y}}$$

$$s.t. \quad \mathbf{y} \in \{c^+, c^-\}^{n \times 1}, \ \mathbf{\Lambda} = diag(1, \dots 1, \underbrace{\lambda, \dots \lambda}_{\mathbf{x}_j \in L}, 1, \dots 1), \qquad (3)$$

$$\tilde{y}_i = \begin{cases} \frac{\gamma_2}{\|\mathbf{y}\|_+}, & y_i = c^+, \\ -\frac{\gamma_3}{\|\mathbf{y}\|_-}, & y_i = c^-, \end{cases}$$

in which $\|\mathbf{y}\|_+ = n_+$ and $\|\mathbf{y}\|_- = n_-$, standing for the number of positive elements and negative elements in vector $\mathbf{y}$ respectively. In our method, we adopt the same soft label assignment for (c^+, c^-) as in [9], i.e. $(\sqrt{\frac{n_-}{n_+}}, -\sqrt{\frac{n_+}{n_-}})$.

3.2 Algorithm

Similar to the UOCL method, solving the proposed model involves a mixed optimization of a continuous variable α and a discrete variable $\mathbf{y}$. One key observation is that if one of the two components is fixed, the optimization problem becomes easy to solve. Here we propose a procedure that alternatingly optimizes α and $\mathbf{y}$ similar to the EM framework by updating α and $\mathbf{y}$ iteratively.

First, for a given label indicator $\mathbf{y}$, computing the optimal α is equivalent to minimization of the following sub-problem:

$$\min_{\alpha} Q(\alpha) := \alpha^{\mathrm{T}} \mathbf{K} (\mathbf{\Lambda} + \gamma_1 \mathbf{L}) \mathbf{K} \alpha - 2\alpha^{\mathrm{T}} \mathbf{K} \mathbf{\Lambda} \mathbf{y} - 2\alpha^{\mathrm{T}} \mathbf{K} \tilde{\mathbf{y}}. \qquad (4)$$

Algorithm 1. SSLM

Input: The kernel and graph Laplacian matrices $\mathbf{K}$, $\mathbf{L}$, model parameters $\lambda, \gamma_1, \gamma_2, \gamma_3 > 0$, Λ and *maxiter*

Initialization

$\quad \alpha_0 = \frac{1}{\sqrt{n}}$, $m_0 = \arg\max\limits_{m} H(q(\mathbf{K}\alpha_0, m))$, $\mathbf{y}_0 = q(\mathbf{K}\alpha_0, m_0)$, $\widetilde{\mathbf{y}}_0 = h(m_0, \mathbf{y}_0)$, $t = 0$;

repeat

$\quad$ Update α_{t+1} by optimizing function (4) using conjugate gradient descent method;

$\quad$ Update m_{t+1}: $m_{t+1} = \arg\max\limits_{m} H(q(\mathbf{K}\alpha_{t+1}, m))$;

$\quad$ Update $\mathbf{y}_{t+1}$ and $\widetilde{\mathbf{y}}_{t+1}$: $\mathbf{y}_{t+1} = q(\mathbf{K}\alpha_{t+1}, m_{t+1})$, $\widetilde{\mathbf{y}}_{t+1} = h(m_{t+1}, \mathbf{y}_{t+1})$;

$\quad t = t + 1$;

until convergence or $t > maxiter$

Output: expansion coefficient $\alpha^* = \alpha_t$ and the soft label assignment $\mathbf{y}^* = \mathbf{y}_t$.

The gradient of the objective function (4) with respect to α is $\delta Q/\delta \alpha = 2\{[\mathbf{K}(\Lambda + \gamma_1 \mathbf{L})\mathbf{K}]\alpha - \mathbf{K}\Lambda\mathbf{y} - \mathbf{K}\widetilde{\mathbf{y}}\}$. By using the gradient, problem (4) can be efficiently solved by the conjugate gradient descent method.

When α is fixed, we need to deal with the $\mathbf{y}$-subproblem, that is

$$\max_{\mathbf{y}} H(\mathbf{y}) := 2\alpha^{\mathrm{T}}\mathbf{K}(\Lambda\mathbf{y} + \widetilde{\mathbf{y}}) - \mathbf{y}^{\mathrm{T}}\Lambda\mathbf{y}$$

$$s.t. \quad \mathbf{y} \in \{c^+, c^-\}^{n \times 1}, \ \widetilde{y}_i = \begin{cases} \frac{\gamma_2}{\|\mathbf{y}\|_+}, & y_i = c^+, \\ -\frac{\gamma_3}{\|\mathbf{y}\|_-}, & y_i = c^-. \end{cases} \tag{5}$$

Here a simpler case is shown to solve this discrete optimization problem. If an integer $m = \|\mathbf{y}\|_+$ is given, then $\mathbf{y}^{\mathrm{T}}\Lambda\mathbf{y}$ and the soft label assignment for labelled data remain the same regardless of the label assignment for unlabelled data. Thus this problem reduces to the same one as in UOCL, i.e., to maximize $(\mathbf{K}\alpha)^{\mathrm{T}}(\mathbf{y} + \widetilde{\mathbf{y}})$ in the unlabelled data set. It has been shown in [9] that an optimal solution satisfies $y_i > 0$ if and only if f_i is among m largest elements of $\mathbf{f}$.

One optimal solution to the Eq. (5) can be simply obtained by sorting $\mathbf{f}$ for unlabelled data in a descending order. Then $y_i > 0$ is assigned to samples before and including the m_U-th element, while $y_i < 0$ to those after the m_U-th element. Here $m_U = m - m_L$, in which m_U and m_L stand for the number of positive samples in the unlabelled and labelled data sets respectively, with m_L a fixed number. Therefore, the solution to the subproblem (5) can be expressed as $\mathbf{y}^*(\alpha) = q(\mathbf{K}\alpha, m^*(\alpha))$, in which $m^*(\alpha) = \arg\max\limits_{m} H(q(\mathbf{K}\alpha, m))$. Note that the known labels are kept unchanged when learning. For simplicity, we further define $\widetilde{\mathbf{y}}$ as a function of m and $\mathbf{y}$, i.e., $\widetilde{\mathbf{y}} = h(m, \mathbf{y})$. The summarization of this method is shown in Algorithm 1.

4 Results

Data used in the preparation of this work consisted of T1 and FLAIR MR images from 280 subjects acquired on a 3T MR scanner. The cohort included 53 subjects with subjective memory complaints (SMC), 155 subjects with probable AD, 34 subjects with fronto-temporal lobe dementia (FTD), 10 subjects with VaD, and 28 subjects with DLB. All images have been rated by an expert in terms of WMH using the Fazekas score.

Here, multichannel information (T1 and FLAIR MR images) is used to identify WMH. To do this, we first applied an automated brain segmentation tool [8] to the T1 scan to remove non-brain tissue and to extract a WM tissue probability map. All T1 and white matter tissue maps were registered to the FLAIR space. Additionally, bias correction and intensity normalization were also applied to both T1 and FLAIR images. The WMH segmentation was then performed for voxels with WM probability larger than 0.1. For each voxel of interest, a feature vector was constructed with intensities of a 3×3 neighborhood from both FLAIR and coregistered T1 images. Here we used 2D patches as FLAIR MR images commonly have slices with low resolution in the through-plane direction.

We have evaluated the performance of the proposed method against the lesion growth algorithm (LGA) [10] and lesion predict algorithm (LPA) as implemented in Lesion Segmentation Toolbox (LST), which is a widely used tool for WM lesion segmentation. LPA is a supervised method which was trained by a logistic regression model with the data of 53 MS patients, and the pre-chosen threshold τ in LGA was set to 0.3 as suggested by [10]. Preliminary experiments showed that UOCL method failed on images with fewer lesions and thus its results were omitted. For the proposed method, labelled data was automatically and conservatively determined based on the distribution of the WM intensities on each subject, which took up a proportion of around 25 %. Note that the number of labelled voxels from normal tissues is much more than that of labelled WMH. Gaussian kernel $\kappa(\mathbf{x}, \mathbf{x}') = \exp(- \|\mathbf{x} - \mathbf{x}'\|^2 /2\sigma^2)$ was used in the classification function in which $\sigma^2 = \sum_{i,j=1}^{n} \|\mathbf{x}_i - \mathbf{x}_j\|^2 /n^2$, and the model parameters $\lambda, \gamma_1, \gamma_2$ and γ_3 were determined empirically based on a subset of the data. A comparison of the WMH segmentation visualization results is shown in Fig. 1.

For a more quantitative assessment of the performance of our method, we have computed the correlation between the segmented WMH volumes and their Fazekas scores. The results are shown in Table 1. Here $Corr$ denotes the correlation coefficient between the Fazekas score and the percentage of WMH volume relative to the WM volume, and $Corr_{(1,2,3)}$ is the same measure but excluding subjects with Fazekas score of 0. From Table 1, it can be seen that our approach achieved higher correlation score than LGA and LPA on both $Corr$ and $Corr_{(1,2,3)}$, which indicates that the segmentation results of the proposed model are more consistent with the the standard clinical measurement. Furthermore, the proposed method can better discriminate WMH voxels from non-WMH voxels on subjects with relatively higher volume of lesions and thus can give a higher correlation value when excluding subjects with lower Fazekas scores. This can be further explained by Fig. 2, which shows the distribution of the segmentation results with Fazekas scores. It can also be seen that the proposed method is able to better classify subjects according to Fazekas score. Overall, from both the visualization results and the correlation score, it can be concluded that the proposed method outperforms both LGA and LPA and has promising results.

FLAIR   LGA   LPA   SSLM

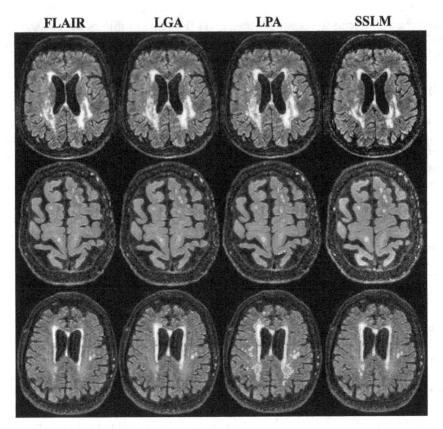

Fig. 1. Example WMH segmentation results compared with LGA and LPA on three different subjects with Fazekas score 1, 2 and 3 (from bottom to top) respectively.

Table 1. Correlation between WMH segmentation results and Fazekas scores

Method	*Corr*	$Corr_{(1,2,3)}$
LGA	0.5902	0.6532
LPA	0.6977	0.7661
SSLM	**0.7540**	**0.8333**

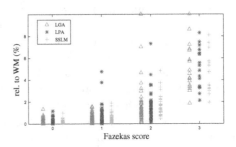

Fig. 2. Results of (WMH volume/WM volume) corresponding to Fazekas scores.

5   Conclusion

In this work, we proposed a novel semi-supervised large margin algorithm. The proposed model can better discover suspicious outliers under the supervision of a limited amount of available labelled data. We have shown that the framework jointly learns a large margin classifier and a label assignment, which can be solved effectively by an iterative algorithm. Experiments for WMH segmentation were implemented on a database of 280 MR images from subjects with SMC or NDs. Encouraging experimental results were obtained on the qualitative visualization results and the quantitative correlation scores, showing the effectiveness and competitiveness of the proposed model against other methods.

References

1. Anbeek, P., Vincken, K.L., van Osch, M.J., Bisschops, R.H., van der Grond, J.: Probabilistic segmentation of white matter lesions in MR imaging. NeuroImage **21**(3), 1037–1044 (2004)
2. Caligiuri, M.E., Perrotta, P., Augimeri, A., Rocca, F., Quattrone, A., Cherubini, A.: Automatic detection of white matter hyperintensities in healthy aging and pathology using magnetic resonance imaging: a review. Neuroinformatics **13**(3), 261–276 (2015)
3. Fazekas, F., Chawluk, J.B., Alavi, A., Hurtig, H.I., Zimmerman, R.A.: MR signal abnormalities at 1.5 T in Alzheimer's dementia and normal aging. Am. J. Neuroradiol. **8**(3), 421–426 (1987)
4. Gibson, E., Gao, F., Black, S.E., Lobaugh, N.J.: Automatic segmentation of white matter hyperintensities in the elderly using FLAIR images at 3T. J. Magn. Reson. Imaging **31**(6), 1311–1322 (2010)
5. Ithapu, V., Singh, V., Lindner, C., Austin, B.P., Hinrichs, C., Carlsson, C.M., Bendlin, B.B., Johnson, S.C.: Extracting and summarizing white matter hyperintensities using supervised segmentation methods in Alzheimer's disease risk and aging studies. Hum. Brain Mapp. **35**(8), 4219–4235 (2014)
6. Kikinis, R., Guttmann, C.R., Metcalf, D., Wells, W.M., Ettinger, G.J., Weiner, H.L., Jolesz, F.A.: Quantitative follow-up of patients with multiple sclerosis using MRI: technical aspects. J. Magn. Reson. Imaging **9**(4), 519–530 (1999)
7. Lao, Z., Shen, D., Liu, D., Jawad, A.F., Melhem, E.R., Launer, L.J., Bryan, R.N., Davatzikos, C.: Computer-assisted segmentation of white matter lesions in 3D MR images using support vector machine. Acad. Radiol. **15**(3), 300–313 (2008)
8. Ledig, C., Heckemann, R.A., Hammers, A., Lopez, J.C., Newcombe, V.F., Makropoulos, A., Lötjönen, J., Menon, D.K., Rueckert, D.: Robust whole-brain segmentation: application to traumatic brain injury. Med. Image Anal. **21**(1), 40–58 (2015)
9. Liu, W., Hua, G., Smith, J.: Unsupervised one-class learning for automatic outlier removal. In: Proceedings of IEEE Conference on Computer Vision and Pattern Recognition, pp. 3826–3833 (2014)
10. Schmidt, P., Gaser, C., Arsic, M., Buck, D., Förschler, A., Berthele, A., Hoshi, M., Ilg, R., Schmid, V.J., Zimmer, C., et al.: An automated tool for detection of FLAIR-hyperintense white-matter lesions in multiple sclerosis. Neuroimage **59**(4), 3774–3783 (2012)
11. Van Leemput, K., Maes, F., Vandermeulen, D., Colchester, A., Suetens, P.: Automated segmentation of multiple sclerosis lesions by model outlier detection. IEEE Trans. Med. Imaging **20**(8), 677–688 (2001)

12. Wardlaw, J.M., Smith, E.E., Biessels, G.J., Cordonnier, C., Fazekas, F., Frayne, R., Lindley, R.I., T O'Brien, J., Barkhof, F., Benavente, O.R., et al.: Neuroimaging standards for research into small vessel disease and its contribution to aging and neurodegeneration. Lancet Neurol. **12**(8), 822–838 (2013)
13. Wu, M., Ye, J.: A small sphere and large margin approach for novelty detection using training data with outliers. IEEE Trans. Pattern Anal. Mach. Intell. **31**(11), 2088–2092 (2009)
14. Yang, F., Shan, Z.Y., Kruggel, F.: White matter lesion segmentation based on feature joint occurrence probability and $\chi2$ random field theory from magnetic resonance (MR) images. Pattern Recogn. Lett. **31**(9), 781–790 (2010)

Deep Ensemble Sparse Regression Network for Alzheimer's Disease Diagnosis

Heung-Il Suk[1]($\boxtimes$) and Dinggang Shen[1,2]

[1] Department of Brain and Cognitive Engineering, Korea University,
Seoul, Republic of Korea
hisuk@korea.ac.kr
[2] Biomedical Research Imaging Center,
University of North Carolina at Chapel Hill, Chapel Hill, USA

Abstract. For neuroimaging-based brain disease diagnosis, sparse regression models have proved their effectiveness in handling high-dimensional data but with a small number of samples. In this paper, we propose a novel framework that utilizes sparse regression models as *target-level representation* learner and builds a deep convolutional neural network for clinical decision making. Specifically, we first train multiple sparse regression models, each of which has different values of a regularization control parameter, and use the outputs of the trained regression models as target-level representations. Note that sparse regression models trained with different values of a regularization control parameter potentially select different sets of features from the original ones, thereby they have different powers to predict the response values, *i.e.*, a clinical label and clinical scores in our work. We then construct a deep convolutional neural network by taking the target-level representations as input. Our deep network learns to optimally fuse the predicted response variables, *i.e.*, target-level representations, from the same sparse response model(s) and also those from the neighboring sparse response models. To our best knowledge, this is the first work that systematically integrates sparse regression models with deep neural network. In our experiments with ADNI cohort, we validated the effectiveness of the proposed method by achieving the highest classification accuracies in three different tasks of Alzheimer's disease and mild cognitive impairment identification.

1   Introduction

One of the main challenges in neuroimaging analysis is the high dimensionality of data in nature but a small number of samples are available. While various methods have been proposed for dimensionality reduction in the literature, due to interpretational requirement in the clinic, it is limited for the applicable methods. In the meantime, the *principle of parsimony* in many areas of science, *i.e.*, the simplest explanation of a given observation should be preferred over more complicated ones, can be associated with the theory of Occam's razor. Motivated this, sparsity-inducing regularization has been considered as one of the key techniques in machine learning and statistics. In light of these, sparse regression

© Springer International Publishing AG 2016
L. Wang et al. (Eds.): MLMI 2016, LNCS 10019, pp. 113–121, 2016.
DOI: 10.1007/978-3-319-47157-0_14

methods with different forms of regularization terms [10,11,13,15] have been proposed and demonstrated their validity for brain disease diagnosis by means of feature selection.

One prevalent step of the sparsity-inducing regularization methods is to find the optimal value of a regularization control parameter, mostly via cross-validation with a grid search strategy. It is, however, possible that for different validation sets, it can be different for the optimal value of a regularization control parameter. Furthermore, many of the previous work in the literature mostly used the sparse regression method for feature selection and then separately trained a classifier. In this work, we propose a novel method that combines sparse regression models with a deep Convolutional Neural Network (CNN) in a unified framework for Alzheimer's Disease (AD) diagnosis. Specifically, instead of selecting a single regularization control parameter, we consider multiple sparse regression models, each of which is learned with a different value of the regularization control parameter. By taking outputs of the sparse regression learners, *e.g.*, a clinical label and clinical scores in our work, as *target-level representations*, we design a deep CNN that systematically integrates the outputs of multiple learners to optimally identify the clinical label of a testing sample. Thus, our deep model can be regarded as deep network that discovers the optimal weights to ensemble multiple sparse regression models, which thus we call 'deep ensemble sparse regression network'.

The main contributions of our work can be two-fold: (1) The different values of the regularization control parameter are used to select different sets of features with different weight coefficients. Hence, different regression models can predict both a clinical status and clinical scores in different feature spaces. Also, the use of target-level representations from multiple sparse regression models has the effect of reducing dimensionality of an observation. (2) Our CNN built on the outputs of the sparse regression models finds the optimal way of combining the regression models in a non-linear manner.

2   Materials and Image Processing

We analyzed a baseline MRI dataset of 805 subjects, including 186 AD, 393 Mild Cognitive Impairments (MCI), and 226 Normal Controls (NC), from the ADNI database. For the MCI subjects, they were clinically further subdivided into 167 progressive MCI (pMCI), who progressed to AD in 18 months, and 226 stable MCI (sMCI), who did not progress to AD in 18 months. Each subject had both Mini-Mental State Examination (MMSE) and Alzheimer's Disease Assessment Scale - Cognition (ADAS-Cog) scores recorded.

We used MIPAV software for anterior commissure - posterior commissure correction, resampled images to $256 \times 256 \times 256$, and applied N3 algorithm [8] to correct intensity inhomogeneity. A skull stripping was performed, followed by cerebellum removal. Then, FAST in FSL package was used for structural MRI image segmentation into three tissue types of Gray Matter (GM), White Matter (WM) and CerebroSpinal Fluid (CSF). We finally parcellated them into 93

Regions Of Interest (ROIs) by warping Kabani *et al.*'s atlas [4] to each subject's space via non-linear registration. Next, we generated the regional volumetric maps, called RAVENS maps, using a tissue preserving image warping method [2]. In this work, we considered only the spatially normalized GM densities, due to its relatively high relevance to AD compared to WM and CSF. For each of the 93 ROIs, we computed the GM tissue volume as feature, *i.e.*, finally 93-dimensional features from an MRI image.

3 Deep Ensemble Sparse Regression Network

3.1 Sparse Linear/Logistic Regression

Assume that we are given a training set $\mathcal{T} = \{\mathbf{X}, \mathbf{T}\}$ with N samples, where $\mathbf{X} \in \mathbb{R}^{D \times N}$ and $\mathbf{T} \in \mathbb{R}^{L \times N}$ denote, respectively, D-dimensional neuroimaging features and the corresponding L-dimensional target values, *i.e.*, clinical label[1] and clinical scores of MMSE and ADAS-Cog in our work. We hypothesize that the target values (*i.e.*, response variables) can be represented by means of a linear combination of the features (*i.e.*, predictors). Under this hypothesis, sparse regression models can be formulated in the form of an optimization problem as follows:

$$\min_{\theta} \mathcal{L}(\mathcal{T}; \theta) + \lambda \Omega(\theta) \qquad (1)$$

where $\mathcal{L}(\mathcal{T}; \theta)$ denotes a loss function, $\Omega(\theta)$ denotes a regularization term over a parameter set θ, and λ is a regularization control parameter, which we regard a hyperparameter throughout the paper.

In terms of sparsity, the regularization term $\Omega(\theta)$ plays the important role of selecting informative features for target tasks, *i.e.*, prediction of clinical label and clinical scores, and also different forms of the regularization term produce different sets of selected features. Motivated by the fact that clinical label and clinical scores are inherently inter-related, it is reasonable to learn the multiple tasks jointly rather than learning each task separately. Among different forms of regularization in the literature, in this paper, we consider an $\ell_{2,1}$-norm regularizer $\|\theta\|_{2,1}$ that induces sparsity in a group-wise manner by following [12,14].

Conventionally, the hyperparameter λ is chosen by means of a cross-validation technique. However, an optimal value of the hyperparameter can be different for different validation sets. In this regard, rather than finding a single optimal value of the hyperparameter, we propose to learn a set of sparse regression models with different values in a predefined space Λ. Since no optimization step is involved in with respect to the hyperparameter, we regard each of the sparse regression models trained with different values of the hyperparameter as a *weak* learner that predicts the response variables, *e.g.*, clinical label and clinical scores. We then build an ensemble classifier that combines the outputs of multiple sparse regression models for clinical status identification. It is noteworthy that different weak learners potentially select different sets of features with their

---

[1] We use a class indicator vector with zero-one encoding.

respective weights. Thus, even though any sparse regression model fails to correctly predict the target response values, there still exists a chance to circumvent such limitation by fusing outputs from other sparse regression models.

For a certain value of the hyperparameter $\lambda_m \equiv \Lambda(m)$, $m = 1, \ldots, M$, where $\Lambda(m)$ denotes the m-th value in a predefine space Λ with M different values, we can then estimate the response values $\hat{\mathbf{t}}_i^{(m)}$ for a feature vector $\mathbf{x}_i$ of the i-th sample in a training set $\mathcal{T}$. A matrix obtained by concatenating the predicted response values $\hat{\mathbf{T}}_i = \left[\hat{\mathbf{t}}_i^{(m)}\right]_{m=1}^{M}$ from M sparse regression models becomes the *high-level* features of the original neuroimaging features and it is fed into our deep network, which will be detailed below.

3.2 Deep Convolutional Neural Network for Classification

Deep architecture models has recently been showing state-of-the-art performance in various fields of computer vision, speech recognition, natural language processing, as well as neuroimaging analysis. Among different network architectures, a Convolutional Neural Network (CNN) is of main stream thanks to its modeling characteristics that help discover local structural relations in an observation and share weight connections, thereby it greatly reduces the number of parameters.

In this work, we propose to utilize a deep CNN for clinical label identification by taking the predicted response values from multiple sparse regression models as input. Note that different values of the hyperparameter λ guide to select different feature sets in regression models learning. Therefore, different sparse regression models produce different target-level representations, predicted from different feature subsets of the original features. Even though different values of λ induce to select different feature sets and thus different sparse regression models produce different target-level representations, it is still likely that sparse regression models trained with slightly different hyperparamter values tend to have similar weight coefficients and select similar feature subsets, thus outputting similar response values. In the meantime, since the target-level representations are basically related to the clinical label and clinical scores jointly predicted from the neuroimaging features, it is obvious that they are highly correlated to each other. In these regards, we couple the target-level representations in the same row and neighboring rows together via kernels in CNN.

Figure 1 illustrates our deep convolutional neural network that takes target-level representations from multiple sparse regression models as input and discovers non-linear relations among them in a hierarchical manner for brain disease diagnosis. From a machine learning standpoint, our deep CNN is an ensemble classifier that systematically finds the relations of different weak learners, *i.e.*, sparse regression models. Thus, we call this network as '*deep Ensemble Sparse Regression Network*' (DeepESRNet) as we already mentioned before.

In our DeepESRNet, we have three types of layers, namely, convolution layer, pooling layer, and fully connected layer. At a convolution layer, the previous layer's feature maps are convolved with learnable kernels and go through a non-linear activation function to form output feature maps as follows:

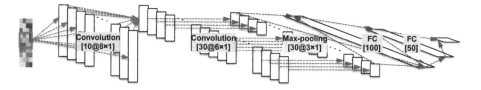

Fig. 1. The proposed convolutional neural network of modelling deep ensemble sparse regressions for brain disorder diagnosis. (FC: Fully Connected)

$$\mathbf{v}_j^\ell = f\left(\sum_{i\in F^{\ell-1}} \mathbf{v}_i^{\ell-1} * \mathbf{k}_{ij}^\ell + b_j^\ell\right) \tag{2}$$

where $*$ is a convolution operator, the superscript ℓ denotes the index of a layer, $\mathbf{v}_j$ is the j-the feature map[2], $F^{\ell-1}$ is the number of feature maps in the $(\ell-1)$-th layer, $\mathbf{k}_{ij}^\ell$ is a learnable kernel between the i-th feature map in the $(\ell-1)$-th layer and the j-th feature map in the current ℓ-th layer, b_j^ℓ denotes a bias, and $f(\cdot)$ is an activation function. As for the activation function, while the logistic sigmoid function or hyperbolic tangent function has been commonly used, in this work, thanks to its great success in recent applications, we use a Rectified Linear Unit (ReLU) [6] defined as $f(a) = \max(0,a)$. The pooling layer is interspersed with the convolution layer for drawing a consensus with a maximal value among neighboring sparse regression models and for reducing the resolution of feature maps. In our DeepESRNet, we design a max-pooling layer that partitions an input feature map into a set of non-overlapping regions and then outputs the maximum value for each region. Lastly, the fully connected layer is the same as the conventional neural network such that the inter-layer units are fully connected but with no units within the same layer connected. With this fully connected layer, we finally integrate all the information from the outputs from multiple sparse regression models, *i.e.*, predicted clinical labels and clinical scores, for decision making at the output layer.

Figure 1 shows an example of applying our DeepESRNet to a target-level representation map obtained from $M = 10$ sparse regression models. Given a target-level representation map $\mathbf{v}_1^0 = \hat{\mathbf{T}}_i \in \mathbb{R}^{10\times4}$, the first convolution layer with 10 feature maps couples the feature values in the same row and neighboring rows in $\mathbf{v}_1^0$ together with a kernel $\mathbf{k}_{1j}^1$ of 3×4 in size according to Eq. (2), resulting in $\{\mathbf{v}_j^1 \in \mathbb{R}^{8\times1}\}_{j=1}^{10}$. A second convolution layer with 30 feature maps follows to find associations among the values within the same feature maps and across different feature maps simultaneously, producing $\{\mathbf{v}_j^2 \in \mathbb{R}^{6\times1}\}_{j=1}^{30}$. We then apply a max-pooling to each feature map of the second layer, which downsamples the feature maps into $\{\mathbf{v}_j^3 \in \mathbb{R}^{3\times1}\}_{j=1}^{30}$. Beyond the max-pooling

---

[2] A target-level representation map from multiple sparse regression models becomes $\mathbf{v}_1^0$.

layer, the network corresponds to a conventional multi-layer neural network with two hidden layers (100 units and 50 units, respectively) and one output layer by taking vectorized values of the 30 feature maps in the max-pooling layer as input. For the output layer, we use a softmax function for classification. In our DeepESRNet, we have trainable network parameters, *i.e.*, kernels $\mathbf{k}_{ij}^{\ell}$ and biases b_j^{ℓ} in convolutional layers and also connection weights and biases in the top three multi-layer neural network. To train our DeepESRNet, we used a backpropagation algorithm [7] with a mini-batch gradient descent method [1].

4   Experimental Settings and Results

4.1   Experimental Settings

With regard to the structure of deep neural networks, *i.e.*, the number of layers and the number of feature maps per layer, there is no golden rule or general guideline for those. In this work, we empirically designed our DeepESRNet with two convolutional layers followed by one max-pooling layer, two fully connected layers, and one output layer as shown in Fig. 1. The kernels for two convolution layers were 3×4 and 3×1 in size, respectively. In the max-pooling layer, a kernel of 2×1 in size was used. For two fully connected layers, we set 100 hidden units and 50 hidden units sequentially. During parameter learning, we applied a batch normalization [3], which helped reducing training time greatly, to all layers except for the max-pooling and output layers. No dropout [9] was involved based on Ioffe *et al.*'s work [3], where they empirically presented that dropout could be removed in a batch-normalized network. The network parameters were trained via a gradient descent method with a mini-batch size of 50, a learning rate of 0.001, a weight decay of 0.005, and a momentum factor of 0.9. We used a MatConvNet toolbox[3] to train our DeepESRNet.

For the sparse regression models, we considered (1) Multi-Output Linear Regression with $\ell_{2,1}$-norm regularization (MOLR) and (2) Joint Linear and Logistic Regression with $\ell_{2,1}$-norm regularization (JLLR) [12]. We defined the hyperparameter space as $\Lambda = \{0.01, 0.042, 0.074, 0.107, 0.139, 0.171, 0.203, 0.236, 0.268, 0.3\}$ equally spaced between 0.01 and 0.3[4] with $M = 10$ empirically determined. By taking the outputs of 10 regression models for each of MOLR and JLLR, we trained MOLR+DeepESRNet and JLLR+DeepESRNet, separately. As the competing methods, we also considered two variant models, namely, MOLR+SVM and JLLR+SVM, which used MOLR and JLLR for feature selection and a linear Support Vector Machine (SVM) as a classifier. The model of MOLR+SVM was earlier proposed by Zhang *et al.* [14] for AD/MCI diagnosis.

---

[3] Available at 'http://www.vlfeat.org/matconvnet/'.

[4] For sparse model training, we used a SLEP toolbox, where it is required for the control parameter to be set between 0 and 1 because its value is internally rescaled [5].

Table 1. Performance comparison with $\ell_{2,1}$-penalized Multi-output Linear Regression (MOLR) as a base sparse regression model.

	Tasks	Accuracy (%)	Sensitivity (%)	Specificity (%)	AUC
MOLR	AD vs. NC	84.93 ± 6.30	83.87	87.05	0.92
	MCI vs. NC	64.66 ± 8.16	**79.40**	51.67	0.72
	pMCI vs. sMCI	63.35 ± 7.88	56.10	71.44	0.68
MOLR+SVM [14]	AD vs. NC	86.87 ± 4.80	88.42	86.35	0.92
	MCI vs. NC	66.62 ± 7.35	72.80	55.26	0.72
	pMCI vs. sMCI	66.66 ± 6.58	62.06	70.02	0.71
MOLR+DeepESRNet	AD vs. NC	**90.28 ± 5.26**	92.65	**89.05**	**0.93**
	MCI vs. NC	**74.20 ± 6.16**	78.74	**66.30**	**0.77**
	pMCI vs. sMCI	**73.28 ± 6.35**	70.61	**75.29**	**0.72**

The boldface denotes the maximal performance in each metric and each task.

4.2 Performance Comparison

In our work, we considered three binary classification tasks of AD vs. NC, MCI vs. NC, and pMCI vs. sMCI. We used GM tissue volumes of 93 ROIs as features $\mathbf{x}_i \in \mathbb{R}^{93}$ and a clinical label and two clinical scores of MMSE and ADAS-Cog as response values $\mathbf{t}_i \in \mathbb{R}^4$. For performance evaluation, we employed a 10-fold cross-validation technique, where the same set of samples per fold was used over all the methods for fair comparison. We considered four metrics for evaluation, namely, accuracy, sensitivity, specificity, and Area Under the receiver operating characteristics Curve (AUC).

The performance of the competing methods as well as our method is presented in Tables 1 and 2, where different sparse regression models, *i.e.*, MOLR and JLLR, were used as base models. First, for the scenario of using MOLR as a base model in Table 1, MOLR achieved the mean accuracies of 84.93 % (AD vs. NC), 64.66 % (MCI vs. NC), and 63.35 % (pMCI vs. sMCI). Compared to these results, MOLR+SVM made improvements by 1.94 % (AD vs. NC), 1.96 % (MCI vs. NC), and 3.31 % (pMCI vs. sMCI) and our MOLR+DeepESRNet enhanced by 5.35 % (AD vs. NC), 9.54 % (MCI vs. NC), and 9.93 % (pMCI vs. sMCI). Noticeably, the proposed method made the highest improvement for the most challenging task of pMCI vs. sMCI, outperforming the two competing methods, *i.e.*, MOLR and MOLR+SVM. Second, for the scenario of using JLLR as a base model in Table 2, the proposed JLLR+DeepESRNet achieved the mean accuracies of 91.02 % (AD vs. NC), 73.02 % (MCI vs. NC), and 74.82 % (pMCI vs. sMCI). Compared to the two competing methods (JLLR/JLLR+SVM), our method improved the accuracies by 6.33 %/4.63 % (AD vs. NC), 4.47 %/6.24 % (MCI vs. NC), and 7.14 %/8.43 % (pMCI vs. sMCI). In terms of the AUC metric, a measure of the overall performance for diagnostic test, the proposed method obtained the highest values over all tasks. In comparison between MOLR+DeepESRNet and JLLR+DeepESTNet, although there is no significant difference, JLLR+DeepESTNet showed slightly higher performance in both accuracy and AUC.

Table 2. Performance comparison with $\ell_{2,1}$-penalized Joint Logistic and Linear Regression (JLLR) as a base sparse regression model.

	Tasks	Accuracy (%)	Sensitivity (%)	Specificity (%)	AUC
JLLR [12]	AD vs. NC	84.69 ± 4.03	84.95	84.95	0.92
	MCI vs. NC	68.55 ± 7.10	73.24	59.42	0.73
	pMCI vs. sMCI	67.68 ± 6.31	64.13	70.24	0.73
JLLR+SVM	AD vs. NC	86.39 ± 5.54	87.62	86.18	0.92
	MCI vs. NC	66.78 ± 7.36	72.87	55.69	0.72
	pMCI vs. sMCI	66.39 ± 6.56	61.94	69.39	0.71
JLLR+DeepESRNet	AD vs. NC	$\mathbf{91.02 \pm 4.29}$	**92.72**	**89.94**	**0.93**
	MCI vs. NC	$\mathbf{73.02 \pm 6.44}$	**77.60**	**68.22**	**0.74**
	pMCI vs. sMCI	$\mathbf{74.82 \pm 6.80}$	**70.93**	**78.82**	**0.75**

The boldface denotes the maximal performance in each metric and each task.

5   Conclusion

In this paper, we proposed a novel method that systematically combines two conceptually different models of sparse regression and convolutional neural network. With an MRI dataset of 805 subjects from the ADNI cohort, we validated the effectiveness of our method by comparing with two types of competing methods in the literature.

Acknowledgement. This research was supported by Basic Science Research Program through the National Research Foundation of Korea (NRF) funded by the Ministry of Education (NRF-2015R1C1A1A01052216) and also partially supported by Institute for Information & communications Technology Promotion (IITP) grant funded by the Korea government (MSIP) (No. B0101-15-0307, Basic Software Research in Human-level Lifelong Machine Learning (Machine Learning Center)).

References

1. Cotter, A., Shamir, O., Srebro, N., Sridharan, K.: Better mini-batch algorithms via accelerated gradient methods. In: Advances in Neural Information Processing Systems, vol. 24, pp. 1647–1655 (2011)
2. Davatzikos, C., Genc, A., Xu, D., Resnick, S.M.: Voxel-based morphometry using the RAVENS maps: methods and validation using simulated longitudinal atrophy. NeuroImage **14**(6), 1361–1369 (2001)
3. Ioffe, S., Szegedy, C.: Batch normalization: accelerating deep network training by reducing internal covariate shift. In: Proceedings of the 32nd International Conference on Machine Learning, pp. 448–456 (2015)
4. Kabani, N., MacDonald, D., Holmes, C., Evans, A.: A 3D atlas of the human brain. NeuroImage **7**(4), S717 (1998)
5. Liu, J., Ji, S., Ye, J.: SLEP: Sparse Learning with Efficient Projections. Arizona State University (2009)

6. Nair, V., Hinton, G.E.: Rectified linear units improve restricted Boltzmann machines. In: Proceedings of the 27th International Conference on Machine Learning, pp. 807–814 (2010)
7. Rumelhart, D.E., Hinton, G.E., Williams, R.J.: Learning representations by back-propagating errors. Nature **323**(6088), 533–536 (1986)
8. Sled, J.G., Zijdenbos, A.P., Evans, A.C.: A nonparametric method for automatic correction of intensity nonuniformity in MRI data. IEEE Trans. Med. Imaging **17**(1), 87–97 (1998)
9. Srivastava, N., Hinton, G., Krizhevsky, A., Sutskever, I., Salakhutdinov, R.: Dropout: a simple way to prevent neural networks from overfitting. J. Mach. Learn. Res. **15**, 1929–1958 (2014)
10. Suk, H.I., Lee, S.W., Shen, D.: Deep sparse multi-task learning for feature selection in Alzheimer's disease diagnosis. Brain Struct. Funct. **221**(5), 2569–2587 (2016)
11. Suk, H.I., Shen, D.: Subclass-based multi-task learning for Alzheimer's disease diagnosis. Front. Aging Neurosci. **6**, 168 (2014)
12. Wang, H., Nie, F., Huang, H., Risacher, S., Saykin, A.J., Shen, L.: Identifying AD-sensitive and cognition-relevant imaging biomarkers via joint classification and regression. In: Fichtinger, G., Martel, A., Peters, T. (eds.) MICCAI 2011. LNCS, vol. 6893, pp. 115–123. Springer, Heidelberg (2011). doi:10.1007/978-3-642-23626-6_15
13. Yuan, L., Wang, Y., Thompson, P.M., Narayan, V.A., Ye, J.: Multi-source feature learning for joint analysis of incomplete multiple heterogeneous neuroimaging data. NeuroImage **61**(3), 622–632 (2012)
14. Zhang, D., Shen, D.: Multi-modal multi-task learning for joint prediction of multiple regression and classification variables in Alzheimer's disease. NeuroImage **59**(2), 895–907 (2012)
15. Zhou, J., Liu, J., Narayan, V.A., Ye, J.: Modeling disease progression via fused sparse group lasso. In: Proceedings of the 18th ACM SIGKDD International Conference on Knowledge Discovery and Data Mining, pp. 1095–1103 (2012)

Learning Representation for Histopathological Image with Quaternion Grassmann Average Network

Jinjie Wu[1], Jun Shi[1(✉)], Shihui Ying[2], Qi Zhang[1], and Yan Li[3]

[1] School of Communication and Information Engineering,
Shanghai University, Shanghai, China
junshi@staff.shu.edu.cn
[2] Department of Mathematics, School of Science,
Shanghai University, Shanghai, China
[3] College of Computer Science and Software Engineering,
Shenzhen University, Shenzhen, China

Abstract. Feature representation is a key step for the classification of histopathological images. The principal component analysis network (PCANet) offers a new unsupervised feature learning algorithm for images via a simple deep network architecture. However, PCA is sensitive to noise and outliers, which may depress the representation learning of PCANet. Grassmann averages (GA) is a newly proposed dimensionality reduction algorithm, which is more robust and effective than PCA. Therefore, in this paper, we propose a GA network (GANet) algorithm to improve the robustness of learned features from images. Moreover, since quaternion algebra provides a mathematically elegant tool to well handle color images, a quaternion representation based GANet (QGANet) is developed to fuse color information and learn a superior representation for color histopathological images. The experimental results on two histopathological image datasets show that GANet outperforms PCANet, while QGANet achieves the best performance for the classification of color histopathological images.

1 Introduction

In recent years, the histopathological image based computer-aided quantitative analysis or diagnosis for cancers has attracted considerable attention, among which, feature representation becomes the critical or even decisive factor. Due to the excellent performance of deep learning (DL) for representation learning, various DL algorithms have been successfully applied to histopathological images.

Recently, a new unsupervised DL algorithm, named principal component analysis network (PCANet), is proposed for representation learning of images [1]. Compared with the commonly used DL algorithms, such as stacked autoencoder (SAE), deep belief networks (DBN) and convolutional neural networks (CNN), PCANet not only has excellent ability to learning feature representation, but also has very simple network

L. Wang et al. (Eds.): MLMI 2016, LNCS 10019, pp. 122–129, 2016.
DOI: 10.1007/978-3-319-47157-0_15

architecture and parameters [1]. However, PCA is extremely sensitive to noise and outliers [2], which may decrease its robustness, and finally affect the performance of PCANet.

Grassmann averages (GA) is a new data transform algorithm, which formulates dimension reduction as the estimation of the average subspace of those spanned by the data on Grassmann manifold [3]. GA coincides with the standard PCA for Gaussian data, but it is inherently more robust than PCA [3]. It has been proved that GA works well on different tasks in computer vision, such as video restoration, background modeling and shadow removal, compared with PCA and its variants [3]. Since the noise and outliers are unavoidable in medical images, effective and robust dimension reduction methods are essential, especially for large-scale data such as medical images. Therefore, GA has the potential to be applied to medical images. Moreover, it is also feasible to develop a GA network (GANet) algorithm.

On the other hand, the color information of histopathological images is very helpful for diagnosis, and hence color descriptors are widely used for histopathological images [4]. However, GA algorithm cannot well handle color information, and color images should be converted to grayscale images. As a result, plenty of useful color information is discarded, leading to reduced performance. Although GANet can be performed on each individual color channel of histopathological images and then concatenate multi-channel features, this way ignores the inherent correlation among different color channels of images [4]. Therefore, it is crucial to integrate color information into GA algorithm so as to learn the representation of color histopathological images.

The recent resurgence of quaternion algebra shows that it is a mathematically elegant tool to handle color images. A quaternion consists of one real and three imaginary parts. The imaginary parts are usually utilized to encode three components of a color image and process them as a vector. The quaternion PCA (QPCA) has been proposed for color images and achieved superior performance [5]. Therefore, it is also feasible to integrate quaternion algebra with GA algorithm to develop the quaternion GA (QGA) algorithm, due to the similarity between PCA and GA [3].

In this work, the QGA is proposed to fuse color information, and then the QGA network (QGANet) is developed for feature representation learning of color histopathological images. The main contributions of this work are twofold: (1) the GANet algorithm is proposed and then applied to learning more effective representative features for histopathological images, relying on the robustness and effectiveness of GA for large-scale data; (2) the QGANet is further developed based on our QGA algorithm to well fuse color information from color histopathological images and then learn more effective feature representation.

2 Quaternion Grassmann Average Network

As shown in Fig. 1, the proposed QGANet model consists of four components, namely, quaternion representation, cascaded QGA, binary hashing and block-wise histograms. In this work, a two-layer cascaded QGA network is constructed as an example. Notably, GANet has a similar architecture to QGANet.

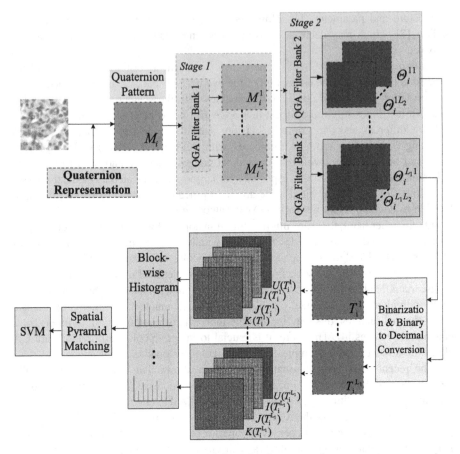

Fig. 1. Schematic diagram of QGANet with four simplest processing components: quaternion representation, cascaded QGA filters, binary hashing and block-wise histogram

2.1 Quaternion Grassmann Average Algorithm

A color image M can be represented in quaternion domain $\mathbf{Q}$ by

$$M = U(M) + I(M)i + J(M)j + K(M)k \tag{1}$$

where $U(M) = 0$, and $I(M), J(M)$ and $K(M)$ are the red, green and blue channels, respectively.

According to the quaternion algebra, three imaginary units i, j and k obey the following rules:

$$i^2 = j^2 = k^2 = ijk = -1, ij = -ji = k, jk = -kj = i, ki = -ik = j \tag{2}$$

The proposed QGA now extends the original GA algorithm from the field of real numbers $\mathbf{R}^D$ to the field of quaternion numbers $\mathbf{Q}^{\bar{D}}$. For a zero-mean dataset $\{x_n\}_{n=1}^N$, the Grassmann manifold $Gr(d, \bar{D})$ is the space of all d-dimensional linear subspaces of $\mathbf{Q}^{\bar{D}}$. Each sample spans a 1-dimensional subspace of $\mathbf{Q}^{\bar{D}}$, which hence is a point in $Gr(1, \bar{D})$. This 1-dimensional subspace can be represented by a unit vector u or its antipode $-u$. Therefore, $Gr(1, \bar{D})$ can be written as the quotient $S^{\bar{D}-1}/\{\pm 1\}$ of the unit sphere with respect to the antipodal action of the group $\{\pm 1\}$. Then, given an observation x_n, we select the representation element of the spanned subspace by

$$[u_n] = U(u_n) + I(u_n)i + J(u_n)j + K(u_n)k := x_n/\|x_n\| \tag{3}$$

The average subspace is now defined corresponding to the first principle component (PC). The weighted averages is defined as the minimizer of the weighted sum-of-squared distances by

$$[u]^* = arg\, min_{[v] \in Gr(1,\bar{D})} \sum_{n=1}^N w_n dist^2_{Gr(1,\bar{D})}([u_n], [v]) \tag{4}$$

where $v = U(v) + I(v)i + J(v)j + K(v)k$, w_n is the weight and $dist_{Gr(1,\bar{D})}$ is a geodesic distance on $Gr(1, \bar{D})$.

Under the distance of Eq. (4), the weighted average of data $u_{1:N} \subset S^{\bar{D}-1}$ is given in closed-form by

$$[u]^* = \frac{\left(\sum_{n=1}^N \omega_n\right)^{-1} \sum_{n=1}^N \omega_n u_n}{\left\|\left(\sum_{n=1}^N \omega_n\right)^{-1} \sum_{n=1}^N \omega_n u_n\right\|} \tag{5}$$

where weight $\omega_n = \|x_n\|$ for normalization.

An average subspace then can be calculated with an iterative scheme by

$$\omega_{n,t} \leftarrow sign\left(u_n^T [u]_{t-1}^*\right)\|x_n\|, \quad [u]_t^* \leftarrow \frac{\left(\sum_{n=1}^N \omega_{n,t}\right)^{-1} \sum_{n=1}^N \omega_{n,t} u_n}{\left\|\left(\sum_{n=1}^N \omega_{n,t}\right)^{-1} \sum_{n=1}^N \omega_{n,t} u_n\right\|} \tag{6}$$

where $[u]_t^* = U(u_t^*) + I(u_t^*)i + J(u_t^*)j + K(u_t^*)k$ is the first PC, and t denotes the iteration number. Notably, Eq. (6) converges to a local optimum in finite time.

With the above algorithm, the leading component of the data is computed. More components then can be calculated in a greedy way by adding a further constraint that these components should be orthogonal. It can be achieved by removing the estimated PC from data and then computing the next component from the residual. Formally, for the data matrix $X \in \mathbf{Q}^{N \times D}$, $\hat{X} \leftarrow X - (Xq)q^T$ is the updated data matrix where the component q is removed [3]. The next component is then calculated on $\hat{X}$ with the same way. Thus, the PCs can successfully be obtained for dimensionality reduction and other applications.

2.2 QGA Network (QGANet)

Cascaded QGA Network. For each pixel in N input training images $\{M_i\}_{i=1}^N$, a $k_1 \times k_2$ patch is taken. Assuming that the number of filters in the jth-layer is L_j, for the first layer of a QGA network, we can achieve L_1 leading components q_{l_1} $(l_1 = 1, 2\ldots, L_1)$ for patches around each pixel by the above-introduced QGA algorithm. The QGA filters of the first stage are expressed as

$$W_{l_1} = mat_{k_1,k_2}(q_{l_1}) \in \mathbf{Q}^{k_1 \times k_2}, \quad l_1 = 1, 2\ldots, L_1 \tag{7}$$

where $mat_{k_1,k_2}(q)$ is a function that maps $q \in \mathbf{Q}^{k_1 k_2}$ to a matrix-form filter $W \in \mathbf{Q}^{k_1 \times k_2}$, and q_{l_1} denotes the l_1th leading eigenvector.

The l_1 th filter output of the first stage is given by

$$M_i^{l_1} = M_i * W_{l_1}, i = 1, 2, \ldots, N \tag{8}$$

where $*$ denotes 2D quaternion convolution. Note that the 2D convolution of quaternion matrices is also linear.

By repeating the same process in the first stage, the next layer network can be easily built. For each input $M_i^{l_1}$ of the second stage, L_2 outputs are generated and each convolves $M_i^{l_1}$ with W_{l_2}

$$\Theta_i^{l_2} = \left\{ M_i^{l_1} * W_{l_2} \right\}_{l_2=1}^{L_2}, \quad l_2 = 1, 2, \ldots, L_2 \tag{9}$$

More QGA stages can be built by simply repeating the above process.

Binary Hashing and Block-Wise Histogram. After filtering by the two-stage cascaded QGA networks, there are totally $L_1 L_2$ quaternion output images. Then a simple binary quantization (hashing) operator, whose value is one for positive entries and zero otherwise, is performed on the four parts of each output quaternion image $\Theta_i^{l_2}$. Here, binary hashing is used as nonlinear layer, and it can also reduce the amount of output images. The binary pixel values at the same location are then regarded as a L_2-bits vector, which belong to the same root image in the first stage of QGA network.

The binary to decimal conversion (B2DC) is then performed on these L_2-bits vectors, namely, each L_2-bit binary vector is converted back into a decimal number. Finally, a new single integer-valued image is generated after B2DC:

$$T_i^{l_1} = \sum_{l_2=1}^{L_2} 2^{l_2-1} \bar{\Theta}_i^{l_2} = U(T_i^{l_1}) + I(T_i^{l_1})i + J(T_i^{l_1})j + K(T_i^{l_1})k, \ i = 1, 2, \ldots, N \tag{10}$$

where every pixel in $U(T_i^{l_1}), I(T_i^{l_1}), J(T_i^{l_1})$ and $K(T_i^{l_1})$ is an integer in the range of $[0, 2^{L_2} - 1]$.

For each of the final images $T_i^{l_1}(l = 1, \ldots, L_1)$, it is partitioned into K blocks. The block-wise histogram (with 2^{L_2} bins) of the integer values is then computed in each block, which can be concatenated as final output feature vector of QGANet. Since T_i has four parts, namely $U(T_i), I(T_i), J(T_i)$ and $K(T_i)$, each part is operated separately.

2.3 QGANet-Based Classification Framework

In the original PCANet, the final output feature is generated by simply concatenating all block histograms, which results in very high feature dimension but a loss of image's spatial information. In this study, the learned local histogram features by the proposed GANet or QGANet will be re-organized by the spatial pyramid matching (SPM) algorithm [6], because it can integrate the spatial information in image by hierarchical pooling local histogram features to generate more efficient image representation. The final feature vector is the concatenation of the pooled features from the $U(T_i), I(T_i), J(T_i)$ and $K(T_i)$ images. The widely used linear support vector machine (SVM) is selected for classification of histopathological images.

3 Experiment and Results

3.1 Experiments

To evaluate the performance of proposed GANet and QGANet algorithms, two histopathological image datasets, namely the hepatocellular carcinoma (HCC) image dataset [7] and the Beth Israel Deaconess Medical Center (BIDMC) breast cancer image dataset [8], are used in this work. There are 66 images with the size of 1024×768 in the HCC dataset, including 21 well differentiated images, 23 moderately differentiated images and 22 poorly differentiated images [7]. The BIDMC image dataset consists of 20 ductal carcinoma in situ (DCIS) images and 31 usual ductal hyperplasia (UDH) images with the image size of 1444×901 [8].

GANet is mainly performed on grayscale histopathological images converted from color cases, which is compared with PCANet, sparse coding (SC) algorithm in [9], SAE and DBN. Both SAE and DBN have three-layer network architectures, and their optimal parameters are set through multiple experiments. For color histopathological images, QGANet is then compared with the quaternion PCANet (QPCANet) algorithm [10], and the classification method directly on the concatenated features of R, G and B images with GANet (named GANet-RGB), that is to say, GANet is performed on R, G and B channels, respectively, and then the SPM-pooled three channel features are concatenated for SVM classifier.

For each dataset, totally 10000 patches are randomly sampled from a training set to learn feature representation models for all the algorithms. The patch size is 17×17 pixels, and all patches are densely sampled without overlapping in each image. The leave-one-out strategy is used to estimate classification performance. We repeat the above experiments five times with randomly selected patches. The averaged classification accuracy, sensitivity and specificity are calculated as evaluation indices.

3.2   Results

Table 1 shows the classification results of different feature learning algorithms on the HCC dataset. It can be found that QGANet outperforms all the compared algorithms with the best mean classification accuracy, sensitivity and specificity of 91.21 ± 0.68 %, 90.99 ± 0.67 % and 95.56 ± 0.34 %, respectively. GANet gets the second overall performance, whose classification accuracy, sensitivity and specificity are 90.00 ± 2.53 %, 89.84 ± 2.63 % and 94.93 ± 1.29 %, respectively. Compared with all the non-GA-based algorithms, namely SC, DBN, SAE, PCANet and QPCA-Net, QGANet achieves at least 2.12 %, 2.20 % and 1.07 % improvements in accuracy, sensitivity and specificity, respectively.

Table 1. Classification results of different algorithms on HCC dataset (unit: %)

	Accuracy	Sensitivity	Specificity
SC	85.45 ± 2.30	85.11 ± 2.21	92.73 ± 1.14
DBN	82.12 ± 2.71	82.22 ± 2.75	91.12 ± 1.38
SAE	85.15 ± 2.71	84.96 ± 2.78	92.57 ± 1.36
PCANet	89.09 ± 0.68	88.79 ± 0.71	94.49 ± 0.34
GANet	$\mathbf{90.00 \pm 2.53}$	$\mathbf{89.84 \pm 2.63}$	$\mathbf{94.93 \pm 1.29}$
GANet-RGB	87.88 ± 1.52	87.65 ± 1.56	93.86 ± 0.77
QPCANet	88.79 ± 2.03	88.51 ± 2.06	94.34 ± 1.02
QGANet	$\mathit{91.21 \pm 0.68}$	$\mathit{90.99 \pm 0.67}$	$\mathit{95.56 \pm 0.34}$

Table 2 gives the classification results of different feature learning algorithms on the BIDMC dataset. It can be seen that QGANet is again superior to all other compared algorithms with the mean accuracy of 85.49 ± 1.07 %, sensitivity of 66.25 ± 2.50 % and specificity of 97.58 ± 1.61 %, and improves at least 3.92 %, 1.25 % and 4.68 % compared with all the non-GA-based algorithms. While for grayscale histopathological images, GANet achieves the best sensitivity of 66.00 ± 5.71 %, and the second best accuracy of 76.08 ± 5.65 %, which are better than the accuracy and sensitivity of PCANet algorithm.

Table 2. Classification results of different algorithms on BIDMC dataset (unit: %)

	Accuracy	Sensitivity	Specificity
SC	72.94 ± 2.56	42.00 ± 5.70	92.90 ± 2.70
DBN	70.20 ± 4.25	52.00 ± 4.47	83.23 ± 1.44
SAE	76.47 ± 3.10	63.00 ± 2.73	85.16 ± 4.89
PCANet	73.33 ± 2.97	54.00 ± 4.47	88.39 ± 3.95
GANet	76.08 ± 5.65	$\mathbf{66.00 \pm 5.71}$	82.59 ± 8.22
GANet-RGB	78.04 ± 2.56	53.00 ± 5.70	94.19 ± 1.44
QPCANet	81.57 ± 1.07	65.00 ± 0.00	92.26 ± 1.77
QGANet	$\mathit{85.49 \pm 1.07}$	$\mathit{66.25 \pm 2.50}$	$\mathit{97.58 \pm 1.61}$

4 Discussion and Conclusion

In summary, we propose a simple DL algorithm, namely GANet, motivated by PCANet. GANet is more robust and effective tan PCANet for feature representation of grayscale histopathological images, because GA is operated on the Grassmann manifold to well represent the intrinsic data manifold. In order to overcome the disadvantage that GANet cannot well represent color images, a novel quaternion GANet (QGANet) is then developed based on our proposed QGA algorithm. QGANet can effectively fuse color by quaternion algebra and then learn feature representation for color histopathological images, which achieves the best performance in this work.

It is worth noting that the results of DBN and SAE are unsatisfactory in current work for grayscale image. One possible reason is that the training samples are not large enough for DBN and SAE, because for fair comparison, we only randomly select 10000 patches as the training set for all algorithms. GANet still performs well on with a non-large-scale training dataset of histopathological images. It is worth noting that medical image dataset generally only has small labeled samples, GANet is more appropriate than DBN and SAE in medical domain. In our future work, QGANet will be compared with the most commonly used supervised CNN algorithm for the representation learning of color histopathological images.

Acknowledgments. This work is supported by the National Natural Science Foundation of China (61471231, 61401267, 11471208, 61201042, 61471245, U1201256), the Projects of Guangdong R/D Foundation and the New Technology R/D projects of Shenzhen City.

References

1. Chan, T.H., Jia, K., Gao, S.H., Lu, J.W., Zeng, Z.N., Ma, Y.: PCANet: a simple deep learning baseline for image classification. IEEE Trans. Image Process. **24**(12), 5017–5032 (2015)
2. Nie, F.P., Yuan, J.J., Huang, H.: Optimal mean robust principal component analysis. In: ICML, pp. 1062–1070 (2014)
3. Hauberg, S., Feragen, A., Black, M.J.: Grassmann averages for scalable robust PCA. In: CVPR, pp. 3810–3817 (2014)
4. Gurcan, M.N., Boucheron, L.E., Can, A., Madabhushi, A., Rajpoot, N.M., Yener, B.: Histopathological image analysis: a review. IEEE Rev. Biomed. Eng. **2**, 147–171 (2009)
5. Le Bihan, N., Sangwine, S.J.: Quaternion principal component analysis of color images. In: ICIP, pp. 809–812 (2003)
6. Lazebnik, S., Schmid, C., Ponce, J.: Beyond bags of features: spatial pyramid matching for recognizing natural scene categories. In: CVPR, pp. 2169–2178 (2006)
7. Shi, J., Li, Y., Zhu, J., Sun, H.J., Cai, Y.: Joint sparse coding based spatial pyramid matching for classification of color medical image. Comput. Med. Imaging Graph. **41**, 61–66 (2015)
8. Dong, F., Irshad, H., Oh, E.Y., et al.: Computational pathology to discriminate benign from malignant intraductal proliferations of the breast. PLoS ONE **9**(12), 0114885 (2014)
9. Yang, J.C., Yu, K., Gong, Y.H., Huang, T.: Linear spatial pyramid matching using sparse coding for image classification. In: CVPR, pp. 1794–1801 (2009)
10. Zeng, R., Wu, J.S., Shao, Z.H., et al.: Color image classification via quaternion principal component analysis network. arXiv:1503.01657 (2015)

Learning Global and Cluster-Specific Classifiers for Robust Brain Extraction in MR Data

Yuan Liu[1,2], Hasan E. Çetingül[2(✉)], Benjamin L. Odry[2],
and Mariappan S. Nadar[2]

[1] Vanderbilt Institute in Surgery and Engineering, Vanderbilt University,
Nashville, TN, USA
[2] Medical Imaging Technologies, Siemens Healthineers, Princeton, NJ, USA
hasan.cetingul@siemens.com

Abstract. We present a learning-based framework for automatic brain extraction in MR images. It accepts single or multi-contrast brain MR data, builds global binary random forests classifiers at multiple resolution levels, hierarchically performs voxelwise classifications for a test subject, and refines the brain surface using a narrow-band level set technique on the classification map. We further develop a data-driven schema to improve the model performance, which clusters patches of co-registered training images and learns cluster-specific classifiers. We validate our framework via experiments on single and multi-contrast datasets acquired using scanners with different magnetic field strengths. Compared to the state-of-the-art methods, it yields the best performance with statistically significant improvement of the cluster-specific method (with a Dice coefficient of $97.6 \pm 0.4\%$ and an average surface distance of $0.8 \pm 0.1\,\mathrm{mm}$) over the global method.

1 Introduction

Accurate segmentation of anatomical structures is crucial in various medical imaging applications. Brain extraction, for instance, has become a standard pre-processing step for subsequent tasks such as tissue characterization and cortical surface reconstruction. Automatic brain extraction is desired for saving time and labor, removing intra- or inter-rater variability, and permitting large-scale studies. Yet, this is challenging due to anatomical variations of the brain in size and shape that are related to age and pathology, and imperfections (e.g., partial volume effects, noise, inhomogeneity) in the data.

Over the last two decades, a number of methods have been proposed to tackle the problem of brain extraction. These could be roughly categorized into boundary/region-based [1–3], atlas-based [4,5], and learning-based [6] approaches, each with its own strengths and weaknesses. In particular, learning-based methods have become increasingly popular for benefiting from the rising

---

This feature is based on research and is not commercially available. Due to regulatory reasons its future availability cannot be guaranteed.

© Springer International Publishing AG 2016
L. Wang et al. (Eds.): MLMI 2016, LNCS 10019, pp. 130–138, 2016.
DOI: 10.1007/978-3-319-47157-0_16

amount of annotated data. Generally speaking, those methods build one classifier at a scale to capture correlations between some features that describe a voxel and its ground truth label from a training dataset.

One research avenue to improve the learning performance is to build several classifiers for different types of training samples at each scale. This originates from the fact that the decision boundary of a classifier is optimized to yield a low within-class variability and a high between-class variability for training samples. If the training samples of the same class have diverse appearances that are interspersed with samples of another class, one needs to have enough training samples with each type of feature representation to determine a decision boundary. In practice, this is limited by the training data size and memory. On the contrary, learning several classifiers for each subgroup of training samples with reduced variabilities simplifies the process. For medical image segmentation, *spatial selection* and *image selection* are two common strategies for choosing those samples. Conventional classification methods do not guide sample selection in the spatial domain; instead, they learn a global model by sampling from the entire image or a region of interest [6]. Because of the large variations among samples, complex features that capture intensity, spatial, gradient, and/or contextual information are often used. Label fusion or patch-based methods, on the other hand, take advantage of structural alignment and identify the label for each voxel according to the voxels at the same location or within a neighborhood in a set of atlases [4,5]. These can be interpreted as building a weighted k-nearest neighbor classifier for each voxel, with simple intensity metrics such as cross correlation as features. Bai et al. [7] propose to bridge the above methods by introducing semi-local classifiers trained on the grid partition of images with augmented features. Contrary to using the full image set, some works select a subset of images with similar appearances. Lombaert et al. [8] define image affinity via manifold learning, build decision trees using nearby images in the manifold, and weigh those trees based on their relevance to the test image. This is useful especially for heterogeneous datasets.

Inspired from the results in [5–8], we herein present a supervised learning framework for brain extraction. It uses single or multi-contrast MR data, builds binary random forests (RF) classifiers [9] at multiple resolutions, hierarchically performs voxelwise classifications for a test subject, and refines the brain boundary by applying level sets on the classification map. Since a brain MR image has varying appearances at different locations, we also propose a data-driven sample selection schema based on spatial selection to learn separate classifiers for different brain regions. This is realized by learning the exemplars as cluster representation from patches of co-registered training images via affinity propagation (AP) [10] and building *cluster-specific* classifiers. During runtime, the relevant classifiers for a test voxel are determined by computing its similarity with the exemplars, which is faster than spectral embedding in [8]. We evaluate our framework on MR data acquired from scanners with different magnetic field strengths.

2   Methods

2.1   Supervised Learning via Global Random Forests

Preprocessing. Intensity inhomogeneity correction (via N4) and standardization (via histogram matching) are performed to normalize the intensity distributions for the input data, followed by affine registration to a fixed template from the same set of data.

Feature Extraction and Training. The training stage is triggered to build binary classifiers at four spatial resolution levels (i.e., the original image, I, and the ones downsampled by 2, 4, and 8, denoted by $I_{\downarrow 2}$, $I_{\downarrow 4}$, and $I_{\downarrow 8}$, respectively) and involves data sampling, feature extraction, and random forests learning at each level. First, a probabilistic group mask is computed by averaging the aligned training masks and serves as a spatial prior at the coarsest level. Next, a sampling region is estimated by morphologically processing the corresponding ground truth mask to highlight a narrow-band along the boundaries of the brain. For each randomly drawn voxel $\mathbf{x}$ from this region, we compute the following.

- *Conventional spatial features:* Spatial coordinates $(x, y, z) \in \mathbb{R}^3$ of each voxel $\mathbf{x}$.
- *Intensity contextual features:* Multi-scale high-dimensional Haar-like features [11] computed as mean intensity difference between two cuboids of varying sizes.
- *Spatial prior features:* Intensity contextual features computed from the probabilistic group mask, capturing a rough spatial pattern of the brain mask at the coarsest level.

We empirically choose a patch size of 7^3, 15^3, 25^3, and 20^3 from the lowest to the highest resolution level to extract the above features. Once concatenated, we feed the features and their corresponding labels into random forests [9] to train them as binary classifiers. Each forest shares the same configuration using 100 trees with a depth of 30.

Testing. For an unseen image, starting with the group mask at the coarsest level, we hierarchically refine the boundary by classifying voxels in a fixed-size region along previous estimations. Specifically, at $I_{\downarrow 8}$ level, we use the sampling region computed from the group mask in the training stage as the test region. Features for each voxel $\mathbf{x}$ in the test region are extracted and fed into the corresponding classifier to calculate a score $s(\mathbf{x})$, i.e., if $s(\mathbf{x}) \geq 0.5$, label of $\mathbf{x}$, $l(\mathbf{x})$, is *brain*, else $l(\mathbf{x})$ is *non-brain*). The resulting classification map, combined together with the eroded inner surface of the group mask, is upsampled by two as initialization for $I_{\downarrow 4}$ level. For the next two resolution levels, the test region (from which new classification scores are computed) is a fixed-sized narrow-band calculated by morphological operations on the map from the previous level.

At the finest level, we couple the voxelwise classification with a narrow-band level set approach to dynamically determine the test region. We first initialize a distance map from the classification scores and evolve the surface according to the standard Chan-Vese region force [12]. As the front propagates, the narrow-band shifts accordingly and classification scores are computed only for the newly appeared voxels. This allows the surface to recover from previous mistakes without examining a large search region. We also induce a curvature term in the front propagation as regularization to maintain a smooth closed surface. Propagation stops when the mean classification score of the zero level set is lower than 0.5 or no longer decreasing after a certain number of iterations.

2.2   Learning Cluster-Specific Classifiers

The global approach above attempts to learn a highly nonlinear model from all training samples over the entire brain. Yet, using diverse samples of the same class with high variability in intensities and shapes may confuse training. One can improve the learning performance by building several classifiers for each subgroup of training samples and enforcing each classifier to focus on the training samples for this subgroup. We do this by clustering image patches centered at voxels in a narrow-band region outlining the boundaries of the brain and training multiple cluster-specific RF classifiers.

Cluster Generation and Training Sample Selection. We employ affinity propagation (AP) [10] to find a subset of training patches, known as exemplars, to represent the clusters. AP considers each patch $p(\mathbf{x})$ centered at $\mathbf{x}$ as a node in a graph and performs message-passing until a good set of exemplars, $\mathcal{C}$, and clusters emerges. It accepts pairwise similarities (of patches within or across images) as input, which we compute as

$$\texttt{sim}(\mathbf{x}, \mathbf{y}) \sim -\alpha \|p(\mathbf{x}) - p(\mathbf{y})\|_F - \beta \|\mathbf{x} - \mathbf{y}\|_2, \tag{1}$$

where $\| \cdot \|_F$ denotes the Frobenius norm, and $\alpha, \beta > 0$ are weights associated with the intensity similarity and spatial affinity terms, respectively. In this work we only consider the spatial affinity by setting $\alpha = 0$ to train/test faster. To reduce the memory burden while loading the similarities, we perform a shallow clustering by sparsely sampling a small set of patches from each training image. We then use a soft-clustering scheme to find the training samples for each exemplar. This is done by computing the similarity score between each $\mathbf{x}$ in the training image and the exemplars, $\mathbf{c} \in \mathcal{C}$, and assigning it to the exemplar whose similarity score is the highest, i.e., $\hat{\mathbf{c}} = \text{argmax}_{\mathbf{c} \in \mathcal{C}} \texttt{sim}(\mathbf{x}, \mathbf{c})$, or no smaller than a tolerance compared to the highest score given by another exemplar, i.e., $\texttt{sim}(\mathbf{x}, \hat{\mathbf{c}}) \geq \texttt{sim}(\mathbf{x}, \bar{\mathbf{c}}) - \nu$, where ν is chosen such that the patches adjacent to multiple clusters are assigned to all those clusters. In this way, we consider not only all the data points for $\hat{\mathbf{c}}$, but also other points located near the boundary of the neighboring clusters. This leads to a large training set from which we randomly select a subset using stratified sampling to ensure equal numbers of positive and negative samples.

Cluster-Specific Training and Testing. We modify the original multi-resolution framework by replacing the single global classifier with several cluster-specific classifiers. This is done only at the full resolution level for boundary refinement. To train the classifiers, we first obtain a sampling region from the ground truth brain mask using morphological operations and sparsely sample from this region the input data points for AP. The diagonal terms of the pairwise similarity matrix are set to a common negative value to produce a small number of clusters, with equal likelihood for each patch to be chosen as an exemplar. We then follow the steps described above to identify the exemplars and their training samples. We finally extract the heterogeneous feature vectors presented in Sect. 2.1 for each training sample in the cluster and build a separate RF classifier per cluster.

For an unseen (preprocessed) image, testing remains the same (see Sect. 2.1) at the levels $I_{\downarrow 8}$, $I_{\downarrow 4}$, and $I_{\downarrow 2}$. When the full resolution level is reached, we identify the voxels that need to be tested in the narrow-band at each iteration of the level set propagation. Those voxels are then associated with the best-matched exemplars and fed into the corresponding classifiers to predict the classification scores. A classification map is thus obtained to compute the region force for propagating the brain surface. Figures 1 and 2 show our training and test pipelines including the cluster-specific classification.

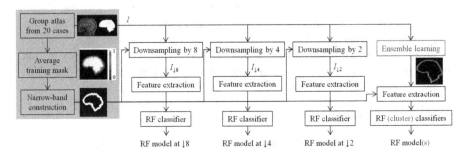

Fig. 1. Training pipeline: preprocessing (blue), cluster-specific analysis (red). (Color figure online)

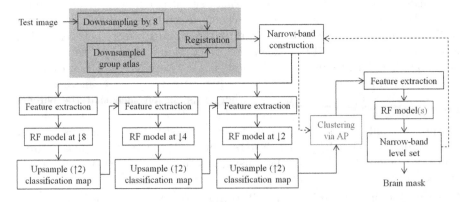

Fig. 2. Test pipeline: preprocessing (blue); cluster-specific analysis (red) with iterative level set refinement (dashed arrows). (Color figure online)

3   Results

We evaluate our framework on multiple datasets acquired with scanners at different magnetic strengths (1.5T, 3T, 7T) using single (T1w) or multi-contrast (T1w and T2w) images. We first show the success of the global random forests (GRF) classifier on 3T multi-contrast and 7T data. We then present the improvement provided by the cluster-specific random forests (CSRF) classifiers on 1.5T data.

Experiments on HCP 3T T1w and T2w Images. We consider a subset of the Human Connectome Project (HCP-500) dataset, which contains 3T T1w and T2w images of 50 healthy subjects.[1] The brain masks given by the HCP minimal processing pipelines are accurate enough to serve as the ground truth. To adapt our framework for multi-contrast data, we extract the contextual features from each co-registered T1w/T2w images and concatenate them to form the entire feature set. We train the GRF classifier with the resulting feature vectors using randomly selected 20 cases and do the testing on the remaining 30 cases. With a Dice coefficient of 98.1 ± 0.25 (%), GRF achieves state-of-the-art accuracy level and hence it naturally extends to multi-contrast data.

Experiments on ATAG 7T T1w Images. We conduct another experiment using "Atlasing of the basal ganglia" (ATAG) dataset [13]. It contains 7T T1w images of 53 normal subjects. We randomly select 20 subjects to train GRF and test on the remaining 33. Since there is no annotation, we use the brain masks produced by the CBS tools [14] for MIPAV in the training. We obtain results that are comparable to, or even better than the ones produced by the CBS tools. Figure 3a shows an example where the mask given by CBS leaks outside the brain and GRF yields a more reasonable result even though the classifiers are trained with data/labels that erroneously include part of the dura mater.

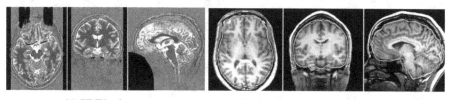

(a) 7T T1w image   (b) 3T T1w image with mTBI lesions

Fig. 3. Examples of brain extraction at 7T and with presence of mTBI: (a) Results given by CBS tools → red, GRF → green; (b) Results given by BET → pink, GRF → green. (Color figure online)

Experiments on LPBA40 1.5T T1w Images. We evaluate our framework on the LPBA40 dataset, which comprises 40 healthy subjects each with a 1.5T T1w image and a manually delineated brain mask [15]. We randomly split the dataset into 20 subjects for training and the other 20 for testing. To train CSRF, we sparsely sample 600 voxels around the brain boundary for each training image

---

[1] http://www.humanconnectome.org/data.

to compute the similarity matrix for AP. This generates 11 clusters, each with its learned RF classifier (see Fig. 4).

Figure 5 shows results for a typical case given by a number of publicly available tools including BET [1], robust BET (BET-R), FreeSurfer (FS) [2], FS with graph cuts refinement (FS+GCUT) [3], and ROBEX [6], as well as our frameworks GRF and CSRF.[2] To quantify the accuracy, we compute the Dice coefficient (%), Jaccard index (%), average surface distance, Hausdorff distance, sen-

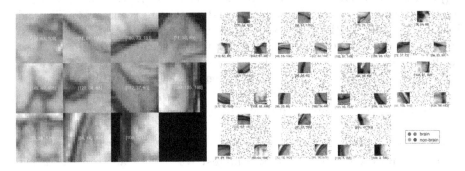

Fig. 4. (Left) 11 exemplars found for the LBPA40 dataset. (Right) Patch embedding: For each cluster, two training patches and one test patch, all randomly selected, are plotted along with their spatial coordinates colored by their labels of being brain tissue or not. (Color figure online)

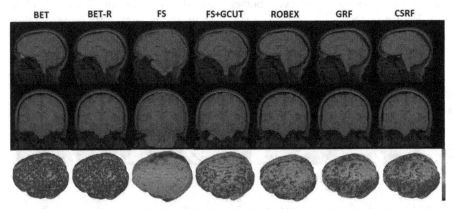

Fig. 5. Typical results using BET, BET-R, FS, FS+GCUT, ROBEX, and our frameworks GRF and CSRF for LPBA40 dataset. Top/middle rows are the sagittal/coronal views, with blue as correctly identified brain tissue (true positive), green as the residual non-brain tissue (false positive), and red as the wrongly removed brain regions (false negative). The bottom row depicts the brain surfaces color coded by errors (blue ~ low, red ~ high). (Color figure online)

---

[2] We run BET, FS, FS+GCUT using default settings; for BET-R, we used *bet* with options *-r -s*. We did not include LABEL [16] due to its long testing time (7 min) for clinical practice.

Table 1. Quantitative brain extraction results for LPBA40 dataset.

Methods	Dice	Jaccard	Avg. dist	Hausdorff	Sensitivity	Specificity
BET	94.4 ± 4.1	89.5 ± 6.7	2.7 ± 2.6	26.7 ± 12.8	98.4 ± 0.7	98.1 ± 1.8
BET-R	94.9 ± 3.5	90.5 ± 5.9	2.5 ± 2.5	25.9 ± 13.8	98.2 ± 0.8	98.4 ± 1.5
FS	89.1 ± 3.1	80.4 ± 4.8	4.4 ± 1.9	24.4 ± 11.4	99.9 ± 0.5	95.5 ± 1.5
FS+GCUT	93.9 ± 4.3	88.8 ± 7.5	2.5 ± 2.4	20.7 ± 14.9	99.5 ± 0.6	97.7 ± 2.0
ROBEX	96.7 ± 0.3	93.6 ± 0.5	1.1 ± 0.1	8.1 ± 1.2	96.3 ± 1.0	99.5 ± 0.2
GRF	97.3 ± 0.4	94.7 ± 0.8	0.9 ± 0.2	6.1 ± 1.8	96.5 ± 1.1	99.6 ± 0.3
CSRF	97.6 ± 0.4	95.2 ± 0.7	0.8 ± 0.1	5.9 ± 1.8	97.0 ± 0.9	99.7 ± 0.2

sitivity, and specificity for the 20 test subjects and present the results in Table 1. While GRF yields better Dice, Jaccard, average surface distance, Hausdorff distance, and specificity compared to all the other tools, CSRF performs even better than GRF in terms of all metrics. In addition, results from Wilcoxon sign-rank tests show that such improvements by CSRF over GRF are statistically significant at the 0.01 level with regard to every metric except for specificity.

4   Discussions

We present a learning framework for automatic brain extraction in MR data, which uses multi-resolution voxelwise classification coupled with narrow-band level set refinement. By operating at varying resolutions, we enhance our ability to describe complex intensity patterns. By constraining the search space by the estimation from the previous levels, we reduce the chances of false positives/negatives while speeding up the runtime, e.g., it takes on average 30 s (for GRF) and 40 s (for CSRF) to strip the skull on a standard preprocessed image. Additionally, by classifying the voxels within the narrow-band and using level sets to evolve the surface based on the classification scores, we allow the surface to recover from previous mistakes without examining a large search region and obtain exactly one connected component. By inducing a curvature term and gradually reducing its weight, we maintain a smooth closed surface fitting to the boundary.

We also propose a fast data-driven approach for spatially selecting the training samples and replace the global classifiers with cluster-specific classifiers. It improves upon the work by [6,7] with increased accuracy and allows the user to focus on problematic region(s), if any, to fine-tune the corresponding classifier(s). This could also be extended to incorporate *image selection*, i.e., intensity similarities in Eq. (1) especially for heterogeneous datasets. In the future, we will explore different measures for clustering, perform further comparisons (e.g., with [17]), and evaluate our framework on datasets with abnormalities (see Fig. 3b for an example on a 3T T1w image with mTBI lesions).

References

1. Smith, S.: Fast robust automated brain extraction. Hum. Brain Mapp. **17**(3), 143–155 (2002)
2. Segonne, F., Dale, A.M., Busa, E., Glessner, M., Salat, D., Hahn, H., Fischl, B.: A hybrid approach to the skull stripping problem in MRI. NeuroImage **22**(3), 1060–1075 (2004)
3. Sadananthan, S., Zheng, W., Chee, M., Zagorodnov, V.: Skull stripping using graph cuts. NeuroImage **49**(1), 225–239 (2010)
4. Leung, K.K., Barnes, J., Modat, M., Ridgway, G.R., Bartlett, J.W., Fox, N.C., Ourselin, S.: Brain maps: an automated, accurate and robust brain extraction technique using a template library. NeuroImage **55**(3), 1091–1108 (2011)
5. Eskildsen, S.F., Coupé, P., Fonov, V., Manjón, J.V., Leung, K.K., Guizard, N., Wassef, S.N., Østergaard, L.R.R., Collins, D.L., Alzheimer's Disease Neuroimaging Initiative: BEaST: brain extraction based on nonlocal segmentation technique. NeuroImage **59**(3), 2362–2373 (2012)
6. Iglesias, J., Liu, C., Thompson, P., Tu, Z.: Robust brain extraction across datasets and comparison with publicly available methods. IEEE Trans. Med. Imaging **30**(9), 1617–1634 (2011)
7. Bai, W., Shi, W., Ledig, C., Rueckert, D.: Multi-atlas segmentation with augmented features for cardiac MR images. Med. Image Anal. **19**(1), 98–109 (2015)
8. Lombaert, H., Zikic, D., Criminisi, A., Ayache, N.: Laplacian forests: semantic image segmentation by guided bagging. In: Golland, P., Hata, N., Barillot, C., Hornegger, J., Howe, R. (eds.) MICCAI 2014. LNCS, vol. 8674, pp. 496–504. Springer, Heidelberg (2014). doi:10.1007/978-3-319-10470-6_62
9. Breiman, L.: Random forests. Mach. Learn. **45**(1), 5–32 (2001)
10. Frey, B., Delbert, D.: Clustering by passing messages between data points. Science **315**(5814), 972–976 (2007)
11. Pauly, O., Glocker, B., Criminisi, A., Mateus, D., Möller, A.M., Nekolla, S., Navab, N.: Fast multiple organ detection and localization in whole-body MR dixon sequences. In: Fichtinger, G., Martel, A., Peters, T. (eds.) MICCAI 2011. LNCS, vol. 6893, pp. 239–247. Springer, Heidelberg (2011). doi:10.1007/978-3-642-23626-6_30
12. Chan, T., Vese, L.: Active contours without edges. IEEE Trans. Image Process. **10**(2), 266–277 (2001)
13. Forstmann, B., Keuken, M., Schafer, A., Bazin, P., Alkemade, A., Turner, R.: Multi-modal ultra-high resolution structural 7-Tesla MRI data repository. Sci. Data **1**, 140050 (2014)
14. Bazin, P.L., Weiss, M., Dinse, J., Schäfer, A., Trampel, R., Turner, R.: A computational framework for ultra-high resolution cortical segmentation at 7 Tesla. NeuroImage **93**, 201–209 (2014)
15. Shattuck, D., Mirza, M., Adisetiyo, V., Hojatkashani, C., Salamon, G., Narr, K., Poldrack, R., Bilder, R., Toga, A.: Construction of a 3D probabilistic atlas of human cortical structures. NeuroImage **39**(3), 1064–1080 (2008)
16. Shi, F., Wang, L., Dai, Y., Gilmore, J., Lin, W., Shen, D.: LABEL: pediatric brain extraction using learning-based meta-algorithm. NeuroImage **62**(3), 1975–1986 (2012)
17. Wang, Y., Nie, J., Yap, P., Li, G., Shi, F., Geng, X., Guo, L., Shen, D., Alzheimer's Disease Neuroimaging Initiative: Knowledge-guided robust MRI brain extraction for diverse large-scale neuroimaging studies on humans and non-human primates. PLoS ONE **9**(1), e77810 (2014)

Cross-Modality Anatomical Landmark Detection Using Histograms of Unsigned Gradient Orientations and Atlas Location Autocontext

Alison O'Neil$^{(\boxtimes)}$, Mohammad Dabbah, and Ian Poole

Toshiba Medical Visualization Systems, Edinburgh EH6 5NP, UK
aoneil@tmvse.com

Abstract. A proof of concept is presented for cross-modality anatomical landmark detection using histograms of unsigned gradient orientations (HUGO) as machine learning image features. This has utility since an existing algorithm trained on data from one modality may be applied to data of a different modality, or data from multiple modalities may be pooled to train one modality-independent algorithm. Landmark detection is performed using a random forest trained on HUGO features and atlas location autocontext features. Three-way cross-modality detection of 20 landmarks is demonstrated in diverse cohorts of CT, MRI T1 and MRI T2 scans of the head. Each cohort is made up of 40 training and 20 test scans, making 180 scans in total. A cross-modality mean landmark error of 5.27 mm is achieved, compared to single-modality error of 4.07 mm.

Keywords: Anatomical landmarks · Random forest · Cross-modality · Histograms of oriented gradients

1 Introduction

This paper is concerned with the *cross-modality* detection and localisation of anatomical landmarks in medical scans of the head. A landmark is defined as a point location which can be described with reference to the anatomical landscape. Landmark detection is an important enabling technology, since landmarks may be used to aid or initialise many image analysis algorithms. Two important examples are deformable image registration [1] and organ segmentation [2].

Cross-modality landmark detection confers the ability to operate where the modality is not known in advance. Further, ground truth from multiple modalities may be pooled to give a larger, richer training set. This is particularly useful when little training data is available for a given modality. There are also practical time savings in ground truth generation and algorithm training. Since image intensities are typically uncalibrated — with CT the notable exception — a feature representation of the data is sought which has invariance to transformations of the data intensities, from simple linear additive and multiplicative transformations, to non-linear monotonic and ultimately bijective transformations.

© Springer International Publishing AG 2016
L. Wang et al. (Eds.): MLMI 2016, LNCS 10019, pp. 139–146, 2016.
DOI: 10.1007/978-3-319-47157-0_17

Table 1. Intensity transformation invariances of a few feature types. The transformations are (L to R): additive, multiplicative, monotonic and bijective. '★' = invariance, '☆' = semi-invariance and '·' = sensitivity.

Feature	Data Intensity Invariances			
	+	×	Mono	Bijective
Intensities	·	·	·	·
Gradients	★	·	·	·
Intensity rankings (LBPs, ranklets)	★	★	★	·
Gradient orientations	★	★	☆	·
Unsigned gradient orientations (HUGO)	★	★	☆	☆
Autocorrelation-based (MIND, ALOST)	★	★	·	·
Magnitude-thresholded gradient orientations (orientation histograms)	★	·	·	·
Magnitude-weighted gradient orientations	★	·	·	·
Normalised magnitude-weighted gradient orientations (HOG, SIFT, Toews et al. [3])	★	★	·	·

Other authors have introduced image features with assorted invariances. Autocorrelation-based measures such as the modality-independent neighbourhood descriptor (MIND) [4] and autocorrelation of local structure (ALOST) [5] do not rely on inter-scan intensity correlations, however they are not invariant to non-linear transformations. Local binary patterns [6] and the ranklet transform [7] both work with intensity *rankings* rather than absolute differences, making them invariant to monotonic intensity differences.

Alternatively, we may switch from the intensity domain to the orientation domain. Orientation refers to the direction of the dominant gradient at any given pixel. Freeman and Roth [8] developed the idea of using orientation histograms for hand gesture recognition in images, characterising spatial regions by their histograms. Gradients were thresholded at some chosen magnitude, below which measurements were assumed to be insignificant. Later variants include the Histogram of Oriented Gradients (HOG) descriptor [9], and the Scale-Invariant Feature Transform (SIFT) [10], which use interpolation and weighting schemes in the spatial and orientation domains to emphasise the contribution of larger and of more centrally located gradients. *Unsigned* orientations (i.e. 180-degree rather than 360-degree range) were originally employed in the context of human detection in images of pedestrians against different backgrounds [9], and this also works well in the case of cross-modality applications where tissue intensities may be inverted in one modality compared to another. For cross-modality image registration, Toews et al. [3] also ranked the bin counts to reduce dependence on the original intensity values. In this paper, we discard the magnitude weighting of gradient orientations altogether to give a descriptor which is semi-invariant to monotonic transformations of the data intensities in the case of signed histograms, and semi-invariant to bijective ("scrambled") intensity transformations for unsigned histograms. Figure 1 gives some visual intuition.

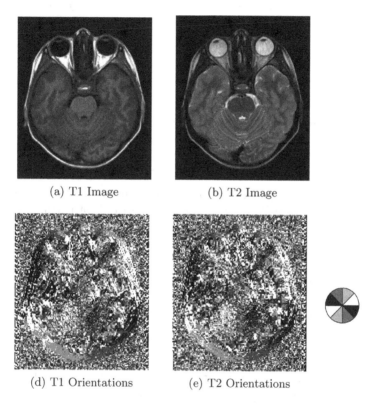

(a) T1 Image   (b) T2 Image

(d) T1 Orientations   (e) T2 Orientations

Fig. 1. Comparison of MRI T1 and MRI T2 slices from the same patient, demonstrating that the unsigned gradient orientation representations are similar. Images courtesy of Dr Subash Thapa, Radiopaedia.org, rID: 40310.

We say *semi*-invariant since the unsigned orientation is only *linearly* invariant within the micro-locality of the pixel i.e. the 4-voxel support over which X and Y gradients are computed by central difference to determine orientation. Compare this to the descriptor of Toews *et al.* [3], which is only linearly invariant within each spatial region over which orientations are binned. If we make the strong assumption that intensities are functions of tissue type, each tissue corresponding to a single intensity value, and further assume spatial coherence, then the invariance to monotonic and bijective intensity transformations holds exactly. Here we define spatial coherence to mean *only two tissues are present* in a micro-locality. See Fig. 2 for illustration. The validity of these assumptions

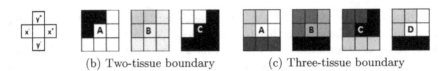

(b) Two-tissue boundary   (c) Three-tissue boundary

Fig. 2. Illustration of the HUGO local sensitivity to nonlinear intensity transforms. Consider the computation of the central pixel's unsigned gradient orientation, $\arctan([y^+ - y^-]/[x^+ - x^-])$. (a) The orientation is identical for A, B and C. (b) The orientation is identical for A, B and C which are linearly related, but different for D which is nonlinearly transformed. Hence, the presence of a three-tissue boundary (which does not satisfy our spatial coherence criterion) would not guarantee invariance to monotonic or bijective transformations.

depends on the voxel resolution and the extent to which noise and texture are absent. We observe that the random property of noise leads to equal distribution of noise gradients within an orientation histogram; a characteristically uniform histogram is observed in homogeneous regions such as air where noise dominates.

Contributions: In this paper we build on previous work with histograms of gradient orientations [3,9,10] by stripping away the gradient magnitude weighting to give a feature descriptor with strong intensity invariance properties which is a natural fit for cross-modality applications.

2   Methodology

A random forest based on [11,12] is used for anatomical landmark detection.

Data Pre-processing: All datasets are first rescaled to a standard resolution D_{Res}, following Gaussian smoothing to avoid aliasing effects.

Histograms of Gradient Orientations: We choose to work with 2D rather than 3D gradients, where gradients are measured in each anatomical plane $\psi \in$ {sagittal, axial, coronal}. Hence anatomical planes can be considered independently, which is useful for (usually MRI) volumes with large slice spacing where gradients are more accurate in the plane of acquisition.

The feature value $f_{\mathrm{HUGO}}(b, v, d, C, \psi)$ denotes the normalised frequency of a bin b, in the histogram of B bins computed over a cuboidal region C with dimensions (s_x, s_y, s_z) centred at a 3D offset d from the voxel of interest v.

$$f_{\mathrm{HUGO}}(b, v, d, C, \psi) = \frac{freq(b|v + d, C, \psi)}{\sum_{i=0}^{B} freq(b_i|v + d, C, \psi)} \quad (1)$$

Random Forest: Landmark detection is treated as classification into n landmark classes $c_i = c_1 \ldots c_n$ and a background class c_0. For each landmark in each of the D training datasets, voxels within a spherical neighbourhood (radius r_{lmk}) of the ground truth landmark position l_i are labelled as landmark samples. These voxels are assigned a Gaussian weighting as a function of the distance from l_i, taking a maximum of 1.0 at l_i. All other voxels are labelled as background with a uniform weighting of 1.0.

The classification forest consists of a set of T binary decision trees. Bagging of the datasets [13] and random feature subspaces [14] are employed, by which we mean that each tree is trained on a different, randomly selected, subset of D_T training datasets and F_T image features respectively. All landmark samples are chosen from the D_T datasets alongside a random selection of background samples at a ratio BG_{Ratio} to the number of landmark samples. Each feature subset consists of F_T HUGO features and a *sagittal displacement* feature $d_{sag}(v)$ comprising the distance of the voxel from the mid-sagittal plane of the volume (on the assumption that scan volumes are approximately centred on the true anatomical mid-sagittal plane). HUGO features are chosen by random selection of offsets between 0 and d_{max}, cuboid dimensions s_x, s_y and s_z between one voxel and C_{max}, and a bin b between 1 and B. To reduce memory usage and to increase tree decorrelation, one anatomical plane ψ is randomly chosen per tree.

Each binary decision tree is grown by recursively splitting the training data samples in two, terminating each branch when either the data has been fully separated into classes or the total sample weight is less than a minimum w_{min}. At each node, the feature is selected which yields a split with greatest information gain over the training data samples. Following training, re-weighting of leaf class samples is performed, in order to apply uniform prior probabilities to the landmark classes, and a greater prior to background (larger by a factor of BG_π).

During detection, test voxels are passed through all T trees and the probabilities are averaged. For each landmark, the voxel v with greatest posterior probability in the volume V is chosen as the landmark location.

$$v^*(c) = \arg\max_{v \in V} P(c | f_{\text{HUGO}}(b, v, d, C, \psi), d_{sag}(v), T_a(v)) \tag{2}$$

Atlas Location Autocontext: Contextual information [12] is learnt to correct spatially spurious detections. Once the random forest classifier has been trained, out-of-bag detection is run on all D training datasets. An affine mapping to a reference landmark atlas $T_a(v)$ is then computed by least squares fitting for each dataset, from those detected landmark locations with posterior probability greater than a threshold p_τ. A subsequent higher-resolution detector is then trained in the same way as the first, except that the x, y and z components of the estimated atlas coordinate $T_a(v)$ for each training voxel are given as scalar features to each tree of the forest in addition to the HUGO features.

During detection, the two classifiers are applied sequentially to each test dataset. Finally, a thin plate spline is fitted from the atlas to those detected landmarks with probability greater than p_τ, followed by iterative elimination of the spline landmark with greatest out-of-spline error ϵ and recomputation of the mapping until all spline landmarks have $\epsilon < \epsilon_\tau$. Excluded landmarks are assigned their interpolated locations according to the spline mapping.

3   Experiments

Datasets: We used three cohorts of 60 head datasets, comprising 40 training and 20 test datasets for each of CT, MRI T1 and MRI T2 data. The population of datasets is diverse. Scans come from Toshiba, Siemens, Phillips and GE scanners. Slice resolutions range between 0.3 and 1.2 mm. Slice thicknesses range between 1 and 8 mm. There are approximately equal splits between male and female subjects and between contrasted and non-contrasted scans. Many contain pathology, inclusive of haemorrhage, tumours and age-related changes.

Landmarks: A set of 20 landmarks were defined: *R. and L. Tragus, Opisthion, Glabella, Nasion, Acanthion, R. and L. top of ear attachment, R. and L. superior aspect of eye globe, R. and L. centre of eye globe, R. and L. attachment of optic nerve to eye, Base of pituitary gland, R. and L. floor of maxillary sinus, R. and L. frontal horn of lateral ventricle, Pineal gland.*

Ground Truth: Ground truth was annotated by anatomically trained experts for all landmarks present in each scan. Where landmarks were present but not visible, they were marked as *uncertain* and excluded from training and from the numerical results.

Algorithm Parameters: The algorithm meta-parameters were empirically chosen through cross-validation experiments to find the best trade-off between speed and accuracy. Values are as follows: $D_{Res} = 4$ / 2 mm voxel^{-1} (classifier 0 / 1), $r_{lmk} = 4.5$ / 2.25 mm (classifier 0 / 1), $T = 80$, $D_T = 20$, $F_T = 2500$, $d_{max} = 50$ mm, $C_{max} = 30$ mm, $B = 4$ (width 45°), $w_{min} = 2.0$, $BG_{Ratio} = 5.0$, $BG_{\pi} = 400$, $p_{\tau} = 0.1$ and $\epsilon_{\tau} = 30$ mm.

Implementation: HUGO was efficiently implemented using B integral volumes per anatomical plane.

Evaluation: Accuracy is measured by the mean error between the detected and ground truth landmark locations.

Results: Three-way cross-validation was performed. Each experiment was run 5 times, each time varying the randomisation of data and feature samples. Figure 4 shows the mean results and 95 % confidence intervals. Table 2 gives summary figures.

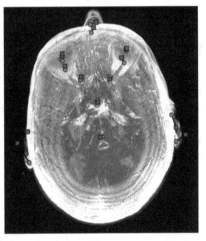

Fig. 3. Axial maximum intensity projection of an example T1 dataset, using CT to T1 detection. Ground truth = green circles. Detected = blue squares. Connecting lines denote correspondences. Image courtesy of Prof. Keith Muir, Glasgow Univ.

Table 2. Overall results averaged across modalities. Error measured in mm.

Experiment	Error
Signed single-modality	4.07
Unsigned single-modality	4.16
Signed cross-modality	11.03
Unsigned cross-modality	5.27

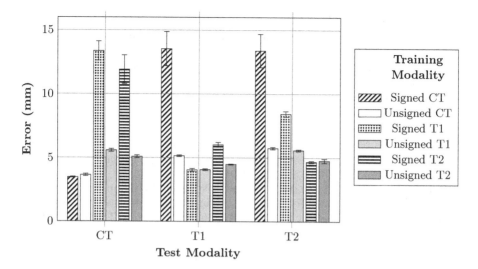

Fig. 4. Histogram of mean errors. The error bars show 95 % confidence intervals.

In the single-modality experiments, there is interestingly no significant advantage to be gained from using signed rather than unsigned orientations, except in the case of CT.

Cross-modality landmark detection lags a little behind single-modality detection, although the results are accurate enough to aid many image analysis algorithms. To refer back to Table 1, we claim only that HUGO is invariant for *bijective* functions where there is a one-to-one correspondence between intensities. Where detail in one modality is not visible in another, there is effectively a many-to-one transform e.g. bone is visible in CT but not in MRI. A second explanation for the performance regression is that there are practical differences in acquisition region and visibility of landmarks between modality cohorts which alters the scope of the anatomical context and the number of training examples.

Run Times: On a dual-core 2.4 GHz machine, the forest training time is approximately 4 hours for the MRI data, and 7 hours for the CT data (larger acquisition regions). Detection time is approximately four seconds per dataset.

4   Conclusion

An analysis of the invariance to intensity transformations of common feature descriptors has been presented, and HUGO features are shown to be invariant to bijective transformations, subject to an assumption of (very) local linearity. In discarding the gradient sign, information about the sense of gradient orientations is traded for robustness to tissue intensity inversion. In discarding the gradient magnitude, information about gradient significance is traded for robustness to nonlinear intensity distortion. To distinguish structural detail from noise, we rely on the aggregation of orientations over a spatial region.

Cross-modality machine learning is demonstrated for anatomical landmark detection, giving a slight decrease in accuracy compared to single-modality learning. There is no need for data normalisation, noise thresholding or bias field correction steps, making HUGO features an efficient and pragmatic solution where time or data is scarce.

References

1. Rohr, K., Stiehl, H.S., Sprengel, R., Buzug, T.M., Weese, J., Kuhn, M.H.: Landmark-based elastic registration using approximating thin-plate splines. IEEE Trans. Med. Imaging **20**(6), 526–534 (2001)
2. Kohlberger, T., Sofka, M., Zhang, J., Birkbeck, N., Wetzl, J., Kaftan, J., Declerck, J., Zhou, S.K.: Automatic multi-organ segmentation using learning-based segmentation and level set optimization. In: Fichtinger, G., Martel, A., Peters, T. (eds.) MICCAI 2011, Part III. LNCS, vol. 6893, pp. 338–345. Springer, Heidelberg (2011)
3. Toews, M., Zöllei, L., Wells, W.M.: Feature-based alignment of volumetric multi-modal images. In: International Conference on Information Processing in Medical Imaging (IPMI), pp. 25–36 (2013)
4. Heinrich, M.P., Jenkinson, M., Bhushan, M., Matin, T., Gleeson, F.V., Brady, S.M., Schnabel, J.A.: MIND: modality independent neighbourhood descriptor for multi-modal deformable registration. Med. Image Anal. **16**, 1423–1435 (2012)
5. Li, Z., Mahapatra, D., Tielbeek, J.A., Stoker, J., van Vliet, L., Vos, F.M.: Image registration based on autocorrelation of local structure. IEEE Trans. Med. Imaging **35**(1), 63–75 (2015)
6. Liu, Y.-Y., Chen, M., Ishikawa, H., Wollstein, G., Schuman, J.S., Rehg, J.M.: Automated macular pathology diagnosis in retinal OCT images using multi-scale spatial pyramid and local binary patterns in texture and shape encoding. Med. Image Anal. **15**, 748–759 (2011)
7. Smeraldi, F.: Ranklets: orientation selective non-parametric features applied to face detection. In: International Conference on Pattern Recognition (ICPR), vol. 3, pp. 379–382. IEEE Press, New York (2002)
8. Freeman, W., Roth, M.: Orientation histograms for hand gesture recognition. In: IEEE International Conference on Automatic Face and Gesture Recognition (FGR), pp. 296–301. IEEE Press, New York (1995)
9. Dalal, N., Triggs, B.: Histograms of oriented gradients for human detection. In: IEEE International Conference on Computer Vision and Pattern Recognition (CVPR), vol. 1, pp. 886–893. IEEE Press, New York (2005)
10. Lowe, D.G.: Object recognition from local scale-invariant features. In: IEEE International Conference on Computer Vision (ICCV). IEEE Press, New York (1999)
11. Dabbah, M.A., Murphy, S., Pello, H., Courbon, R., Beveridge, E., Wiseman, S., Wyeth, D., Poole, I.: Detection, location of 127 anatomical landmarks in diverse CT datasets. In: Medical Imaging: Image Processing. Proceedings of the SPIE, vol. 9034, p. 903415 (2014)
12. O'Neil, A., Murphy, S., Poole, I.: Anatomical landmark detection in CT data by learned atlas location autocontext. In: Lambrou, T., Ye, X. (eds.) Proceedings of the 19th Conference on Medical Image Understanding and Analysis, pp. 189–194 (2015)
13. Breiman, L.: Bagging predictors. Mach. Learn. **24**(2), 123–140 (1996)
14. Ho, T.K.: The random subspace method for constructing decision forests. IEEE Trans. Pattern Anal. Mach. Intell. **20**, 832–844 (1998)

Multi-label Deep Regression and Unordered Pooling for Holistic Interstitial Lung Disease Pattern Detection

Mingchen Gao$^{(\boxtimes)}$, Ziyue Xu, Le Lu, Adam P. Harrison, Ronald M. Summers, and Daniel J. Mollura

Department of Radiology and Imaging Sciences,
National Institutes of Health (NIH), Bethesda, MD 20892, USA
mingchen.gao@nih.gov

Abstract. Holistically detecting interstitial lung disease (ILD) patterns from CT images is challenging yet clinically important. Unfortunately, most existing solutions rely on manually provided regions of interest, limiting their clinical usefulness. In addition, no work has yet focused on predicting more than one ILD from the same CT slice, despite the frequency of such occurrences. To address these limitations, we propose two variations of multi-label deep convolutional neural networks (CNNs). The first uses a deep CNN to detect the presence of multiple ILDs using a regression-based loss function. Our second variant further improves performance, using spatially invariant Fisher Vector encoding of the CNN feature activations. We test our algorithms on a dataset of 533 patients using five-fold cross-validation, achieving high area-under-curve (AUC) scores of 0.982, 0.972, 0.893 and 0.993 for Ground Glass, Reticular, Honeycomb and Emphysema, respectively. As such, our work represents an important step forward in providing clinically effective ILD detection.

Keywords: Interstitial lung disease detection · Convolutional neural network · Multi-label deep regression · Unordered pooling · Fisher vector encoding

1 Introduction

Interstitial lung disease (ILD) refers to a group of more than 150 chronic lung diseases that causes progressive scarring of lung tissues and eventually impairs breathing. The gold standard imaging modality for diagnosing ILD patterns is high resolution computed tomography (HRCT) [1,2]. Figure 1 depicts examples of the most typical ILD patterns.

This research was supported by the NIH Intramural Research Program, the Center for Infectious Disease Imaging, the Imaging Biomarkers and Computer-Aided Diagnosis Laboratory, the National Institute of Allergy and Infectious Diseases and the Clinical Center. We also acknowledge Nvidia Corp. for the donation of a Tesla K40 GPU.

L. Wang et al. (Eds.): MLMI 2016, LNCS 10019, pp. 147–155, 2016.
DOI: 10.1007/978-3-319-47157-0_18

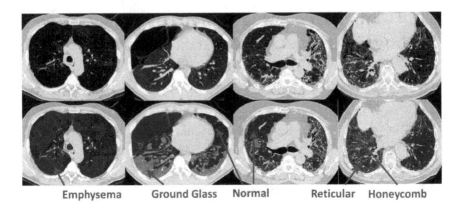

Fig. 1. Examples of ILD patterns. Every voxel in the lung region is labeled as healthy or one of the four ILDs: ground glass, reticular, honeycomb or emphysema. The first row is the lung CT images. The second row is their corresponding labelings.

Automatically detecting ILD patterns from HRCT images would help the diagnosis and treatment of this morbidity. The majority of previous work on ILD detection is limited to patch-level classification, which classifies small patches from manually generated regions of interest (ROIs), into one of the ILDs. Approaches include restricted Boltzmann machines [3], convolutional neural networks (CNNs) [4], local binary patterns [5,6] and multiple instance learning [7]. An exception to the patch-based approach is the recent work of Gao et al. [8], which investigated a clinically more realistic scenario for ILD classification, assigning a *single* ILD label to any holistic two-dimensional axial CT slice without any pre-processing or segmentation. Although holistic detection is more clinically desirable, the underlying problem is much harder without knowing the ILD locations and regions *a priori*. The difficulties lie on several aspects, which include the tremendous amount of variation in disease appearance, location, and configuration and also the expense required to obtain delicate pixel-level ILD annotations of large datasets for training.

Despite of its importance, this challenge of detecting multiple ILDs simultaneously without the locations has not been addressed by previous studies [3,4,8,9], including that of Gao et al. [8], which all treat ILD detection as a single-label classification problem. When analyzing the Lung Tissue Research Consortium (LTRC) dataset [2], the most comprehensive lung disease image database with detailed annotated segmentation masks, we found that there are significant amounts of CT slices associated with two or more ILD labels. For this reason, and partially inspired by the recent natural image classification work [10], we model the problem as multi-label regression and solve it using a CNN. We note that multi-label regression has also been used outside of ILD contexts for heart chamber volume estimation [11,12]. However, this prior work used hand-crafted features and random-forest based regression, whereas we employ learned CNN-based features, which have enjoyed dramatic success in recent years over hand-crafted variants [13]. Thus, unlike prior ILD detection work [3–6,8], our goal is to detect multiple ILDs on holistic CT slices simultaneously, providing a more clinically useful tool.

While CNNs are a powerful tool, their feature learning strategy is not invariant to the spatial locations of objects or textures within a scene. This order-sensitive feature encoding, reflecting the spatial layout of the local image descriptors, is effective in object and scene recognition. However, it may not be beneficial or even be counter-productive for texture classification [14]. The spatial encoding of order-sensitive image descriptors can be discarded via unordered feature encoders such as Bag of Visual Words (BoVW), Fisher Vectors (FV) [15], or aggregated by order-sensitive spatial pyramid matching (SPM). Given the above considerations, we enhance our CNN-regression approach using spatial-invariant encodings of feature activations for multi-label multi-class ILD detection.

Thus, in this work, we propose two variations of multi-label deep convolutional neural network regression (MLCNN-R) models to address the aforementioned challenges. First, an end-to-end CNN network is trained for multi-label image regression. The loss functions are minimized to estimate the actual pixel numbers occupied per ILD class or the binary [0,1] occurring status. Second, the convolutional activation feature maps at different network depths are spatially aggregated and encoded through the FV [15] method. This encoding removes the spatial configurations of the convolutional activations and turns them into location-invariant representations. This type of CNN is also referred as FV-CNN [14]. The unordered features are then trained using a mutlivariate linear regressor (Mvregress function in Matlab) to regress the numbers of ILD pixels or binary labels. Our proposed algorithm is demonstrated using the LTRC ILD dataset [2], composed of 533 patients. Our experiments use five-fold cross-validation (CV) to detect the most common ILD classes of Ground Glass, Reticular, Honeycomb and Emphysema. Experimental results demonstrate the success of our approach in tackling the challenging problem of multi-label multi-class ILD classification.

2   Methods

Our algorithm contains two major components: (1) we present a squared $L2$ loss function based multi-label deep CNN regression method to estimate either the observable ILD areas (in the numbers of pixels), or the binary [0,1] status of "non-appearing" or "appearing". This regression-based approach allows our algorithm to naturally preserve the co-occurrence property of ILDs in CT imaging. (2) CNN activation vectors are extracted from convolutional layers at different depths of the network and integrated using a Fisher Vector feature encoding scheme in a spatially unordered manner, allowing us to achieve a location-invariant deep texture description. ILD classes are then discriminated using multivariate linear regression.

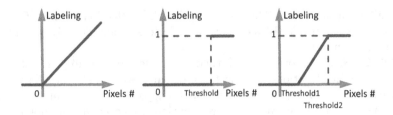

Fig. 2. Three functions for mapping the number of pixels to the regression label.

2.1 CNN Architecture for Multi-label ILD Regression

Deep CNN regression is used to calculate the presence or the area of spatial occupancy for IDL in the image, where multiple pathology patterns can co-exist. The squared $L2$ loss function is adopted for regression [10] instead of the more widely used softmax or logistic-regression loss for CNN-based classification [4,8,13]. There are multiple ways to model the regression labels for each image. One straightforward scheme is to count the total number of pixels annotated per disease to represent its severity, *e.g.*, Fig. 2 **left**. We can also use a step function to represent the presence or absence of the disease, as shown in Fig. 2 **middle**, where the stage threshold T may be defined using clinical knowledge. For any ILD in an image, if its pixel number is larger than T, the label is set to be 1; otherwise as 0. A more sophisticated model would have a piecewise linear transform function, mapping the pixel numbers towards the range of [0,1] (Fig. 2 **right**). We test all approaches in our experiments.

Suppose that there are N images and c types of ILD patterns to be detected or classified, the label vector of the ith image is represented as a c-length multivariate vector $\boldsymbol{y}_i = [y_{i1}, y_{i2}, ..., y_{ic}]$. An all-zero labeling vector indicates that the slice is healthy or has no targeted ILD found based on the ground truth annotation. The $L2$ cost function to be minimized is defined as

$$L(\boldsymbol{y}_i, \hat{\boldsymbol{y}}_i) = \sum_{i=1}^{N} \sum_{k=1}^{c} (y_{ik} - \hat{y}_{ik})^2, \tag{1}$$

There are several successful CNN structures from previous work, such as AlexNet [13] and VGGNet [16]. We employ a variation of AlexNet, called **CNN-F** [17], for a trade-off between efficiency and performance based on the amount of available annotated image data. **CNN-F** contains five convolutional layers, followed by two fully-connected (FC) layers. We set the last layer to the squared $L2$ loss function. Four classes of ILDs are investigated in our experiments: Ground Glass, Rosticular, Honeycomb and Emphysema (other classes have too few examples in the LTRC database [2]). The length of $\boldsymbol{y}_i$ is $c = 4$ to represent these four ILD classes. Based on our experience, random initialization of the CNN parameters worked better than ImageNet pre-trained models. Model parameters were optimized using stochastic gradient descent.

2.2   Unordered Pooling Regression via Fisher Vector Encoding

In addition to CNN-based regression, we also test a spatially invariant encoding of CNN feature activations. We treat the output of each k-th convolutional layer as a 3D descriptor field $\boldsymbol{X_k} \in \mathbb{R}^{W_k \times H_k \times D_k}$, where W_k and H_k are the width and height of the field and D_k is the number of feature channels. Therefore, the whole deep feature activation map is represented by $W_k \times H_k$ feature vectors and each feature vector is of dimension D_k.

We then invoke FV encoding [15] to remove the spatial configurations of total $W_k \times H_k$ vectors per activation map. Following [15], each descriptor $x_i \in \boldsymbol{X_k}$ is soft-quantized using a Gaussian Mixture Model. The first- and second-order differences $(u_{i,m}^T, v_{i,m}^T)$ between any descriptor x_i and each of the Gaussian cluster mean vectors $\{\boldsymbol{\mu_m}\}, m = 1, 2, ..., M$ are accumulated in a $2MD_k$-dimensional image representation:

$$\boldsymbol{f_i^{FV}} = [u_{i,1}^T, v_{i,1}^T, ..., u_{i,M}^T, v_{i,M}^T]^T. \tag{2}$$

The resulting FV feature encoding results in very high $2MD_k$ (e.g., $M = 32$ and $D_k = 256$) dimensionality for deep features of $\boldsymbol{X_k}$. For computational and memory efficiency, we adopt principal component analysis (PCA) to reduce the $\boldsymbol{f_i^{FV}}$ features to a lower-dimensional parameter space. Based on the ground-truth label vectors $\boldsymbol{y_i}$, multivariate linear regression is used to predict the presence or non-presence of ILDs using the low-dimensional image features $PCA(\boldsymbol{f_i^{FV}})$.

3   Experiments and Discussion

There are two main publicly available datasets for CT imaging based ILD classification [1,2]. Out of these, only the LTRC [2] enjoys complete ILD labeling at the CT slice level [18]. As a result, we use the LTRC dataset for method validation and performance evaluation. Every pixel in the CT lung region is labeled as healthy or one of the four tissue types: Ground Glass, Reticular, Honey-comb or Emphysema. Only 2D axial slices are investigated here, without taking successive slices into consideration. Many CT scans for ILD study have large inter-slice distances (for example 10 mm in [1]) between axial slices, making direct 3D volumetric analysis implausible. The original resolution of the 2D axial slices are 512×512 pixels. All images are resized to the uniform size of 214×214 pixels.

To conduct holistic slice based ILD classification [8], we first convert the pixelwise labeling into slice-level labels. There are 18883 slices in total for training and testing. Without loss of generality, if we set T = 6000 pixels as the threshold to differentiate the presence or absence of ILDs, there are 3368, 1606, 1247 and 2639 positive slices for each disease, respectively. In total there are 11677 healthy CT images, 5675 images with one disease, 1410 images with two diseases, 119 images with three diseases, and 2 images with four diseases. We treat the continuous values after regression (in two types of pixel numbers or binary status) as "classification confidence scores". We evaluate our method by comparing against ground truth ILD labels obtained from our chosen threshold.

Each ILD pattern is evaluated separately by thresholding the "classification confidence scores" from our regression models to make the binary presence or absence decisions. Classification receiver operating characteristic (ROC) curves can be generated in this manner. We experimented with Fig. 2's three labeling converting functions. Regression using the ILD occupied pixel numbers or the binary status labels produced similar quantitative ILD classification results. However, the piecewise linear transformation did not perform well.

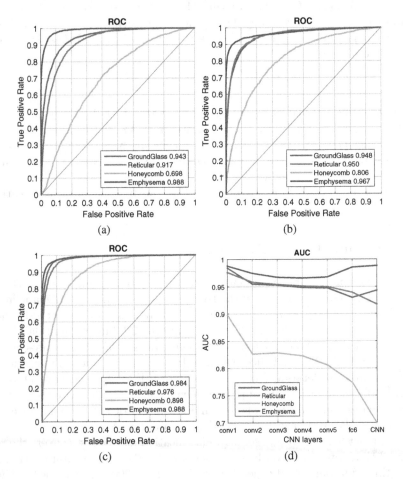

Fig. 3. ILD detection results shown in ROC curves. Both CNN and FV-CNN regression are used to regress to the numbers of pixels. (a) Detection results of CNN regression. (b)(c) Detection results of FV-CNN via the unordered feature pooling using conv5 and conv1 layer, respectively. (d) AUC versus FV pooling at different convolutional layers.

When constructing the FV-encoded features, f_i^{FV}, the local convolutional image descriptors are pooled into 32 Gaussian components, producing dimensionalities as high as 16 K dimensions [15]. We further reduce the FV features to 512 dimensions using PCA. Performance was empirically found to be insensitive to the number of Gaussian kernels and the dimensions after PCA.

All quantitative experiments are performed under five-fold cross-validation. The training folds and testing fold are split at the patient level to prevent overfitting (i.e., no CT slices from the same patient are used for both training and validation). CNN training was performed in Matlab using MatConvNet [19] and was run on a PC with an Nvidia Tesla K40 GPU. The training for one fold takes hours. The testing could be accomplished in seconds per image.

We show the ROC results directly regressed to the numbers of ILD pixels in Fig. 3. The area-under-the-curve (AUC) values are marked in the plots. In Fig. 3(d), AUC scores are compared among configurations using FV encoding on deep image features pooled from different CNN convolutional layers. Using activations based on the first fully-connected layer (fc6) are also evaluated. Corresponding quantitative results are shown in Table 1. Both deep regression models achieve high AUC values for all four major ILD patterns. FV unordered pooling operating on the first CNN convolutional layer **conv1** produces the overall best quantitative results, especially for Honeycomb. Despite residing in the first layer, the filters and activations on **conv1** are still part of a deep network since they are learned through back-propagation. Based on these results, this finding indicates that using FV encoding with deeply-learned **conv1** filter activations is an effective approach to ILD classification.

Table 1. Quantitative results comparing the AUC between different layers. Both CNN and multi-variant linear regression regress to pixel numbers.

Disease	Area under curve (AUC)						
	Conv1	Conv2	Conv3	Conv4	Conv5	Fc6	CNN
Ground glass	**0.984**	0.955	0.953	0.948	0.948	0.930	0.943
Reticular	**0.976**	0.958	0.954	0.951	0.950	0.939	0.917
Honeycomb	**0.898**	0.826	0.828	0.823	0.806	0.773	0.698
Emphysema	**0.988**	0.975	0.967	0.966	0.967	0.985	0.988

Figure 4 presents some examples of successful and misclassified results. In (a), our algorithm successfully detects all three types of ILD patterns appearing on that slice. In (b), although it is marked as misclassified (compared to the ground truth binary labels with T = 6000 pixels), our method finds and classifies emphysema and ground glass correctly that do occupy some image regions. (c) and (d) are misclassified examples. These qualitative results visually confirm the high performance demonstrated by our quantitative experiments.

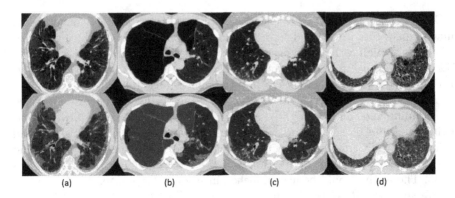

Fig. 4. Examples of correctly detected and misclassified ILD slices. (a) is a correctly classified case. All three diseases, ground glass, reticular and honeycomb are detected. (b) detects two types of diseases, ground glass and emphysema. Emphysema is correctly detected. However, ground glass is labeled as negative during the ground truth binary labeling conversion since its pixel number is less than 6000. (c) and (d) are misclassified. In (c), ground glass and emphysema are detected, reticular is labeled. In (d), ground glass is detected, honeycomb is labeled.

4   Conclusion

In this work, we present a new ILD pattern detection algorithm using multi-label CNN regression combined with unordered pooling of the resulting features. In contrast to previous methods, our method can perform multi-label multi-class ILD detection. Moreover, this is performed without the manual ROI inputs needed by much of the state-of-the-art [3–5]. We validate on a publicly available dataset of 533 patients using five-fold CV, achieving high AUC scores of 0.982, 0.972, 0.893 and 0.993 for GroundGlass, Reticular, Honeycomb and Emphysema, respectively. Future work includes performing cross-dataset learning and incorporating weakly supervised approaches to obtain more labeled training data. Nonetheless, as the first demonstration of effective multi-class ILD classification, this work represents an important contribution toward clinically effective CAD solutions.

References

1. Depeursinge, A., Vargas, A., Platon, A., Geissbuhler, A., Poletti, P.A., Müller, H.: Building a reference multimedia database for interstitial lung diseases. CMIG **36**(3), 227–238 (2012)
2. Bartholmai, B., Karwoski, R., Zavaletta, V., Robb, R., Holmes, D.: The lung tissue research consortium: an extensive open database containing histological, clinical, and radiological data to study chronic lung disease (2006). http://hdl.handle.net/1926/221

3. van Tulder, G., de Bruijne, M.: Combining generative and discriminative representation learning for lung CT analysis with convolutional restricted boltzmann machines. IEEE Trans. Med. Imag. **35**(5), 1262–1272 (2016)
4. Anthimopoulos, M., Christodoulidis, S., Ebner, L., Christe, A., Mougiakakou, S.: Lung pattern classification for interstitial lung diseases using a deep convolutional neural network. IEEE Trans. Med. Imag. **35**(5), 1207–1216 (2016)
5. Song, Y., Cai, W., Huang, H., Zhou, Y., Feng, D.D., Wang, Y., Fulham, M.J., Chen, M.: Large margin local estimate with applications to medical image classification. IEEE Trans. Med. Imag. **34**(6), 1362–1377 (2015)
6. Song, Y., Cai, W., Zhou, Y., Feng, D.D.: Feature-based image patch approximation for lung tissue classification. IEEE Trans. Med. Imag. **32**(4), 797–808 (2013)
7. Hofmanninger, J., Langs, G.: Mapping visual features to semantic profiles for retrieval in medical imaging. In: Proceedings of the IEEE Conference on Computer Vision and Pattern Recognition, pp. 457–465 (2015)
8. Gao, M., Bagci, U., Lu, L., Wu, A., Buty, M., Shin, H.-.C., Roth, H., Papadakis, G.Z., Depeursinge, A., Summers, R.M., et al.: Holistic classification of CT attenuation patterns for interstitial lung diseases via deep convolutional neural networks. Comput. Meth. Biomech. Biomed. Eng. Imag. Vis. 1–6 (2016). Taylor & Francis
9. Gong, Y., Wang, L., Guo, R., Lazebnik, S.: Multi-scale orderless pooling of deep convolutional activation features. In: Fleet, D., Pajdla, T., Schiele, B., Tuytelaars, T. (eds.) ECCV 2014. LNCS, vol. 8695, pp. 392–407. Springer, Heidelberg (2014). doi:10.1007/978-3-319-10584-0_26
10. Wei, Y., Xia, W., Huang, J., Ni, B., Dong, J., Zhao, Y., Yan, S.: CNN: Single-label to multi-label. arXiv preprint arXiv:1406.5726 (2014)
11. Zhen, X., Islam, A., Bhaduri, M., Chan, I., Li, S.: Direct and simultaneous four-chamber volume estimation by multi-output regression. In: Navab, N., Hornegger, J., Wells, W.M., Frangi, A.F. (eds.) MICCAI 2015. LNCS, vol. 9349, pp. 669–676. Springer, Heidelberg (2015). doi:10.1007/978-3-319-24553-9_82
12. Zhen, X., Wang, Z., Islam, A., Bhaduri, M., Chan, I., Li, S.: Direct estimation of cardiac bi-ventricular volumes with regression forests. In: Golland, P., Hata, N., Barillot, C., Hornegger, J., Howe, R. (eds.) MICCAI 2014. LNCS, vol. 8674, pp. 586–593. Springer, Heidelberg (2014). doi:10.1007/978-3-319-10470-6_73
13. Krizhevsky, A., Sutskever, I., Hinton, G.E.: Imagenet classification with deep convolutional neural networks. In: NIPS, pp. 1097–1105 (2012)
14. Cimpoi, M., Maji, S., Kokkinos, I., Vedaldi, A.: Deep filter banks for texture recognition, description, and segmentation. Int. J. Comput. Vis. **118**(1), 65–94 (2016)
15. Perronnin, F., Sánchez, J., Mensink, T.: Improving the fisher kernel for large-scale image classification. In: Daniilidis, K., Maragos, P., Paragios, N. (eds.) ECCV 2010. LNCS, vol. 6314, pp. 143–156. Springer, Heidelberg (2010). doi:10.1007/978-3-642-15561-1_11
16. Simonyan, K., Zisserman, A.: Very deep convolutional networks for large-scale image recognition. arXiv preprint arXiv:1409.1556 (2014)
17. Chatfield, K., Simonyan, K., Vedaldi, A., Zisserman, A.: Return of the devil in the details: delving deep into convolutional nets. arXiv preprint arXiv:1405.3531 (2014)
18. Gao, M., Xu, Z., Lu, L., Wu, A., Summers, R., Mollura, D.: Segmentation label propagation using deep convolutional neural networks and dense conditional random fields. In: IEEE ISBI (2016)
19. Vedaldi, A., Lenc, K.: MatConvNet: convolutional neural networks for matlab. In: Proceedings of the 23rd Annual ACM Conference on Multimedia Conference, pp. 689–692. ACM (2015)

Segmentation-Free Estimation of Kidney Volumes in CT with Dual Regression Forests

Mohammad Arafat Hussain[1]([✉]), Ghassan Hamarneh[2],
Timothy W. O'Connell[3], Mohammed F. Mohammed[3],
and Rafeef Abugharbieh[1]

[1] Department of Electrical and Computer Engineering,
University of British Columbia, Vancouver, BC, Canada
{arafat,rafeef}@ece.ubc.ca
[2] School of Computing Science, Simon Fraser University, Burnaby, BC, Canada
hamarneh@sfu.ca
[3] Division of Emergency and Trauma Radiology,
Vancouver General Hospital, Vancouver, BC, Canada
tim.oconnell@gmail.com, mohammed.f.mohammed@gmail.com

Abstract. Accurate estimation of kidney volume is essential for clinical diagnoses and therapeutic decisions related to renal diseases. Existing kidney volume estimation methods rely on an intermediate segmentation step that is subject to various limitations. In this work, we propose a segmentation-free, supervised learning approach that addresses the challenges of accurate kidney volume estimation caused by extensive variations in kidney shape, size and orientation across subjects. We develop dual regression forests to simultaneously predict the kidney area per image slice, and kidney span per image volume. We validate our method on a dataset of 45 subjects with a total of 90 kidney samples. We obtained a volume estimation accuracy higher than existing segmentation-free (by 72 %) and segmentation-based methods (by 82 %). Compared to a single regression model, the dual regression reduced the false positive area-estimates and improved volume estimation accuracy by 41 %. We also found a mean deviation of under 10 % between our estimated kidney volumes and those obtained manually by expert radiologists.

1 Introduction

The economic burden of chronic kidney disease (CKD) is significant, estimated in Canada in 2007 at $1.9 Billion just for patients with end-stage renal disease (ESRD) [1]. In 2011, about 620,000 patients in United States received treatment for ESRD either by receiving dialysis or by receiving kidney transplantation [2]. ESRD is the final stage of different CKDs, e.g. Autosomal dominant polycystic kidney disease (ADPKD), renal artery atherosclerosis (RAS), which are associated with the change of kidney volume. However, detection of CKDs are complicated; multiple tests such as the estimated glomerular filtration rate (eGFR) and serum albumin-to-creatinine ratio may not detect early disease and may be poor

© Springer International Publishing AG 2016
L. Wang et al. (Eds.): MLMI 2016, LNCS 10019, pp. 156–163, 2016.
DOI: 10.1007/978-3-319-47157-0_19

at tracking progression of disease [3]. Recent works [2,4] have suggested kidney volume as the potential surrogate marker for renal function and is thus useful for predicting and tracking the progression of different CKDs. In fact, the *total kidney volume* has become the gold-standard image biomarker for the ADPKD and RAS progression at early stages of this disease [4]. In addition, the renal volumetry has recently emerged as the most suitable alternative to renal scintigraphy in evaluating the *split renal function* in kidney donors as well as the best biomarker in follow-up evaluation of kidney transplants [2]. Consequently, estimation of the 'volume' of a kidney has become the primary objective in various clinical analyses of kidney.

Traditionally, the kidney volume is estimated by means of segmentation. However, existing kidney segmentation algorithms have various limitations (e.g. requiring user interaction, sensitivity to parameter setting, heavy computation). For example, Yan et al. [5] proposed a simple intensity thresholding-based method, which is often inaccurate and was limited to 2D. Other intensity-based methods have used graph cuts [6] and active contours/level sets [7]. But these methods are sensitive to the choice of parameters [8], which often need to be tweaked for different images. In addition, the graph cuts [6] and level sets-based [7] methods are prone to leaking through weak anatomical boundaries in the image, and often require considerable computation [8]. The method proposed by Lin et al. [9] relies extensively on prior knowledge of kidney shapes. However, building a realistic model of kidney shape variability and balancing the influence of the model on the resulting segmentation are non-trivial tasks.

To overcome the aforementioned limitations of the traditional methods, a number of kidney segmentation methods have been proposed based on supervised learning [10–12]. Cuingnet et al. [10] used a classification forest to generate a kidney spatial probability map and then deformed a ellipsoidal template to approximate the probability map and generate the segmentations. Due to this restrictive template-based approach, it is likely to fail for kidneys having abnormal shape due to disease progression and/or internal tumors. Therefore, crucially, [10] did not include the truncated kidneys (16 % of their data) in their evaluation. Even then, their proposed method did not correctly detect/segment about 20 % of left and 20 % of right, and failed for another 10 % left and 10 % right kidneys of their evaluation data set. Glocker et al. [11] used a joint classification-regression forest scheme to segment different abdominal organs, but their approach suffers from leaking, especially for kidneys, as evident in their results. Thong et al. [12] showed promising kidney segmentation performance using convolutional networks, however, it was designed only for 2D contrast-enhanced computed tomography (CT) slices.

Recently, supervised learning-based direct volume estimation methods, which eliminate the segmentation step altogether, have become attractive and shown promise in cardiac bi-ventricular volumetry [8,13]. These methods can effectively bypass the computation complexities and limitations of segmentation-based approaches while producing accurate volume estimates. Although these methods require manual segmentation during the training phase; once deployed, the trained algorithm can respond to quick clinical queries by skipping the segmentation step. This idea of direct volume estimation can be effectively adapted to kidneys, when inferring the scalar-valued kidney volume (e.g. in mm^3) is the ultimate goal. But kidney anatomy varies more extensively across patients than that of the target anatomy in [8,13]. Therefore, a more robust learning-based direct approach is necessary for accurate estimation of kidney volumes.

In this paper, we propose a novel method for direct estimation of kidney volumes for 3D CT images with dual regression forests that omits the error-prone segmentation step. Given an approximate kidney location within the 3D CT images, our method uses dual random forests, one to predict the kidney area in each axial image plane, and another to enhance the results by removing outliers from the initially estimated areas. We adopt a smaller subpatch-based approach instead of a full 2D patch (as in [8,13]) in order to increase the number of observations, which ultimately improved our results. Using this novel combination of 'dual regression' and 'subpatch', our method outperforms the single forest+full patch-based method [13]. We use kidney appearance, namely intensity and texture information to generate features. Note that kidney localization (i.e. locating a 3D kidney bounding box inside the full CT volume) is not the aim of our work since quick manual localization is acceptable for the clinical workflow, as confirmed by our clinical collaborators. Nevertheless, existing localization methods may be applied prior to using our method, e.g. [10]. Even if only a crude auto-localization is available, our method performs inference on a generously bigger bounding box to avoid any kidney truncation.

2   Methods

Our volume estimation technique is divided into three steps as shown in Fig. 1. In Sect. 2.1, we discuss the 2D image patch representation. Then, in Sect. 2.2, we discuss the training of regression forests and subsequent prediction of kidney areas. Finally, in Sect. 2.3, we discuss the estimation of kidney volumes based on predictions by the dual regression forests.

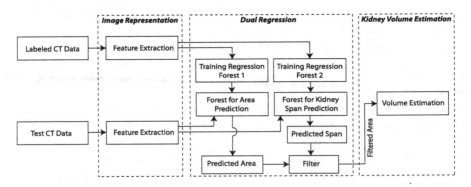

Fig. 1. Flowchart showing different components of the proposed method.

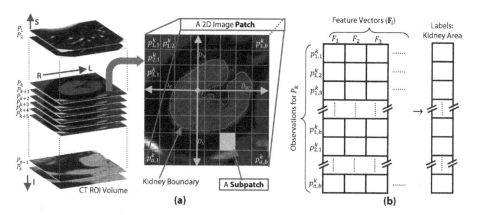

Fig. 2. Illustration of (a) the representation of our 2D image patch containing kidney, and (b) the formation of feature vectors from its subpatches.

2.1   Image Representation

We divide each image patch into square subpatches (Fig. 2(a)). Then, in order to obtain the prediction of the kidney area for each of the sub-patches, we train a regression forest with these sub-patches as observations. We use various features $\mathbf{F}_i$ for each subpatch p: (1) the sum of image intensities $\sum_p I$; (2) sum of non-overlapped binned intensities $\sum_p I_b$, where b stands for different bin numbers and $\min(I) \leq I_b \leq \max(I)$; (3) entropy $E = -\sum h \times log_2(h)$, where h are the histogram counts of I; (4) sum of image intensity ranges $\sum_p R$, which is (max value - min value) in a 3×3 pixel neighborhood around the corresponding pixel; (5) sum of standard deviations $\sum_p SD$, where SD is estimated in a 3×3 neighborhood pixels around the corresponding pixel; and (6) axially aligned distances D_E, D_W, D_N and D_S of the interrogated subpatch center from the east, west, north and south boundaries of the 2D image patch, respectively (Fig. 2(a)). Features (3)–(5) capture the texture information in each subpatch.

2.2   Learning and Prediction

Regression forest 1 (Fig. 1) learns the correspondence between input features and kidney areas for training subpatches, and then predicts kidney areas in unseen subpatches. For feature matrix $v = (\mathbf{F}_1, \mathbf{F}_2, ..., \mathbf{F}_d)$, where $\mathbf{F}_i$ is a feature vector (Fig. 2(b)) and d is the total number of features, forest 1 learns to associate observations $\mathbf{F}_i(r, s)$, $(i = 1, .., d)$ with a continuous scalar value $y^k(r, s)$ which is the estimated kidney area in the corresponding subpatch $p_{r,s}^k$. Here, k is the patch index, and r and s are the subpatch indices along the posterior-anterior (P-A) and right-left (R-L) directions, respectively. The distribution of estimated kidney area values $D(\tilde{y})$ vs. subpatches for a kidney sample is shown in Fig. 3(b). However, due to extensive variation in kidney shapes, sizes and orientations across subjects, we observed that non-zero volumes are predicted for areas devoid of

160   M.A. Hussain et al.

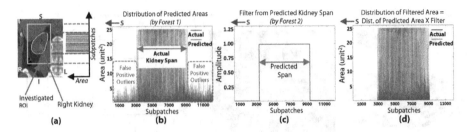

Fig. 3. (a) Schematic diagram showing an example investigated ROI and its most likely kidney-area *vs.* subpatches distribution. (b) A typical distribution of predicted kidney-area *vs.* subpatches (red), overlaid on the actual kidney-area *vs.* subpatches (deep blue). Predicted areas include false positive outliers as shown with the light-blue dashed-boxes. (c) An example plot of a predicted kidney span. (d) The final distribution of the filtered kidney-area *vs.* subpatches, overlaid on the actual kidney-area *vs.* subpatches where most of the outliers are removed. (Color figure online)

kidney tissue (Figs. 3(a) and (b)). These false positives are removed using a spatial filter (Fig. 3(c)) having an extent (or bandwidth) equal to a spatial kidney span measure (along superior-inferior direction). This important span parameter is learnt by forest 2. For training forest 2, we rearrange (i.e. negligible extra computations) the feature vectors as $\hat{\mathbf{F}}_i^k = \sum_{m=1}^{a \times b} \mathbf{F}_i^k(m)$, where a and b are the total number of subpatches along the P-A and R-L directions, respectively. We define a unit step function $U(\tilde{u})$ whose spatial bandwidth is equivalent to the span $\tilde{u}$ predicted by forest 2 for a particular kidney sample (Fig. 3(c)). We approximate the most probable kidney span in the false positives-corrupted D by calculating the cross-correlation between D and U defined as $\rho(l) = \sum_{q=1}^{Q} D(q) \cdot U(q + l)$, where Q is the total number of subpatches in an investigated ROI containing kidney. The lag corresponding to the maximum of $\rho(l)$, $l_{max} = \mathrm{argmax}_l\{\rho(l)\}$ is then used to align U with D. Finally, an element-wise multiplication $D \cdot U$ generates the filtered area distribution (D_f), where almost all of the false positives are removed (Fig. 3(d)). Note that although we use subpatches, we are not labeling every pixel, as done for classification-based segmentation in [10–12], but rather inferring a scalar area for every subpatch.

2.3 Kidney Volume Estimation

There are some subpatches that completely lie inside the kidney cross-section, and we expect the predicted kidney areas for those subpatches to be the maximum, S_A (area of a subpatch). However, we observed that almost no predicted-subpatch-area (by forest 1) reaches this obvious maximum value S_A. On the other hand, there are few false positives still left inside the filtered area distribution D_f. We therefore choose an empirical threshold g and fine tune D_f as: $D_f(p) = 0$, if $D_f(p) < g$, and $D_f(p) = S_A$, if $S_A - D_f(p) < g$. Finally, we estimate the volume of a kidney by integrating the areas in D_f in the axial direction.

3   Validation Setup

We acquired abdominal CT images from 45 patients using the CT scanner Siemens SOMATOM Definition Flash (Siemens Healthcare GmbH, Erlangen, Germany) at Vancouver General Hospital, Vancouver, BC, Canada with all ethics review board approvals in place. Prior to image acquisition, 30 of the patients were injected with a contrast agent. We were able to use a total of 90 kidney samples (both left and right kidneys) from which 46 samples (from 23 randomly chosen patients) were used for training and the rest as unseen. The in-plane pixel size ranged from 0.67 to 0.98 mm and the slice thickness ranged from 1.5 to 3 mm. The ground truth kidney volumes (referred to as 'actual volumes') were calculated from kidney delineations performed by expert radiologists. We used a leave-one-kidney-sample-out cross-validation approach on the training set to choose suitable tree and leaf sizes. We use the subpatch size 5×5 pixels, and $g = S_A/5$ throughout the paper.

4   Results

We provide comparative results of our proposed method with those obtained by four generic approaches: two segmentation algorithms, a naïve clinical method, a deep learning method, and three forest-based approaches. But first, we show the performance of the proposed method visually in Fig. 4(a) where we illustrate the correlation between the actual and estimated kidney volumes. This figure shows that, aside from few exceptions, almost all of the estimates are close to their corresponding ground truth measurements.

We also show the performance comparison of the execution time, volume estimation accuracy, and extra-time requirements for parameter optimization for different methods in Fig. 4(b). We see in Fig. 4(b): rows 1 & 2 that it was necessary to use extra-time for kidney-sample-wise parameter optimization for both

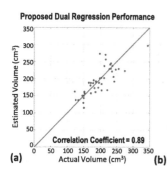

(a)

Row	Generic Methods	Method Tools	Execution Time per Run per Sample (seconds)	Extra-time for Parameter Optimization	Mean Volume Error (%)
1	Segmentation	Intensity Thresholding	1.10 ± 0.06	Moderate	67.57 ± 114.10
2		3D Active Contour [7]	70.10 ± 10.19	Extensive	55.91 ± 98.17
3	Naïve Clinical Approach	Manual Ellipsoid Fitting	~180	None	14.20 ± 13.56
4	Deep Learning	Convolutional Neural Network (CNN) + 2D Patches	0.15 ± 0.0089 §	None	16.42 ± 13.56
5	Regression Forests	Single Regression + 2D Patches [13]	1.57 ± 0.09	None	36.14 ± 20.86
6		Single Regression + 2D Subpatches	1.88 ± 0.12	None	16.88 ± 10.82
7		Single Regression + 3D Subpatches	1.02 ± 0.04	None	26.88 ± 20.11
8		Proposed Dual Regression	3.75 ± 0.23	None	9.97 ± 8.69

(b)   § With Nvidia GeForce GTX 460 v2 GPU with 1GB of GDDR5 VRAM

Fig. 4. (a) Scatter plot showing the volume correlations between the actual and proposed dual regression-based estimates, and (b) a table showing a comparison of volume estimation accuracies, estimation speeds, and requirements of extra-time for parameter optimization during the execution for different types of methods. Execution time is the Matlab(R) runtime on Intel(R) Xeon(R) CPU E3 @ 3.20GHz with 8 GB RAM.

segmentation-based approaches. Although it is possible to find optimal settings of parameters for active contours and other energy-minimizing segmentation methods through cross-validation, the pursuit for optimal parameters is computationally expensive and near infeasible. We also see in row 1 that the estimated mean volume error (MVE) for the intensity thresholding-based method is the highest since it cannot differentiate between two different organs if the intensities associated with these organs fall inside the same user-defined/automatically chosen range. On the other hand, the 3D active contours-based method [7] produces kidney surface which leaks through the weaker boundaries even with the most optimal empirical parameter configuration. As a result, the MVE performance is poor (Fig. 4(b): row 2). Moreover, it is time inefficient as well.

Then we consider a manual approach which is typically used by the radiologists in the clinical settings. The experts obtain three major axes on a kidney, which correspond to a 3D ellipsoid that approximates that particular kidney. In Fig. 4(b): row 3, we see that the estimated MVE (computed by expert radiologists) for this approach is approximately 15 % with high standard deviations. In addition, it takes around 3 min per kidney sample.

Next we consider a segmentation-free convolutional neural network-based deep learning method, where a particular 2D image patch (see Fig. 2(a)) is used as a single observation domain. We see in Fig. 4(b): row 4, that the estimated MVE is similar to that of single forest+2D subpatch-based approach (row 6) but is worse, however, than the manual clinical approach (row 3).

Finally, we consider four segmentation-free approaches using regression forests. The first approach [13] uses single forest+2D patch and the corresponding MVE performance is poor as seen in row 5. This approach works well for cardiac bi-ventricles but fails for kidney, since sizes, shapes and orientations of kidneys vary more extensively across subjects. Subsequently, we adopt an efficient approach of learning using image subpatches (5×5 pixels). This subpatch-based approach improves the MVE performance than that of the patch-based approach (see rows 5 & 6). However, these subpatch-based results are still corrupted by the false positive estimates. We also tested using 3D subpatches ($5 \times 5 \times 2$ voxels). Since CT axial resolution is lower than those of the coronal and sagittal, $5 \times 5 \times 2$ closely resembles a cube shape. However, we see in row 7 that the corresponding MVE is worse than that of 2D subpatches (row 6). We suspect that this poor performance may be caused by the reduced number of training samples. The proposed method (dual regression+2D subpatch) combines the 2D subpatch-based area prediction and patch-based kidney span prediction, which ultimately gives the best improvement of volume estimation. While the mean accuracy of the forest 2-based kidney span prediction is approximately 95.5 % alone, the Table (row 8) shows that the MVE by the proposed method falls below 10 %, with the cost of a prediction time of ~4 sec per kidney sample, which can be further accelerated via a GPU-implementation.

5   Conclusions

In this paper, we proposed an effective method for direct estimation of kidney volumes from 3D CT images. We formulated our volume estimation problem as a 2D subpatch learning-based regression problem and were able to avoid the problematic segmentation step. Though kidney shapes, sizes and orientations vary extensively across subjects, we addressed this challenge by adopting a dual regression forest formulation that were trained by making use of the same extracted image features and their combined predictions resulted in satisfactory kidney volume estimates. Our experimental results showed that the proposed method can estimate kidney volumes with high correlation compared with those obtained manually by expert radiologists (89 %) and reported the MVE of 10 %.

References

1. Zelmer, J.L.: The economic burden of end-stage renal disease in canada. Kidney Int. Masson SAS. **72**(9), 1122–1129 (2007)
2. Diez, A., Powelson, J., et al.: Correlation between CT-based measured renal volumes and nuclear-renography-based SRF in living kidney donors. clinical diagnostic utility and practice patterns. Clin. Transplant. **28**(6), 675–682 (2014)
3. Connolly, J.O., Woolfson, R.G.: A critique of clinical guidelines for detection of individuals with chronic kidney disease. Neph. Clin. Pract. **111**(1), c69–c73 (2009)
4. Widjaja, E., Oxtoby, J.W., et al.: Ultrasound measured renal length vs. low dose CT volume in predicting single kidney GFR. Br. J. Radiol. **77**, 759–764 (2014)
5. Yan, G., Wang, B.: An automatic kidney segmentation from abdominal CT images. IEEE Intell. Comput. Intell. Syst. **1**, 280–284 (2010)
6. Li, X., Chen, X., Yao, J., Zhang, X., Tian, J.: Renal cortex segmentation using optimal surface search with novel graph construction. In: Fichtinger, G., Martel, A., Peters, T. (eds.) MICCAI 2011. LNCS, vol. 6893, pp. 387–394. Springer, Heidelberg (2011). doi:10.1007/978-3-642-23626-6_48
7. Zhang, Y., Matuszewski, B.J., Shark, L.K., Moore, C.J.: Medical image segmentation using new hybrid level-set method. In: BioMedical Visualization, pp. 71–76 (2008)
8. Zhen, X., Wang, Z., Islam, A., Bhaduri, M., Chan, I., Li, S.: Multi-scale deep networks and regression forests for direct bi-ventricular volume estimation. Med. Image Anal. **30**, 120–129 (2016)
9. Lin, D.T., Lei, C.C., Hung, S.W.: Computer-aided kidney segmentation on abdominal CT images. IEEE Trans. Inf. Tech. Biomed. **10**(1), 59–65 (2006)
10. Cuingnet, R., Prevost, R., Lesage, D., Cohen, L.D., Mory, B., Ardon, R.: Automatic detection and segmentation of kidneys in 3D CT images using random forests. In: Ayache, N., Delingette, H., Golland, P., Mori, K. (eds.) MICCAI 2012. LNCS, vol. 7512, pp. 66–74. Springer, Heidelberg (2012). doi:10.1007/978-3-642-33454-2_9
11. Glocker, B., Pauly, O., Konukoglu, E., Criminisi, A.: Joint classification-regression forests for spatially structured multi-object segmentation. In: European Conference on Computer Vision, pp. 870–881 (2012)
12. Thong, W., Kadoury, S., Piche, N., Pal, C.J.: Convolutional networks for kidney segmentation in contrast-enhanced CT scans. Comput. Methods Biomech. Biomed. Eng.: Imaging Visual., 1–6 (2016)
13. Zhen, X., Wang, Z., Islam, A., Bhaduri, M., Chan, I., Li, S.: Direct estimation of cardiac bi-ventricular volumes with regression forests. In: Golland, P., Hata, N., Barillot, C., Hornegger, J., Howe, R. (eds.) MICCAI 2014. LNCS, vol. 8674, pp. 586–593. Springer, Heidelberg (2014). doi:10.1007/978-3-319-10470-6_73

Multi-resolution-Tract CNN with Hybrid Pretrained and Skin-Lesion Trained Layers

Jeremy Kawahara$^{(\boxtimes)}$ and Ghassan Hamarneh

Medical Image Analysis Lab, Simon Fraser University, Burnaby, Canada
{jkawahar,hamarneh}@sfu.ca

Abstract. Correctly classifying a skin lesion is one of the first steps towards treatment. We propose a novel convolutional neural network (CNN) architecture for skin lesion classification designed to learn based on information from multiple image resolutions while leveraging pretrained CNNs. While traditional CNNs are generally trained on a single resolution image, our CNN is composed of multiple tracts, where each tract analyzes the image at a different resolution *simultaneously* and learns interactions across multiple image resolutions using the *same* field-of-view. We convert a CNN, pretrained on a single resolution, to work for multi-resolution input. The entire network is fine-tuned in a fully learned end-to-end optimization with auxiliary loss functions. We show how our proposed novel multi-tract network yields higher classification accuracy, outperforming state-of-the-art multi-scale approaches when compared over a public skin lesion dataset.

1 Introduction

The World Health Organization estimates that globally each year, between two and three million nonmelanoma skin cancers are diagnosed, and 130,000 melanoma skin cancers occur [16]. Classifying different types of skin lesions is needed to determine appropriate treatment, and computerized systems that classify skin lesions from skin images may serve as an important screening or second opinion tool. While considerable research has focused on computerized diagnosis of melanoma skin lesions [9], less work has focused on the more common nonmelanoma skin cancers and on the general multi-class classification of skin lesions. In this work, we focus on predicting multiple types of skin lesions that includes both melanoma and nonmelanoma types of cancers.

To classify skin lesions, Ballerini et al. [1] performed 5-class classification, and Leo et al. [12] performed 10-class classification over images that included nonmelanoma and melanoma skin lesions. They segmented lesions, extracted color and texture based features, and used K-nearest neighbours to classify the images. To perform 5- and 10-class skin lesion classification of nonmelanoma and melanoma skin lesions, Kawahara et al. [8] performed a two step process: first, using a Convolutional Neural Network (CNN) pretrained over ImageNet [13], they extracted image features at two different image resolutions, and second, these features were concatenated and used to train a linear classifier.

© Springer International Publishing AG 2016
L. Wang et al. (Eds.): MLMI 2016, LNCS 10019, pp. 164–171, 2016.
DOI: 10.1007/978-3-319-47157-0_20

CNNs generally learn based on an image of a single fixed resolution (e.g., Krizhevsky et al. [10]). However, this single resolution may not be optimal and depends on the scale of the objects within the image. Information from multiple image resolutions may be critical in capturing fine details, especially in the domain of medical images (e.g., to discriminate pathology). As such, other works have proposed different multi-scale approaches. During testing, Sermanet et al. [14] used a fully convolutional neural network to extract predictions over multiple image resolutions and spatial locations and aggregated the predictions using a spatial max and averaging of scales. This simple aggregation approach, however, does not *learn* interactions across different resolutions (i.e. multi-resolution only applied during testing, not training). He et al. [5] proposed a spatial pyramid pooling layer applied after the last convolutional layer to produce fixed-sized responses regardless of the image size. The CNN is trained on images of multiple resolutions *sequentially*, causing the CNN to learn parameters that generalize across image resolutions. However, each prediction is based only on a single input resolution, and interactions across multiple input image resolutions are not considered. Bao et al. [2] proposed a multi-scale CNN trained and tested on image patches of different sizes (i.e. *different* field-of-view) simultaneously for segmentation, but did not explore multi-resolution input (i.e. *same* field-of-view at different resolutions) for whole image classification. Kamnitsan et al. [7] proposed a multi-scale dual-path 3D CNN for brain segmentation that, like the prior approach, considers *different* field-of-views. While the previously mentioned approach by Kawahara et al. [8] does consider multiple image resolutions, only a final linear classifier learns interactions across different image resolutions, and the CNN itself does not learn based on the input images.

In this work, we propose a CNN for skin lesion classification that *learns interactions across multiple image resolutions* of the same image simultaneously through multiple network tracts. Unlike prior multi-scale architectures [2,7], our network keeps the *same* field-of-view for image classification, uses auxiliary loss functions, and leverages parameters from existing pretrained CNNs. Leveraging pretrained CNN parameters (i.e. transfer learning) is especially useful with limited training images, and has resulted in consistent improvements in other medical image analysis tasks when compared to starting from random initialization [15]. Thus a key contribution of our work is to extend pretrained CNNs for multiple image resolutions, optimized end-to-end with a single objective function. We demonstrate that our proposed multi-tract CNN outperforms competing approaches over a public skin dataset.

2   Methods

We design a CNN to predict the true lesion class label y, given a skin lesion image x. Our CNN is composed of multiple tracts where each tract considers the same image at a different resolution using the same field-of-view. An end layer combines the responses from multiple resolutions into a single layer. We attach a *supervised loss layer* (i.e. layer with a loss function that compares predicted with true class labels) to these combined responses, thus making the final prediction a learned function of multiple resolutions of the same image. This loss is backpropagated through all tracts causing the entire network to be optimized with respect to multiple image resolutions. We add auxiliary supervised loss layers to each tract, motivated by the work of Lee et al. [11], who found that adding additional "companion"/"auxiliary" supervised layers regularize the responses learned. In this work, auxiliary losses cause each tract to learn parameters that classify well at that particular resolution. At test time, we ignore the auxiliary classifiers and only use the final end classifier.

Converting a Pretrained CNN to Multi-tract CNN. In order to train large CNNs with a limited skin dataset, we use a hybrid of the pretrained AlexNet [4,10] architecture and parameters θ_p, (omitting the 1000-d ImageNet-specific output layer) for early network layers, and additional untrained layers for later network layers that learn only from skin images. To pass images of different resolutions through all the layers pretrained on a single resolution, we convert (keeping the trained parameters) fully-connected layers to convolutional layers, as convolutional layers allow for variable sized inputs [14].

For practical considerations (e.g., limited GPU memory), we limit our discussion and experiments to two tracts, although this approach is applicable to additional tracts/resolutions. We refer to the two tracts as the *upper tract*, which takes in a low-resolution image, and the *lower tract*, which takes in a high-resolution image. Our full proposed network is shown in Fig. 1.

We pass an image $x^{(0)}$, of the same image resolution that the pretrained network (AlexNet) was trained on to the *upper tract* of our network. This produces responses of size $1 \times 1 \times 4096$. We add an additional convolutional layer with untrained (i.e. randomly initialized) parameters $\theta_t^{(0)}$, which produces responses of lower dimensionality $1 \times 1 \times 256$. To the *lower tract*, we pass an image $x^{(1)}$ with an image resolution greater than that of $x^{(0)}$. After being convolved with the pretrained parameters, the lower tract produces responses of $m \times m \times 4096$ (Fig. 1 *lower green box*). Other works have reduced this $m \times m$ dimensionality through pooling [5,8,14], but in this work, we add additional untrained $1 \times 1 \times 4096$ and $m \times m \times 64$ convolutional filters, $\theta_t^{(1)}$, that *learn* to reduce the dimensionality to $1 \times 1 \times 256$. Using these two layers instead of a single fully-connected layer, we significantly reduce the amount of needed parameters. Auxiliary supervised loss layers with untrained parameters, $\theta_l^{(0)}, \theta_l^{(1)}$, are added to the upper and lower tract responses.

An untrained convolutional layer takes as input the 256-dimensional responses from both tracts. We add a supervised loss layer to these combined responses making the final prediction a function of the image taken at two different resolutions. In order to reduce the total number of independent parameters in our model, we are inspired by the work on Siamese nets [3] to share the AlexNet weights θ_p, across the upper and lower tracts. This means that updates to θ_p will be based on both image resolutions. Finally, rather than storing separate image resolutions of the same image, we only store the highest desired resolution.

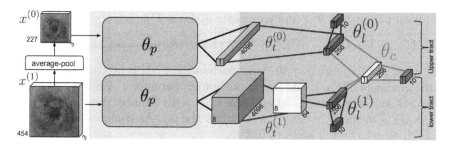

Fig. 1. The proposed two-tract fully convolutional multi-resolution neural network. The highest resolution image $x^{(1)}$, is averaged-pooled to create a low-resolution image $x^{(0)}$, as input to the *upper tract*. $x^{(1)}$ is fed to the *lower tract* to extract responses at a finer scale. As all layers are convolutional layers, a larger input produces larger responses (*green lower box*). After the layers with pretrained parameters θ_p, additional layers with unshared trainable parameters θ_t, are added. Each tract has a supervised auxiliary loss layer (*blue box*). The responses from both image resolutions are combined and an output layer makes the final prediction (*pink box*). Spatial dimensions (e.g., 8 mean 8×8) are given inside each box, and the number of channels are shown alongside each box. (Color figure online)

Within the network architecture itself, we average-pool the high-resolution image to the desired low-resolution scale, allowing for more efficient storage.

Multi-tract Loss and Optimization. Our network has a supervised data loss that considers the combined high and low resolution images, as well as auxiliary data losses that each only considers the responses from a single image resolution. These equally weighted losses are averaged over n mini-batches of training instances along with a regularization over the parameters,

$$\mathcal{L}(\boldsymbol{x}, \boldsymbol{y}, \boldsymbol{\theta}) = \frac{\lambda}{n} \sum_i^n \left(\ell(x_i, y_i; \theta_p, \theta_t, \theta_c) + \sum_{j=0}^{n_{\text{aux}}} \ell(x_i^{(j)}, y_i; \theta_p, \theta_t^{(j)}, \theta_l^{(j)}) \right) + \gamma ||\boldsymbol{\theta}|| \tag{1}$$

where $\ell(.)$ is the cross-entropy loss using a softmax activation function; the ith image is transformed into the jth resolution $x_i^{(j)}$; y_i is the ground truth class label of x_i; the parameters $\boldsymbol{\theta} = \{\theta_p, \theta_t, \theta_c, \theta_l\}$ are composed of the shared pretrained parameters θ_p, the unshared tract parameters $\theta_t = \{\theta_t^{(j)}\}$ where j indicates the tract, the parameters connecting the j auxiliary loss $\theta_l = \{\theta_l^{(j)}\}$, and the parameters connecting the tracts together θ_c; $||\boldsymbol{\theta}||$ is the L2 regularization over the parameters; and, λ, γ weight the terms where $\lambda = \frac{1}{n_{\text{aux}}+1}$ and n_{aux} is the number of auxiliary supervised layers in the network (e.g., 2).

We update our network parameters $\boldsymbol{\theta}$ using stochastic gradient descent with mini-batches. Thus, for the $k+1$ iteration, we compute $\boldsymbol{\theta}_{(k+1)}$, from the previous

k iteration parameters $\boldsymbol{\theta}_{(k)}$ and parameter updates $\boldsymbol{U}_{(k)}$ as,

$$\boldsymbol{U}_{(k+1)} = \mu \boldsymbol{U}_{(k)} - \alpha \nabla \mathcal{L}(\boldsymbol{\theta}_{(k)}) \quad \text{and} \quad \boldsymbol{\theta}_{(k+1)} = \boldsymbol{\theta}_{(k)} + \boldsymbol{U}_{(k+1)}, \quad (2)$$

using a low learning rate $\alpha = 10^{-4}$, as much of the CNN is pretrained; $\nabla \mathcal{L}(\boldsymbol{\theta}_{(k)})$ are the gradients of Eq. 1; and μ is a momentum parameter. We use Caffe [6] to implement our architecture and optimize Eq. 1 with mini-batches of size $n = 15$ (lowers GPU memory to allow for multiple tracts). As common in the literature [10], we set $\mu = 0.9$ and $\gamma = 0.0005$.

3   Results

We used the Dermofit Image Library[1] to test our proposed method. This dataset contains 1300 skin lesion images from 10 classes: Actinic Keratosis (AK), Basal Cell Carcinoma (BCC), Melanocytic Nevus/Mole (ML), Squamous Cell Carcinoma (SCC), Seborrhoeic Keratosis (SK), Intraepithelial Carcinoma (IEC), Pyogenic Granuloma (PYO), Haemangioma (VSC), Dermatofibroma (DF), and Malignant Melanoma (MEL). We randomly divided the dataset into three subsets of approximately the same number of images and class distributions. One subset is used to train (i.e. optimize Eq. 1), validate (e.g., test design decisions), and test. We resized the $x^{(0)}$ image to 227×227 and $x^{(1)}$ to 454×454. Each image was normalized by subtracting the per-image-mean intensity as in [8].

For our first experiments (Table 1 rows a-c), we implemented the two-step approach of Kawahara et al. [8] by extracting responses from the sixth layer (FC6) of the pretrained AlexNet for images $x^{(0)}$ and $x^{(1)}$, and max-pool the spatial responses of $x^{(1)}$. As in [8], these extracted responses are used to train a logistic regression classifier. We report the accuracy for classifying $x^{(0)}$ and $x^{(1)}$ individually, and on the concatenated responses from the two image resolutions (note this experimental setup only uses half of the training images that [8] did).

Our next experiments (rows d,e) show that our hybrid use of pretrained and additional skin-lesion trained layers improved classification accuracy. We split the two-tract network into upper and lower tracts and train each separately on a single resolution. For a fair comparison, we doubled the number of nodes in the layer before the auxiliary loss layer (i.e. Fig. 1 *orange layer*) to closely match the number of independent parameters within the two-tract model. The accuracy of the one-tract single-resolution model (rows d,e) improved over rows a,b, but is less than our proposed model (row i), indicating that considering multiple resolutions within our two-tract architecture improves accuracy.

Row f details the results of applying the classification approach of Sermanet et al. [14] to aggregate the CNN responses from multiple image resolutions. To implement their classification approach, we pass high-resolution $x^{(1)}$ images through the one-tract model (row d) trained on low-resolution $x^{(0)}$ images to produce class responses with spatial dimensions. We take the maximum spatial response and average it with the class responses computed from the low-resolution image to compute a class unnormalized probability vector.

---

[1] https://licensing.eri.ed.ac.uk/i/software/dermofit-image-library.html.

Table 1. Experimental results. *image res.* shows the image resolution in the train/test phase (e.g., 227/454 means image size 227×227 and 454×454). We report the averaged classification accuracy for the *valid* and *test* datasets. Rows *a-i* use multi-resolution versions of an image spanning the same field-of-view. Rows *j,k* use augmented image views, where row *k* combines the multi-resolution approach with augmented views.

	method	image res.	valid	test	
(a)	FC6+LogReg	227	0.674	0.705	
(b)	FC6+LogReg	454	0.649	0.700	
(c)	Kawahara et al. 2015 [8]	227/454	0.684	0.741	
(d)	1-tract (*ours*)	227	0.733	0.741	single
(e)	1-tract (*ours*)	454	0.737	0.759	view
(f)	1-tract + Sermanet et al. 2014 [14]	227/454(test)	0.719	0.748	
(g)	He et al. 2014 [5] (SPP)	224/448	0.688	0.711	
(h)	2-tract 0-aux-losses (*ours*)	227/454	0.723	0.755	
(i)	2-tract 2-aux-losses (*ours*)	227/454	**0.751**	**0.773**	
(j)	1-tract (*ours*)	454	0.760	0.775	aug.
(k)	2-tract 2-aux-losses (*ours*)	227/454	**0.781**	**0.795**	view

Row *g* uses He et al. [5]'s Spatial Pyramid Pooling (SPP) approach, which learns CNN parameters from multiple image resolutions. To implement, we use the pretrained Zeiler-Fergus (ZF) SPP network He et al. [5] provided (similar architecture to AlexNet) and replace their final output layer with our own. We train over ≈11 epochs before switching between 224×224 and 448×448 image resolutions, repeating 20 times for 9000 iterations (more iterations did not improve results). Each image resolution is fine-tuned for 1000 iterations. During testing, we averaged the CNN's output class responses from both resolutions.

Rows *h,i* show results using our two-tract multi-resolution architecture. Without auxiliary losses (row *h*), the two-tract model performs worse than the single tract (row *e*), highlighting the need to include the auxiliary loss functions (Eq. 1) to achieve the highest accuracy (row *i*). Note that we outperform [8], which was shown to outperform [1,12], and that [1,12] were non-CNN based approaches specifically designed for this dataset. The confusion matrix over the test data is shown in Fig. 2 (*right*). We ran additional experiments to cross-validate over the two other folds and obtained a statistically significant difference between the baseline of [8] (using the approach from row *c*) and our two-tract approach (row *i*) with a mid-p McNemar's test, $p = 0.0155$.

We compare the accuracy of the final output classifier with the accuracy of the auxiliary classifiers (Fig. 2 (*left*)). Generally, the final classifier has a higher accuracy, indicating that this classifier (which considers the same responses as each auxiliary classifier) has learnt to combine responses from multiple image resolutions, and that this improves classification accuracy. This plot also highlights the advantage of pretrained parameters, as high accuracy occurs within 5000 iterations (1 hour of training), using a low number (430) of training images.

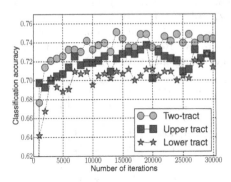
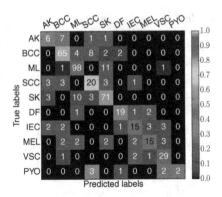

Fig. 2. (*left*) A comparison of the classification accuracy of the individual upper and lower single resolution-tracts with the two-tracts. Integrating multiple image resolutions yields higher accuracy. By using pretrained parameters, we reach a high accuracy within a short number of iterations. (*right*) The confusion matrix over the 10-classes from our test data using our proposed multi-tract CNN (heatmap indicates class-specific classification accuracy normalized across rows).

In order to focus on the effects of our proposed architecture and multi-resolution input, the experiments in rows *a-i* did not use data augmentation. Our final set of experiments demonstrates that our multi-resolution approach is *complementary* to the commonly used approach of training using different image views. We augment the training images with left-right flips, and rotations. Row *k* combines augmented image views with multi-resolution input, resulting in further accuracy improvements when compared to using only augmented views (row *j*) and using only multiple resolutions (row *i*), highlighting that the proposed multi-resolution input complements existing image augmentation approaches.

We did not compare to [2,7] as their approach was designed for 3D segmentation, and while their approach of taking as input different amount of spatial context is well motivated for patch-based segmentation of 3D volumes, it is less applicable to whole image classification. Further contributions we make that differ with their work include: pretrained CNNs for multiple resolutions, the use of auxiliary losses, and multi-resolution input.

Finally, we discuss possible reasons why successful approaches used in *computer vision datasets* (e.g., ImageNet [13] where images are captured at widely different scales), were found less effective for our skin diagnosis application (where dermatology images are captured at a similar scale). When the scale of objects widely differs, the SPP approach [5] to learn parameters that *generalize* over multiple scales, and the approach to *aggregate* responses over different scales [14], are desirable. However, in our case, where the objects' scale are roughly fixed, the different CNN-tracts learn to respond to characteristics that are *specific* to that resolution. This highlights how our proposed architecture is well designed for skin images captured at relatively fixed scales.

4   Conclusions

We presented a novel multi-tract CNN that extends pretrained CNNs for multi-resolution skin lesion classification using a hybrid of pretrained and skin-lesion trained parameters. Our approach captures interactions across multiple image resolutions simultaneously in a fully learned end-to-end optimization, and outperforms related competing approaches over a public skin lesion dataset.

Acknowledgments. Thanks to the Natural Sciences and Engineering Research Council (NSERC) of Canada for funding and to the NVIDIA Corporation for the donation of a Titan X GPU used in this research.

References

1. Ballerini, L., Fisher, R.B., Aldridge, B., Rees, J.: A color and texture based hierarchical K-NN approach to the classification of non-melanoma skin lesions. In: Celebi, M.E., Schaefer, G. (eds.) Color Medical Image Analysis, vol. 6, pp. 63–86. Springer Netherlands, New York (2013)
2. Bao, S., Chung, A.C.S.: Multi-scale structured CNN with label consistency for brain MR image segmentation. Comput. Methods Biomech. Biomed. Eng.: Imaging Visual. 1–5 (2016). doi:10.1080/21681163.2016.1182072
3. Chopra, S., Hadsell, R., LeCun, Y.: Learning a similiarty metric discriminatively, with application to face verification. In: IEEE CVPR, pp. 349–356 (2005)
4. Donahue, J., et al.: DeCAF: a deep convolutional activation feature for generic visual recognition. ICML **32**, 647–655 (2014)
5. He, K., Zhang, X., Ren, S., Sun, J.: Spatial pyramid pooling in deep convolutional networks for visual recognition. In: Fleet, D., Pajdla, T., Schiele, B., Tuytelaars, T. (eds.) ECCV 2014. LNCS, vol. 8691, pp. 346–361. Springer, Heidelberg (2014)
6. Jia, Y., et al.: Caffe: convolutional architecture for fast feature embedding. In: ACM Conference on Multimedia, pp. 675–678 (2014)
7. Kamnitsas, K., et al.: Multi-scale 3D convolutional neural networks for lesion segmentation in brain MRI. In: ISLES Challenge (2015)
8. Kawahara, J., BenTaieb, A., Hamarneh, G.: Deep features to classify skin lesions. In: IEEE ISBI, pp. 1397–1400 (2016)
9. Korotkov, K., Garcia, R.: Computerized analysis of pigmented skin lesions: a review. Artif. Intell. Med. **56**(2), 69–90 (2012)
10. Krizhevsky, A., Sutskever, I., Hinton, G.E.: ImageNet classification with deep convolutional neural networks. In: NIPS, pp. 1097–1105 (2012)
11. Lee, C.Y., Xie, S., Gallagher, P.W., Zhang, Z., Tu, Z.: Deeply-supervised nets. AISTATS **38**, 562–570 (2015)
12. Leo, C.D., et al.: Hierarchical classification of ten skin lesion classes. In: Proceedings SICSA Dundee Medical Image Analysis Workshop (2015)
13. Russakovsky, O., et al.: ImageNet large scale visual recognition challenge. IJCV **115**(3), 211–252 (2015)
14. Sermanet, P., et al.: OverFeat: integrated recognition, localization and detection using convolutional networks. In: ICLR (2014)
15. Shin, H.C., et al.: Deep convolutional neural networks for computer-aided detection. IEEE TMI **35**(5), 1285–1298 (2016)
16. World Health Organization: INTERSUN: the global UV project (2003). http://who.int/uv/publications/en/Intersunguide.pdf. Accessed 13 Feb 2016

Retinal Image Quality Classification Using Saliency Maps and CNNs

Dwarikanath Mahapatra$^{(\boxtimes)}$, Pallab K. Roy, Suman Sedai, and Rahil Garnavi

IBM Research, Melbourne, Australia
{dwarim,pallroy,ssedai,rahilgar}@au1.ibm.com

Abstract. Retinal image quality assessment (IQA) algorithms use different hand crafted features without considering the important role of the human visual system (HVS). We solve the IQA problem using the principles behind the working of the HVS. Unsupervised information from local saliency maps and supervised information from trained convolutional neural networks (CNNs) are combined to make a final decision on image quality. A novel algorithm is proposed that calculates saliency values for every image pixel at multiple scales to capture global and local image information. This extracts generalized image information in an unsupervised manner while CNNs provide a principled approach to feature learning without the need to define hand-crafted features. The individual classification decisions are fused by weighting them according to their confidence scores. Experimental results on real datasets demonstrate the superior performance of our proposed algorithm over competing methods.

1 Introduction

Image quality assessment (IQA) of retinal fundus images is an important step in screening systems for diseases like diabetic retinopathy (DR). Automated analysis requires retinal images to be of a minimum quality that would facilitate feature extraction. Figures 1(a)-(b) shows examples of ungradable images that hamper reliable feature extraction.

Reliable factors for IQA identified by the Atherosclerotic Risk in Communities (ARIC) [1] study are grouped into two major categories: generic image quality parameters (e.g. contrast, clarity, etc.) and structural quality parameters (such as visibility of the optic disc and macula). Methods using generic image information include histogram matching [10] and distribution of edge magnitudes [9]. Despite low computational complexity, they do not always capture diversity of conditions affecting image quality. Other IQA methods use retinal landmarks like the vasculature [15] and multi scale filter banks [12]. They require anatomical landmark segmentation which is complex and error prone, especially for poor quality images. Paulus et al. [14] combined generic and structural image features but rely heavily on accurate landmark segmentation.

Humans rely on the human visual system (HVS) to identify poor quality images. IQA is subjective as it depends on a user's perception of good quality.

© Springer International Publishing AG 2016
L. Wang et al. (Eds.): MLMI 2016, LNCS 10019, pp. 172–179, 2016.
DOI: 10.1007/978-3-319-47157-0_21

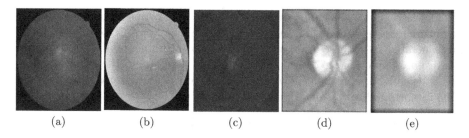

Fig. 1. (a)-(c) Examples of ungradable images; (d)-(e) example outputs of convolving learned kernels with original image.

Current approaches to IQA use hand crafted features which do not generalize well to new datasets. Neither do they leverage the functioning of the HVS to improve IQA. This necessitates solving the problem using computational principles behind the working of the HVS, thus minimizing subjectivity and bias of existing algorithms. We propose a method for retinal IQA that uses computational algorithms imitating the working of the HVS. Our objective is achieved through the following novelties: (1) We propose a novel 'local saliency map' that calculates saliency values for every image pixel across different scales, and captures local and global image information that is relevant for IQA; (2) we leverage learned supervised information from convolutional neural networks (CNNs) thus avoiding hand crafted features. We combine supervised (trained CNNs) and unsupervised (local saliency maps) models using Random forest (RF) classifiers and the associated confidence scores, and demonstrate their superior performance over competing methods.

2 Methods

2.1 Saliency Model

The original 8 bit color images are intensity normalized to $[0, 1]$ and resized to 512×512 pixels. Saliency defines the degree to which a particular region is different from its neighbors with respect to image features. The original model by Itti-Koch [7] gives a global saliency map highlighting attractive regions in the image. Visual input is first decomposed into a set of multiscale feature maps and different spatial locations compete for saliency within each map. These feature maps are combined to form a final saliency map that highlights the most salient regions in an image. The limitation of state of the art saliency algorithms [5–7] is they highlight a single region that is most salient and pixels outside the salient region have no importance. We propose a 'local' saliency map method that calculates the saliency value of each pixel by incorporating principles of neurobiology into the algorithm. Since image quality assessment should incorporate both local and global features, our saliency maps incorporate them by taking multiple scales (neighborhoods) of each pixel.

The resized color image is converted to gray scale intensity, and texture and curvature maps are obtained from this grayscale image. Multiscale saliency maps are generated from these 3 feature maps. According to neurobiological studies, the response function of cortical cells is Gaussian [2], i.e., further away a point, less is its influence on the central pixel. Thus, to calculate a pixel's uniqueness from its surroundings a sum of weighted difference of feature values is calculated,

$$D_F(s) = \sum_i \exp\left(-\|s - s_i\|\right) |F(s) - F(s_i)|, \tag{1}$$

where D_F indicates the difference map for feature F; s_i is the ith pixel in the $N \times N$ neighborhood of pixel s; $\|s - s_i\|$ denotes the Euclidean distance between s and s_i. $F(s_i)$ denotes the feature value at pixel s_i. This gives a saliency value for each pixel. We use different values of N (5×5, 11×11, 19×19, 31×31 and 41×41) to get saliency maps for intensity, texture and curvature at varying scales for capturing local and global information.

Figure 2 shows the 'global' saliency maps generated by different methods and the local saliency maps obtained by our method at different scales for an original 'gradable image'. Figure 2 also shows the corresponding saliency maps for an ungradable image. A comparative study of the maps highlights the following points: (1) our local saliency maps provide more discriminative information than the global saliency maps which only highlights the optic disc region as the most salient region. (2) the local saliency maps are able to capture different levels of local and global information by varying the operation scale. (3) local saliency maps are more effective than global saliency maps in discriminating between gradable and ungradable images. These set of results justify our proposed local saliency maps instead of using the conventional saliency maps.

5 different scales for the 3 saliency maps gives a total of 15 saliency maps. Each map is divided into non-overlapping 64×64 blocks, giving a total of 64 blocks. The mean pixel value of each block is calculated to give 64 feature values for one map. The total number of features from the 15 maps is ($64 \times 15 =$)960 which is the feature vector obtained from saliency maps.

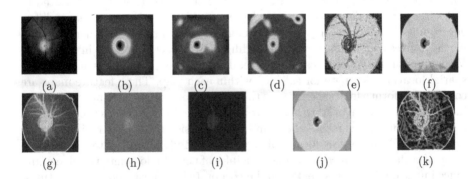

Fig. 2. (a) original gradable image; (b)-(d) global saliency maps obtained using [5–7]; (e)-(g) local saliency maps from our method at different scales; (h) ungradable image; (i)-(k) corresponding local saliency maps by our method.

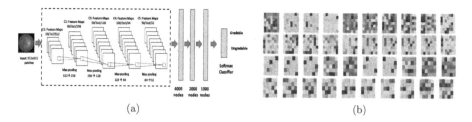

(a)   (b)

Fig. 3. (a) Illustration of the CNN architecture used for our proposed method; (b) Examples of learned filters from the final convolutional layer.

2.2 CNN Architecture

Figure 3(a) shows the architecture of our proposed network. The input patches are of size 512×512 which are put through 5 layers of convolution and max pooling operations. The first convolution layer $C1$ takes as input the 512×512 patch and convolves it with 10 11×11 kernels to return a 512×512 output. The patches are symmetrically padded to ensure that the convolution output is of the same size as the input. The details of the number of kernels and their sizes are depicted in Fig. 3(a). $C1$ 10/11/512 denotes that layer $C1$ has 10 kernels of size 11×11 and outputs a 512×512 patch. The max pooling layer is 2×2 with $512 \rightarrow 256$ indicating the input 512×512 patch is downsampled to 256×256 using max pooling. Following $C5$ (the fifth convolution layer) we have 3 fully connected layers of $4000, 2000, 1000$ nodes followed by a soft-max classifier that outputs the class label as either gradable or ungradable. We refer to this architecture as CNN_5, i.e., a CNN with 5 convolution layers. The soft-max layer has a logistic regression that calculates the probability of each class as,

$$P\left(y = i | \mathbf{W}, \mathbf{b}\right) = \frac{\exp^{W_i x + b_i}}{\sum_{j=1}^{M} \exp^{W_i x + b_i}}, \tag{2}$$

where x is the output of the second fully connected layer, W_i and b_i are the weights and biases of the ith neuron in this layer. The class with maximum probability is the predicted class.

Instead of traditional sigmoid or tanh neurons, we use Rectified Linear Units (ReLUs) [11] in the different layers since recent research [8] has demonstrated the speedup in training compared to using tanh units. An ReLU has an output of $f(x) = max(0; x)$ where x denotes the input. ReLUs enable the training to complete several times faster and are not sensitive to the scale of input.

2.3 Training the CNN

We use negative log-likelihood as the loss function and perform Stochastic Gradient Descent (SGD) using dropout where the neuron outputs are masked out with probability of 0.5, and at test time their outputs are halved. Dropout alleviates overfitting by introducing random noise to training samples and boosts the performance of large networks. Since applying dropout to all layers significantly increases the training time, we only apply dropout at the second fully connected layer, i.e., half of the outputs of the second fully connected layer are randomly masked out in training, and in testing the weights of the logistic regression layer are divided by 2, which is equivalent to halving the outputs of the second fully connected layer. Figure 3(b) shows example learned filters from the final convolutional layer.

2.4   Image Quality Classification

The feature vector from saliency maps (f_1) and the 1000 dimensional feature vector from the last fully connected layer of the CNN (f_2) are used to train two different Random forest (RF) classifiers [3] (denoted as RF_1 and RF_2). RF_1 and RF_2 are both trained on the image labels. A given test image is resized to 512×512 and put through the process of saliency map generation and CNN classification to output two class labels (0/1 for ungradable/gradable images) alongwith probabilty scores. Thus for every test image we have two probability values (for gradable/ungradable) each from RF_1 and RF_2.

The probability values act as confidence scores for each classifier which is used to calculate the final label (C) as,

$$C = \frac{w_{1,1} + w_{2,1}}{2}, \tag{3}$$

where $w_{1,1}$ is the confidence score (probability) of RF_1 predicting class 1 and $w_{2,1}$ is the confidence score of RF_2 predicting class 1. If $C > 0.5$ then the final prediction is class 1 (gradable), else the image is deemed ungradable. The advantage of this approach is the combination of supervised (RF_1) and unsupervised (RF_2) image features. Note that the CNN has a probabilistic classifier which also outputs probability score, and in principle, there is no need to train a separate RF_2 classifier. However we do that for the sake of continuity with saliency features, although our experiemntal results show there is no significant performance difference if we use the soft max classifier instead of RF_2.

3   Experiments and Results

3.1   Dataset Description

We use a dataset acquired from a DR screening initiative. The dataset ($D1$) has 9653 ungradable retinal images and 11347 gradable images. All of the images are non-mydriatic, have a $45°$ FOV and a resolution of 2812×2442 pixels. All the images have been graded by human graders, thus confirming their gradability labels.

Data Augmentation: Since the dataset size is not large enough to train a robust CNN we apply data augmentation by image translation and horizontal reflections to increase the number of images. All image intensities were normalized between $[0, 1]$ and then resized to 512×512 pixels. These resized images were subject to different operations like horizontal and vertical flipping, rotation, translation and contrast changes. Using these operations the size of our dataset was increased 50 times, which is large enough to avoid overfitting. Henceforth further references to any dataset refers to the augmented version. $400,000$ images from each class of the augmented dataset are used to train the CNN. We use a $5-$ fold cross validation approach where the training data consists of 80 % of the total images. We ensure that the augmented versions of an image are either in the training or test set.

Classification Results: Results of our method (denoted RF_{1+2}) are compared with the following methods: RF_{All} where the feature vectors f_1, f_2 are concatenated to train a RF; SVM_{All} - support vector machines using f_1, f_2 with linear kernels for classification; $RF_1 + SM$ - weighted combination of outputs of RF_1 and the CNN softmax classifier for predicting the gradability. To perform a comparative study, we have tested the methods proposed in [4,12,14]. We re-implement these algorithms by closely following the details given in the respective works.

Table 1 shows Sensitivity (Sen), Specificity (Spe) and Accuracy (Acc) obtained using $5-$fold cross validation. We obtain high sensitivity (correctly identified gradable images), specificity (correctly identified ungradable images) and accuracy values which outperforms current state-of-the-art methods for our dataset. These values are higher than those reported in the original works of [4,12] and significantly better than [14]. A significant achievement of our method is that it has been tested on a much larger dataset than previous works. The dataset covers a wide range of images acquired under different conditions and provides a much stricter evaluation of different algorithms. The $p-$values from a paired $t-$test with the results of RF_{1+2} show the significant improvement brought about by neurobiological models of the HVS. $p < 0.05$ indicates that the two sets of results being compared are statistically significant.

The kernel sizes in different layers were decided based on extensive experiments where effect of different kernel sizes on final accuracy was studied. We have used progressively smaller kernel sizes in different layers in order to capture information at different scales. The first layer has 7×7 kernels which captures more global information. From the second convolution layer onwards the kernel size is fixed at 3×3. Since the image dimensions are progressively halved in each layer, the fixed size kernels capture a mix of local and global information.

Results from Table 1 also show the advantages of fusing the decisions of RF_1, RF_2 instead of concatenating them in a single feature vector (RF_{All}, SVM_{All}). It also shows that the softmax classifier ($RF_1 + SM$) performs as good as the RF classifiers. Figures 4(a)-(b) show examples of gradable images which were correctly classified by RF_{1+2} as gradable but incorrectly classified by [4,12,14]. This was probably due to uneven illumination and intensity saturation at some parts. Figures 4(c)-(d) show the opposite case where ungradable images were classified as gradable by [4,12,14] but not by RF_{1+2}.

Table 1. Sensitivity (*Sen*), Specificity (*Spe*), Accuracy (*Acc*) and p−values for different methods compared to CNN.

	RF_{1+2}	RF_{All}	SVM_{All}	Paulus [14]	Dias [4]	Niemeijer [12]	RF_1+SM	RF_1	SM
Sen	98.2	95.4	95.1	94	96.1	96.7	97.9	92.2	93.4
Spe	97.8	94.6	94.2	90.1	95.4	96.0	97.8	91.8	92.4
Acc	97.9	94.7	94.5	91.4	95.6	96.2	97.9	91.9	92.8
$p-$	-	0.0012	0.0018	0.00009	0.0017	0.0024	0.56	0.0001	0.0001

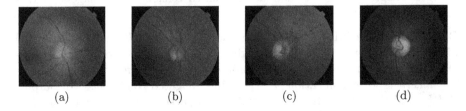

(a)   (b)   (c)   (d)

Fig. 4. (a)-(b) Gradable images which were classified incorrectly by other algorithms except RF_{1+2} as ungradable; (c)-(d) ungradable images classified as gradable by all algorithms except RF_{1+2}.

Computation Time: The average computation time for classifying a test image is 8.2 s with our method using non-optimized MATLAB code on a Intel Core 2.3 GHz $i5$ CPU running Windows 7 with 8 GB RAM. Although not real time, classification time is small enough to make a quick decision about repeat scans. The CNN architecture was trained using the MATLAB Deep Learning Toolbox [13]. The average training time for 400,000 patches from each class is 22 h. Feature extraction from saliency maps and its classification takes 3.2 s while feature extraction from CNNs and classification takes 4.7 s with a further 0.3 s for fusing the two decisions.

4   Conclusion

We have proposed a novel method to determine image quality of acquired retinal scans by combining unsupervised information from visual saliency maps and supervised information from trained CNNs. Our key contribution is the use of computational models of HVS for IQA, and an algorithm for local saliency map computation. We also extract additional information from trained CNNs. Combining these two sources of information leads to high sensitivity and specificity of our method which outperforms other approaches. The low computation time is an added benefit for a quick assessment of image quality in settings which require a quick decision to determine whether the patients would need a repeat scan.

References

1. The atherosclerosis risk in communities (ARIC) study: design and objectives. The ARIC investigators. Am J Epidemiol, 129(4), 687–702, April 1989
2. Goldstein, E.: Sensation and Perception. Thomson Wadsworth, Belmont (2007)
3. Breiman, L.: Random forests. Mach. Learn. **45**(1), 5–32 (2001)
4. Dias, J., Oliveira, C., Cruz, L.: Retinal image quality assessment using generic image quality indicators. Inf. Fusion **19**, 73–90 (2014)
5. Harel, J., Koch, C., Perona, P.: Graph-based visual saliency. In: Advances in Neural Information Processing Systems (NIPS), pp. 545–552 (2006)
6. Hou, X., Harel, J., Koch, C.: Image signature: highlighting sparse salient regions. IEEE Trans. Pattern Anal. Mach. Intell. **34**(1), 194–201 (2012)
7. Itti, L., Koch, C., Niebur, E.: A model of saliency-based visual attention for rapid scene analysis. IEEE Trans. Pattern Anal. Mach. Intell. **20**(11), 1254–1259 (1998)
8. Krizhevsky, A., Sutskever, I., Hinton, G.: Imagenet classification with deep convolutional neural networks. In: Advances in Neural Information Processing Systems (NIPS), pp. 1106–1114 (2012)
9. Lalonde, M., Gagnon, L., Boucher, M.: Automatic visual quality assessment in optical fundus images. In: Proceedings of Vision Interface, pp. 259–264 (2001)
10. Lee, S., Wang, Y.: Automatic retinal image quality assessment and enhancement. In: Proceedings of SPIE Medical Imaging, pp. 1581–1590 (1999)
11. Nair, V., Hinton, G.E.: Rectified linear units improve restricted Boltzmann machines. In: International Conference on Machine Learning, pp. 807–814 (2010)
12. Niemeijer, M., Abramoff, M., van Ginneken, B.: Image structure clustering for image quality verification of color retina images in diabetic retinopathy screening. Med. Imag. Anal. **10**(6), 888–898 (2006)
13. Palm, R.B.: Prediction as a Candidate for Learning Deep Hierarchical Models of Data. Masters Thesis, Technical University of Denmark (2012)
14. Paulus, J., Meier, J., Bock, R., Hornegger, J., Michelson, G.: Automated quality assessment of retinal fundus photos. Int. J. Comp. Assist. Radiol. Surg. **10**(6), 888–898 (2006)
15. Usher, D., Himaga, M., Dumskyj, M.: Automated assessment of digital fundus image quality using detected vessel area. In: Proceedings of Medical Image Understanding and Analysis, pp. 81–84 (2003)

Unsupervised Discovery of Emphysema Subtypes in a Large Clinical Cohort

Polina Binder[1]([✉]), Nematollah K. Batmanghelich[2], Raul San Jose Estepar[2], and Polina Golland[1]

[1] Computer Science and Artificial Intelligence Lab, EECS, MIT, Cambridge, USA
polinab@mit.edu
[2] Brigham and Womens Hospital, Harvard Medical School, Boston, USA

Abstract. Emphysema is one of the hallmarks of Chronic Obstructive Pulmonary Disorder (COPD), a devastating lung disease often caused by smoking. Emphysema appears on Computed Tomography (CT) scans as a variety of textures that correlate with disease subtypes. It has been shown that the disease subtypes and textures are linked to physiological indicators and prognosis, although neither is well characterized clinically. Most previous computational approaches to modeling emphysema imaging data have focused on supervised classification of lung textures in patches of CT scans. In this work, we describe a generative model that jointly captures heterogeneity of disease subtypes and of the patient population. We also describe a corresponding inference algorithm that simultaneously discovers disease subtypes and population structure in an unsupervised manner. This approach enables us to create image-based descriptors of emphysema beyond those that can be identified through manual labeling of currently defined phenotypes. By applying the resulting algorithm to a large data set, we identify groups of patients and disease subtypes that correlate with distinct physiological indicators.

1 Introduction

Chronic Obstructive Pulmonary Disorder (COPD) is a chronic lung disease characterized by poor airflow. One of the hallmarks of COPD is emphysema, i.e., destruction of lung alveoli and permanent enlargement of airspaces [1]. Several subtypes of emphysema have been identified and are commonly used for diagnosis and prediction of patient prognosis [2]. The disease subtypes have also been shown to correlate with genetic data and physiological indicators [1].

Emphysema appears on Computed Tomography (CT) scans as a variety of textures which are associated with clinically defined disease subtypes. However, there is substantial intra-reader and inter-reader variability when identifying subtypes in CT images [2]. Computational approaches to the classification of textures in CT scans promise to identify subtle textural differences beyond those that are visible to human readers. This nuanced information can be harnessed to produce well-defined, reproducible disease subtypes. Beyond fully 3D texture

© Springer International Publishing AG 2016
L. Wang et al. (Eds.): MLMI 2016, LNCS 10019, pp. 180–187, 2016.
DOI: 10.1007/978-3-319-47157-0_22

analysis, the additional benefits of computational approaches include the possibility of providing novel insights into the disease once the heterogeneity of the patient population is characterized.

We present a method that simultaneously detects distinct patient clusters and disease subtypes. The algorithm is based on a generative model that captures the underlying hypothesis about population structure and distributions of disease subtypes. We assume that each cluster of patients is associated with a distinct distribution of disease subtypes, which are based on features extracted from Computed Tomography scans [3]. We derive an inference algorithm that is based on variational Expectation-Maximization [4]. We apply the algorithm to a data set of 2457 thoracic CT scans and observe notable associations between physiological indicators and patient clusters and disease subtypes identified by the method. Further, we examine associations in simplified models that omit either patient clusters or disease subtypes to demonstrate the clinical advantage of the hierarchical model that includes both patient clusters and disease subtypes. We compare associations that are identified in the generative model to those found in a model where disease subtypes are discovered in a supervised manner.

Our approach departs from the majority of prior research that has focused on supervised classification of patches extracted from CT scans based on examples labeled by clinical experts [5,6]. An exception is a method for joint modeling of imaging and genetic data in the same clinical population [7]. By contrast, our work models only imaging data, but we explicitly detect and characterize homogeneous sub-populations defined by similar groups of disease subtypes, which opens directions for future analysis. An additional work similar to ours is found in [8], which discovers disease subtypes in an unsupervised manner. However, it was conducted on a smaller data set and does not model patient clusters.

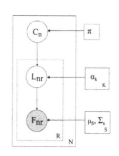

Fig. 1. Graphical representation of the generative model.

2   Model

Our generative model relies on the assumption that there are K underlying patient clusters, each characterized by a different distribution of disease subtypes. We use N to denote the total number of CT scans in the study. When processed, each scan is represented by R non-overlapping patches. Let S_{nr} be the patch around voxel r in patient n. Patches are entirely contained within a lung. We apply a chosen feature extraction method to S_{nr} to construct a feature vector F_{nr}. The feature vectors $\{F_{nr}\}$ serve as the input into our algorithm. In our experiments we use a combination of Grey Level Co-Occurrence Matrix (GLCM) [6] features and intensity histograms as feature descriptors which are both extracted from three-dimensional patches; the modeling approach readily accepts a broad range of descriptors.

The distribution of cluster assignments for any patient in the study is parametrized by π and is represented by a vector C_n for patient n. $C_{nk} = 1$ if patient n belongs to cluster k; $C_{nk} = 0$ otherwise. For all patients in cluster k the distribution of disease subtypes is parametrized by α_k and is represented by L_{nr} for patch r in patient n. Each patch belongs to one of S disease subtypes. $L_{nrs} = 1$ if the patch belongs to subtype s; $L_{nrs} = 0$ otherwise. We use a Gaussian distribution $\mathcal{N}(\cdot; \mu, \Sigma)$ with mean μ_s and covariance Σ_s to model feature vectors in the disease subtype s. The generative model can be summarized as follows (Fig. 1):

$$C_n \sim \prod_{k=1}^{K} \pi_k^{C_{nk}},$$

$$L_n | C_n \sim \prod_{k=1}^{K} \prod_{r=1}^{R} \prod_{s=1}^{S} (\alpha_{ks})^{L_{nrs} C_{nk}},$$

$$F_n | L_n \sim \prod_{s=1}^{S} \prod_{r=1}^{R} \mathcal{N}(F_{nr}; \mu_s, \Sigma_s)^{L_{nrs}}.$$

Each subject is viewed as an independent and identically distributed sample from this distribution, giving rise to the full likelihood model:

$$p(F, C, L; \alpha, \pi, \mu, \Sigma) = \prod_{n=1}^{N} \prod_{k=1}^{K} \prod_{r=1}^{R} \prod_{s=1}^{S} \left(\pi_k \alpha_{ks}^{L_{nrs}}\right)^{C_{nk}} \mathcal{N}(F_{nr}; \mu_s, \Sigma_s)^{L_{nrs}}.$$

Inference Algorithm. We set the number of patient clusters K and the number of disease subtypes S. The observed data consists of feature vectors $\{F_{nr}\}$ of N patients for whom we extracted features from R patches each. We aim to infer the most likely subtype L_{nr} for each patch r in patient n and the most likely cluster C_n for each patient n. Additionally, we estimate the parameters: the mixing proportions of the patient clusters π, the mixing proportions of the disease subtypes $\{\alpha_k\}$ for each patient cluster, and the means and variances $\{\mu_s, \Sigma_s\}$ of the image features for each disease subtype.

We perform inference via variational Expectation-Maximization (EM) [4]. Since computing expectation with respect to the full posterior distribution $p(L, C | F, \alpha, \pi, \mu, \Sigma)$ is intractable due to coupling between C and L, we approximate the posterior distribution with a product of two categorical distributions:

$$q(C, L; \psi, \theta) = q_C(C; \psi) q_L(L; \theta) = \prod_{n=1}^{N} \prod_{k=1}^{K} \psi_{nk}^{C_{nk}} \prod_{r=1}^{R} \prod_{s=1}^{S} \theta_{nrs}^{L_{nrs}}, \tag{1}$$

where ψ and θ are variational parameters. This simplifies the computation of the expectations.

In the variational approach, we iteratively optimize a lower bound for $\ln(p(F; \alpha, \pi, \mu, \Sigma))$ with respect to the parameters $\{\pi_k, \alpha_{ks}, \mu_s, \Sigma_s, \psi_{nk}, \theta_{nrs}\}$. This lower bound can be expressed as:

$$\ln(p(F; \alpha, \pi, \mu, \Sigma)) \geq E_q \left[\ln \frac{p(F, C, L; \alpha, \pi, \mu, \Sigma)}{q(C, L; \psi, \theta)} \right]. \tag{2}$$

We randomly initialize π and α, and then iterate between two steps until convergence. In the expectation step, we hold π, α, μ and Σ fixed and estimate the variational parameters ψ and θ to maximize the lower bound in Eq. (2) by iteratively applying the updates:

$$\psi_{nk} \propto \prod_{s=1}^{S} \prod_{r=1}^{R} \alpha_{ks}^{\theta_{nrs}}, \quad \text{s.t.} \quad \sum_{k=1}^{K} \psi_{nk} = 1,$$

$$\theta_{nrs} \propto \prod_{k=1}^{K} \alpha_{ks}^{\psi_{nk}}, \quad \text{s.t.} \quad \sum_{s=1}^{S} \theta_{nrs} = 1.$$

In the maximization step, we hold the values of ψ and θ fixed and estimate the model parameters, π, α, μ and Σ, that maximize the lower bound in Eq. (2) via the following update equations:

$$\pi_k = \frac{1}{N} \sum_{n=1}^{N} \psi_{nk},$$

$$\alpha_{ks} \propto \sum_{n=1}^{N} \psi_{nk} \sum_{r=1}^{R} \theta_{nrs}, \quad \text{s.t.} \quad \sum_{s=1}^{S} \alpha_{ks} = 1,$$

$$\mu_s = \frac{1}{N_s} \sum_{n=1}^{N} \sum_{r=1}^{R} \theta_{nsr} \cdot F_{nr}, \quad \text{where} \quad N_s = \sum_{n=1}^{N} \sum_{r=1}^{R} \theta_{nsr},$$

$$\Sigma_s = \frac{1}{N_s} \sum_{n=1}^{N} \sum_{r=1}^{R} \theta_{nsr} \cdot (F_{nr} - \mu_s) \cdot (F_{nr} - \mu_s)^T.$$

Once the parameter estimation process is complete, we determine C_n and L_{nr} by maximizing the approximate posterior distributions $q_C(C_n; \psi_n)$ and $q_L(L_{nr}; \theta_{nr})$ respectively.

3   Empirical Results

Data. We investigated the proposed method in the context of an imaging study that includes 2457 thoracic CT scans of smokers diagnosed with COPD [1]. COPDGene is a multi-center study that acquired CT scans, genetic data, and physiological indicators in COPD patients. The data was collected by 21 sites across the United States. The volumetric CT scans were obtained at full inhalation and at relaxed exhalation. Image reconstruction produces sub-millimeter slice thickness, and employs edge and smoothness enhancing filtering [1]. In addition, we have 1525 patches from the CT scans of 267 patients from this cohort that were manually assigned to clinically defined disease subtypes by an expert.

Parameter Selection. We randomly sampled 1000 non-overlapping patches from each patient. Emphysema has been described at the level of the secondary pulmonary lobules [5], therefore we select $11 \times 11 \times 11$ patches, which are approximately the size of this structure. There have been between four and 12 disease subtypes and between three and 10 patient clusters described in clinical literature [3,5]. We examine models with the number of patient clusters and disease subtypes in this range. We chose to further analyze the model with eight patient clusters and six disease subtypes, as this was the largest number of disease subtypes and patient clusters for which each patient cluster and disease subtype received at least five percent probability.

Feature Vectors. We employed 11-dimensional feature vectors, which were chosen based on their classification accuracy on the labeled patches in our data set when using the features as a texture descriptor. The first nine dimensions correspond to Grey Level Co-Occurrence Matrix (GLCM) features [6]. GLCMs represent the joint probability distribution of intensity values of pixel pairs in a given patch [6]. To construct this descriptor, the image is discretized into eight gray levels. The value of the entry at position (i, j) in the GLCM captures the proportion of pixel pairs at a given offset with the corresponding intensity pair values for $i, j \in \{1...8\}$. To obtain a degree of rotational invariance, we averaged the GLCMs over uniformly distributed directions in three dimensions. We extracted nine features from these matrices to construct the descriptor: contrast, dissimilarity, homogeneity, correlation, entropy, energy, cluster shade, cluster prominence and maximum probability [6]. The next two dimensions of the feature vector correspond histogram bins of the voxel intensities within the patch.

3.1 Results

Disease Subtypes. Figure 2 illustrates example patches for each of the identified disease subtypes. A confusion matrix between the disease subtypes and the clinical labels is shown in Table 1. On the labeled portion of our data set, we found that 67 % of patches that were labeled as clinically normal were placed in the same dis-

Table 1. Confusion matrix between clinically defined subtypes and automatically detected subtypes. The values in the table correspond to the number of patches with the corresponding clinical label and detected subtype.

Clinical label	ST 1	ST 2	ST 3	ST 4	ST 5	ST 6
Normal lung tissue	339	0	1	103	7	61
Panlobular emph.	1	146	9	0	0	0
Paraseptal emph.	16	53	100	48	20	6
Mild centrilobular emph.	96	3	11	68	3	30
Mod. centrilobular emph.	69	74	112	28	4	2
Sev. centrilobular emph.	8	57	49	0	0	0

ease subtype by our algorithm, and clinically normal patches represent 64 % of all labeled patches within this disease subtype. Panlobular and paraseptal emphysema correspond to disease subtype 2 and subtype 3 respectively. Our results suggest that centrilobular emphysema is a mixture of identified disease subtypes 1, 2, 3 and 4.

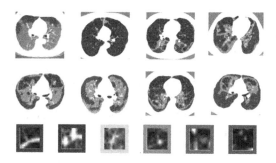

Fig. 2. Top two rows: example CT scans from each of the eight patient clusters identified by our algorithm. Colors correspond to disease subtypes identified by our algorithm. Bottom row: patches from the six disease subtypes identified by our algorithm. (Color figure online)

Spatial Contiguity. Emphysema clusters spatially in the lungs, as do the disease subtypes our algorithm identifies, as can be seen in Fig. 2. Each voxel in every lung was labeled independently based on the most likely subtype it would belong to under our model, without any enforced smoothing. We evaluated spatial contiguity by permutation testing [9]. For each voxel labeled by our algorithm we compute the proportion of neighboring voxels that belong to the same disease subtype. We average this value over the entire lung to obtain a spatial contiguity score. To obtain a distribution of the score under the null hypothesis we assigned voxels within the lungs to random disease subtypes 1000 times for each scan while maintaining the proportion of disease subtypes for each lung. We found that across all CT scans, the spatial contiguity scores produced by our algorithm are greater than the maximal values in the corresponding null distribution, corresponding to rejecting the null hypothesis with $p < 0.001$.

Associations with Physiological Indicators. We emphasize that the physiological indicators are not available to the algorithm when fitting the generative model to the image data and therefore provide an indirect validation of the model's clinical relevance. We quantify the associations between the structure detected by our method and physiological indicators relevant to COPD: six minute walking distance, body mass index (BMI), forced vital capacity (FVC), forced expiratory volume (FEV), change in FVC value from treatment, the ratio between the FEV and FVC values, and the number of years smoked. We ran our algorithm on a randomly selected half of our scans and labeled the remaining scans based on the estimated model parameters. In particular, we assigned each patient to the most likely cluster and constructed an empirical distribution of disease subtypes for the patient based on the image patches. We repeated this procedure 100 times to estimate variability in the results.

We constructed three baseline models by eliminating patient clusters $(K = 1)$ or disease subtypes $(S = 1)$ or both $(K = 1, S = 1)$. In the last case, we extract feature vectors from patches in each patient, and then average and normalize the feature vectors in each patient to produce a single patient-specific feature vector. A fourth baseline method was constructed by identifying the disease subtypes in a supervised manner. In this case, we utilized the same feature vectors as previously described, and performed classification with Support Vector Machines (SVMs) trained on the labeled patches to assign 1000 random patches in each lung to one of six clinically identified subtypes. We learned the patient clusters in an unsupervised manner as in the fully unsupervised model.

To quantify the associations between distributions of disease subtypes or the averaged normalized feature vector for a patient and a physiological indicator we perform linear regression. The strength of the correlation is quantified via the R^2 value. The association between patient clusters and physiological indicators is quantified via the normalized mutual information score [10]. Different metrics are used to quantify the associations between patient clusters and proportions of disease subtypes or feature vectors, as the former is a discrete label while the last two are continuous quantities. These associations were identified on the portion of the data set that was not used to construct the model.

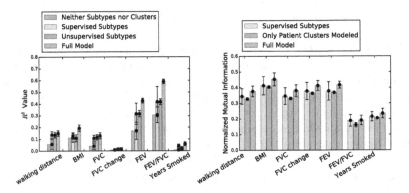

Fig. 3. Left: R^2 value between the distributions of disease subtypes (1st, 3rd, and 4th model) or feature vectors (2nd model) and physiological indicators. Right: Normalized Mutual Information between patient clusters and physiological indicators.

Figure 3 reports the associations for all models. These results demonstrate the advantage of modeling both patient clusters and disease subtypes. We observe that there is a stronger association between physiological indicators and patient clusters in the full model than in the model with only clusters. For all physiological indicators, there is a higher association with the distributions of disease subtypes in the full model than in the model with only disease subtypes. This demonstrates that modeling patient clusters produces more clinically relevant distributions of disease subtypes in each patient. The model without patient clusters or disease subtypes exhibits even weaker associations than a model with only disease subtypes.

Figure 3 demonstrates the advantage of discovering the disease subtypes in an unsupervised manner. In the full model, we obtain stronger associations than in the model where disease subtypes are found in a supervised manner. This is partially explained by the fact that feature selection was performed to optimize classification performance on supervised patches and additional structure is obtained in the unsupervised discovery of patient clusters and disease subtypes.

4   Conclusions

We presented an unsupervised framework for the discovery of disease subtypes within emphysema and of patient clusters that are characterized by distinct distributions of such subtypes. We built a generative model that parametrizes the assignment of voxels in CT scans to disease subtypes and the assignment of patients to clusters. The associations between the patient clusters and physiological indicators and distributions of disease subtypes and physiological indicators illustrate the clinical relevance of the detected heterogeneity in the patient cohort.

The patient clusters that our model produces merit further exploration. It would be worthwhile to examine their correlations to genetic markers. An additional extension is to directly examine whether different patient clusters exhibit distinct clinical prognoses or respond differently to clinical interventions.

References

1. Regan, E.A., Hokanson, J.E., et al.: Genetic epidemiology of COPD (COPDGene) study design. COPD **7**(1), 32–43 (2010)
2. Aziz, Z., Wells, A., et al.: HRCT diagnosis of diffuse parenchymal lung disease: inter-observer variation. Thorax **59**(6), 506–511 (2004)
3. Raghunath, S., Rajagopalan, S., et al.: Quantitative stratification of diffuse parenchymal lung diseases. PloS ONE **9**, e93229 (2014)
4. Blaiotta, C., Cardoso, M.J., et al.: Variational inference for image segmentation. Comput. Vis. Image Underst. (2016)
5. Mendoza, C., Washko, G., et al.: Emphysema quantification in a multi-scanner HRCT cohort using local intensity distributions. In: 2012 9th IEEE International Symposium on Biomedical Imaging (ISBI), pp. 474–477 (2012)
6. Prasad, M., Sowmya, A., et al.: Multi-level classification of emphysema in HRCT lung images. Pattern Anal. Appl. **11**(1), 9–20 (2006)
7. Batmanghelich, N.K., Saeedi, A., Cho, M., Estepar, R.S.J., Golland, P.: Generative method to discover genetically driven image biomarkers. In: Ourselin, S., Alexander, D.C., Westin, C.-F., Cardoso, M.J. (eds.) IPMI 2015. LNCS, vol. 9123, pp. 30–42. Springer, Heidelberg (2015). doi:10.1007/978-3-319-19992-4_3
8. Hame, Y., Angelini, E.D., et al.: Sparse sampling and unsupervised learning of lung texture patterns in pulmonary emphysema: MESA COPD study. In: 2015 IEEE 12th International Symposium on Biomedical Imaging (ISBI), pp. 109–113. IEEE (2015)
9. Efron, B., Tibshirani, R.J.: An Introduction to the Bootstrap. Chapman & Hall, New York (1993)
10. Vinh, N.X., Epps, J., et al.: Information theoretic measures for clusterings comparison: variants, properties, normalization and correction for chance. J. Mach. Learn. Res. **11**, 2537–2854 (2010)

Tree-Based Transforms for Privileged Learning

Mehdi Moradi[1]([✉]), Tanveer Syeda-Mahmood[1], and Soheil Hor[2]

[1] IBM Almaden Research Center, San Jose, CA, USA
mmoradi@us.ibm.com
[2] University of British Columbia, Vancouver, Canada

Abstract. In many machine learning applications, samples are characterized by a variety of data modalities. In some instances, the training and testing data might include overlapping, but not identical sets of features. In this work, we describe a versatile decision forest methodology to train a classifier based on data that includes several modalities, and then deploy it for use with test data that only presents a subset of the modalities. To this end, we introduce the concept of cross-modality tree feature transforms. These are feature transformations that are guided by how a different feature partitions the training data. We have used the case of staging cognitive impairments to show the benefits of this approach. We train a random forest model that uses both MRI and PET, and can be tested on data that only includes MRI features. We show that the model provides an 8 % improvement in accuracy of separating of progressive cognitive impairments from stable impairments, compared to a model that uses MRI only for training and testing.

1 Introduction

One of the basic assumptions of supervised learning is that samples in the training and testing data are described by the same set of features. If a small number of samples randomly miss a number of features, then imputation methods such as K nearest neighbors or statistical modeling can be used to satisfy the need for consistency of samples. However, imputation fails if the discrepancy of the feature vectors is systematic. Consider this example: positron emission tomography (PET) and magnetic resonance tomography (MRI) have both been studied for staging of cognitive impairments. There is a consensus that PET is a more accurate indicator of the kind of cognitive impairment that will progress to Alzheimer's disease and dementia. Nevertheless, MRI is more routinely prescribed and performed due to the high cost of PET imaging which has primarily remained in research domain. As a result, although training data on PET and MRI is available from large research institutions, a classifier trained with the traditional assumptions of machine learning on PET and MRI data will not be useful in most cases that present only the MRI data.

The central goal of our work is to use all the features available for samples in the training phase, even those that are systematically missing in the testing/deployment environment, and find a solution to test the resulting model

© Springer International Publishing AG 2016
L. Wang et al. (Eds.): MLMI 2016, LNCS 10019, pp. 188–195, 2016.
DOI: 10.1007/978-3-319-47157-0_23

on only a subset of features. Using the Alzheimer's disease example, this would mean that the patients in clinical practice would go through MRI imaging only, but could benefit from a model that was trained on PET and MRI, and is more accurate in disease characterization than a model trained on MRI data alone.

The problem of missing data in the context of random forests has been addressed for randomly missing features in methods such as CART algorithm [4] and rfImpute [1], but not in the context of complete lack of one modality at test time. In this paper we report a method for transfer of knowledge from one set of features to another, in the context of decision forests. This method is based on building functions in form of shallow decision trees that map feature values to a categorical space, guided by a different group of features. We call these mapping functions tree feature transforms. The resulting features are used along with the subset of features shared between test and training stages to train a decision forest. Using decision trees as feature generators is not common. Recently, the idea of stacked random forests was introduced. This uses the probability distributions at the leaf level of one tree as features for a second decision tree [2]. That work, however, does not provide any recourse for mapping a specific subset of features. Other recent work in this area includes a methodology to build a tree that mimics the divisions of another tree, from root to leaf, using a different set of features [3]. That work addresses the problem of limited data from one modality at the time of training. The current work solves the inverse of that problem. In the area of general machine learning, the lack of a modality at testing time has been dealt with under the topic of "privileged learning" mainly for support vector machines [6]. To the best of our knowledge, we are the first to address this problem within the paradigm of decision forests.

2   Method

Let us first formally describe the problem. We assume that the training data, M, consists of samples $M = (m_1, m_2, \ldots, m_{N_m})$, each described by the feature vectors of form F_m of size N_m, and each assigned a label C_i. Within F_m, there is a subset of features, $F_s \in F_m$ that is available in the testing stage. Also in most practical situations, the features that are in F_m, but not in F_s, are among the most discriminating features. We need to train a classifier using F_m, which is capable of predicting C for a given test sample that is only described by F_s features. For this to be of any practical value, the classifier should be more accurate than one trained and tested on F_s in predicting the label. Before describing the solution, note that the training data too could include features that only present F_s and lack the rest of features in F_m. Our method provides a way to benefit from this data as well. As Fig. 1 illustrates, the proposed methodology builds feature transforms that map one feature type inspired by other feature types, using the concept of scandent tree proposed in [3].

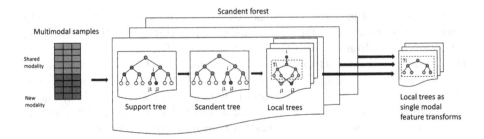

Fig. 1. Forming cross-modality tree-based feature transforms.

2.1   Building a Support Forest Using F_m

Similar to [3], we start by building a random forest based on bagging from the full feature set, F_m, and optimizing through leave-one-out cross-validation in training data. We call this a "support forest". As an advantage of having all the important features, trees formed by the full feature set are expected to partition the feature space very effectively. The method used in this paper for growing of the support trees is based on the implementation of CART algorithm in the package "rpart" in R language [5].

2.2   Growing Cross-Modality Tree-Based Feature Transforms

The process of feature space division in the support trees can be considered as grouping the training data set M to different subsets. Let us define the subset of the samples of M in the i_{th} node as M_i and the feature used for sample space division at node i as f_i. Intuitively, the idea of the scandent tree algorithm is to break the support tree into subtrees that partition the sample space either using only the missing modalities or only the shared modality. And then replace these sub-trees with a shared modality local tree that divides the samples in a similar way. In order to reduce the number of consecutive estimations, it is critical that the shared modality local trees estimate the largest subtrees in the support tree that hold these assumptions. We name the nodes that define the boundaries of such trees as "link nodes". In other words, given the F_s subset feature of interest for testing phase, we define node i of a support tree as a link node if it is either the root node, or f_i belongs to a different feature set from f_{i-1}. Node i is a link node if and only if:

Node i is the root node,

or

$$f_i \in F_s \quad \text{and} \quad f_{i-1} \notin F_s$$

or

$$f_i \notin F_s \quad \text{and} \quad f_{i-1} \in F_s$$

For each division node i in the set of the link nodes of the support tree, there exists a set of nearest child link nodes and child leaves $j_1, j_2, \dots j_{ki}$. We define

T_i as an optimum tree that can divide the set of training samples at node i (M_i) to the set of training samples at each child node (M_j) using only the feature set F_s. The pseudo-code for forming all these trees is as follows:

For each link node i in the support tree,
{

       For each sample n in M_i and each node j in set of
       nearest child link nodes and child leaves of node i
       {

              if $n \in M_j$,
              $C'_{i,n} = j$

       }
       Grow T_i, as optimum tree that for each sample n in M_i,
       predicts $C'_{i,n}$ using only F_s.

}

The above algorithm forms local trees T_i for each node i that divide M_i to the child subsets M_j, using only the shared modality features F_s. Here C' is a new categorical label-set defined for the corresponding local tree. For each sample in the parent node, the C' is assigned in a way that the samples belonging to a specific child node j are mapped to the same category within C'. For each node i, if $f_i \notin F_s$, then T_i is optimized to form the smallest tree that can divide the sample space in a similar manner to the support tree. The set of T_i's are critical for transfer of knowledge in our framework.

It is notable that by replacing all divisions within the support trees where $f_i \notin F_s$ with their equivalent T_i's, one can obtain a new tree/forest that can be tested on F_s features only. In a recent work, reported in [3], this has been used to form a tree that mimics the support tree. To obtain a forest that transfers the value of the multimodal dataset into the shared modality environment, it is tempting to simply replace all the trees in a forest trained on the available multimodal training data with their corresponding shared modality trees. However, this approach fails in practice. This is because many of the divisions of the support trees predicted by F_m features might not be accurately predictable by the F_s feature-set.

Instead, we choose an approach inspired by the use of decision trees as feature maps. We use the set of local trees (T_i's) from all the trees of the support forest as tree-based feature-maps. *Each T_i is a tree which maps F_s to a new space defined by the corresponding C' set. This means that each T_i yields a categorical feature to describe each sample. Then we use F_s along with the extended tree-based features, to grow an improved forest.*

This method has a few advantages. First, because at each split of each tree in the enhanced forest, the tree growth algorithm searches for the best division feature among both the F_s features and the new transform features, the resulting tree is expected to be equally or more accurate than a tree grown using only the F_s features. Second, it is commonly difficult to build a large dataset with F_m.

Therefore, the T_i's are formed by a potentially small training dataset. However, in the third stage of training in our method, when transform features are combined with F_s, one can use a larger training dataset that only presents F_s. This means that in building the final forest, the feature selection criteria (Gini impurity or information gain) is calculated based on a large training, albeit with fewer features. In other words, the final model uses the features inspired by a potentially small training dataset that includes all F_m, but it is completely randomized and optimized based on a large dataset with only F_s features.

Why does cross-modality transform work? Assuming that two features are dependent over the whole sample space (unconditional dependence) also guarantees that they are predictable by each other over a sub-space of the sample space. But if the dependence is conditional, they cannot be universally predicted by each other. Since each cross-modality transform is built to replace a small part of the support tree, we rely on local dependence of the two feature sets and do not require a global dependence. In other words, the idea of cross-modality tree transforms works because at each node, the tree asks a fairly simple question from the training data. Therefore, the second modality could potentially answer that question the same way, even though they two modalities might not be in global agreement. However, if the training data size is very small, the local predictions at the nodes of the support tree are based on a small number of samples. As a result, many of the produced transforms could be unhelpful. The bagging in the final stage can partially weed out these. But one can also rank them based on a measure of discrimination and perform thresholding.

2.3   Implementation Details

For building the support trees, we randomly bagged 2/3 of the training data and randomly selected the square root of the dimension of the feature set as the feature bag. Considering the large number of trees in the support forest, we obtain a large number of transform trees. This can flood the original shared modality features during the training of the final forest. So we filter the new features by a conventional feature selection algorithm, namely based on the feature importance measure in a decision forest. We apply feature bagging separately to the set of the original F_s features and the transform features, and then merge them together to form the feature bag used for training the final model. If M is small, the T_i's could be prone to overfitting if only the few samples in the corresponding link nodes are used for training T_i. To avoid this issue, we use all of the available samples (M) for training of each transform tree by running all of them through the corresponding sub-tree of the support tree. This will give each sample in M a label from the set C'. The F_s part of all samples in M can then be used to optimize the T_i transform.

3   Evaluation Data and Methods

We test the proposed method on a dataset from Alzheimer's Disease Neuroimaging Initiative (ADNI) database (adni.loni.usc.edu). We have access to 218 cases with both MRI and PET, and 508 cases consisting of patients with MRI data. This includes the MRI data from the 218 multimodal samples. The MRI features are volume measurements of six ROIs in the human brain (ventricles, hippocampus, whole-brain, entorhinal, fusiform and mid-temporal) and intracranial volume (ICV) in mm^3. The PET feature set consists of FluoroDeoxyGlucose (FDG) measurement and AV45 uptake measurement. The outcome labels include cognitively normal patients (NL), patients with confirmed dementia (AD) and patients with mild cognitive impairment (MCI). The MCI group is divided into progressive (pMCI) that eventually converts to dementia and, stable MCI (sMCI). MCI is considered progressive if it converts to dementia in less than 36 months.

The distribution of different outcome classes in the two datasets is as follows: for the normal class we have 178 samples with MRI only and 18 samples with MRI and PET. For the dementia class we have 108 MRI only and 29 MRI and PET cases, for the sMCI class we have 126 MRI cases and 144 MRI and PET samples. And for the pMCI class we have 96 MRI cases versus 27 MRI plus PET samples. In other words, the MRI+PET dataset is smaller than the MRI only dataset, and it also does not have the same distribution of outcome classes. This makes the data fusion between the two datasets extremely difficult with traditional approaches such as imputation. We examine the performance of the proposed method by reporting AUC for three classification scenarios: NL versus pMCI, sMCI versus AD, and sMCI versus pMCI. In all experiments, we use all of the PET+MRI data for training, plus 80 % of the MRI only data. The test data is 20 % of the MRI only data and the results are reported on five-fold partitioning of the MRI only data between test and training.

We compare the performance of our method first with a baseline method of training and testing only on MRI, keeping a similar partitioning of the samples between training and testing. Another potential comparison of performance could be between the proposed method and imputation of the missing features at test time. This is vastly inferior in performance. For a more reasonable comparison in the context of decision forest methods, consider that our method is a tree-based feature transform. Therefore, we compare it with other similar decision forest methods that involve a transformation. These include (1) PC-forest: using principal components (PCs) of the shared modality (MRI) features used along with the original shared modality features for training an enhanced-forest baseline, and (2) shared modality (MRI) transform forest: uses tree-based transforms generated using only F_s features. This is similar to stacking forests. However, we use categorical, as opposed to continuous probability features unlike [2]. In this approach, decision trees are used as transform generators, but the PET features are ignored.

4   Results

The performance of the proposed and compared methods are evaluated for three classification tasks: discrimination of normal samples from progressive MCI

(NL vs. pMCI), discrimination of stable MCI from progressive MCI (sMCI vs. pMCI) and stable MCI from dementia (sMCI vs. AD).

Table 1. Accuracy (Acc), sensitivity (Sens), specificity (Spec) and area under ROC curve (AUC) of the proposed methods and the baseline forest for the NL vs. pMCI

	Acc	Sens	Spec	AUC
Single modal forest using MRI only	0.74	0.66	0.79	0.78
PC forest	0.77	0.88	0.75	0.78
Tree-based transforms using only the MRI	0.78	0.69	0.84	0.82
Cross-modality transform	0.79	0.75	0.81	0.84

Five-fold cross-validated results for the baseline single modal forest, PC forest, single modal transform forest, and the cross-modality transform forest for NL vs. pMCI classification task are shown in Table 1. The transform-based forests significantly outperform the baseline single modal forest and the PC forest. The difference between the baseline and the transform methods is statistically significant for both the shared modality (MRI) transform and for the cross-modality transform ($p < 0.01$). However, the improvement in the performance achieved by the PC-based features compared to baseline is not statistically significant. The cross-modality transforms are more effective compared to the single modal transforms. This difference is significant ($p < 0.05$). As listed in Table 2, for the classification task of stable MCI versus dementia, the same trends hold ($p < 0.01$).

Table 2. Accuracy (Acc), sensitivity (Sens), specificity (Spec) and area under ROC curve (AUC) of the proposed methods and the baseline forest for the sMCI vs. AD

	Acc	Sens	Spec	AUC
Single modal forest using MRI only	0.73	0.82	0.70	0.81
PC forest	0.75	0.76	0.75	0.84
Tree-based transforms using only the MRI	0.78	0.73	0.86	0.87
Cross-modality transform	0.80	0.74	0.90	0.89

The third classification task which separates sMCI from pMCI cases is potentially the most clinically relevant model. As Table 3 shows, the tree-based transforms outperform a simple single modal forest ($p < 0.01$) and the PC forest provides an insignificant enhancement. Similar to the previous experiments, the cross-modality transforms yield a larger AUC than single modal ones ($p < 0.01$). The accuracy improves from 74 % to 82 % with the introduction of the cross-modality transforms compared to the baseline method (Table 3).

Table 3. Accuracy (Acc), sensitivity (Sens), specificity (Spec) and area under ROC curve (AUC) of the proposed methods and the baseline forest for the sMCI vs. pMCI

	Acc	Sens	Spec	AUC
Single modal forest using MRI only	0.74	0.71	0.74	0.81
PC forest	0.76	0.77	0.75	0.82
Tree-based transforms using only the MRI	0.78	0.82	0.75	0.85
Cross-modality transform	0.82	0.83	0.80	0.87

5 Conclusions and Future Work

In this paper we addressed the problem of inconsistency between training and testing data in decision forest learning algorithms in a scenario where test samples are non-randomly missing a large portion of the most discriminating features. We described a novel learning method for training on multiple modalities and testing on one modality. We investigated the performance of the proposed method for classification on the ADNI dataset. We used samples with both MRI and PET features for training a classifier that only needs the MRI features at test time. The solution presented here relies on the new concept of cross-modality tree-based transforms. We showed that in all clinically relevant questions related to the ADNI dataset, the use of cross-modality tree-based transforms results in an improved performance in comparison with methods that rely only on MRI features. In other words, we have effectively transferred the value of PET imaging to an MRI only dataset through our methodology.

While we have described our method here for a bimodality situation, the extension to more complicated and flexible arrangements can be easily achieved. If a sample is described with a variety of modalities, one can build transforms that map any given modality to a new categorical space, guided by a number of other modalities. A part of our future work will be focused on streamlining this process in multimodal situations.

References

1. Breiman, L.: Random forests. Mach. Learn. **45**(1), 5–32 (2001)
2. Cao, Y., Wang, H., Moradi, M., Prasanna, P., Syeda-Mahmood, T.F.: Fracture detection in X-ray images through stacked random forests feature fusion. In: IEEE ISBI, pp. 801–805 (2015)
3. Hor, S., Moradi, M.: Scandent tree: a random forest learning method for incomplete multimodal datasets. In: Navab, N., Hornegger, J., Wells, W.M., Frangi, A.F. (eds.) MICCAI 2015. LNCS, vol. 9349, pp. 694–701. Springer, Heidelberg (2015). doi:10. 1007/978-3-319-24553-9_85
4. Steinberg, D., Colla, P.: Cart: classification and regression trees. Top Ten Algorithms Data Min. **9**, 179 (2009)
5. Therneau, T.M., Atkinson, B., Ripley, B.: RPART: recursive partitioning. R package version 3.1-46. Ported to R by Brian Ripley. 3 (2010)
6. Vapnik, V., Izmailov, R.: Learning using privileged information: similarity control and knowledge transfer. J. Mach. Learn. Res. **16**, 2023–2049 (2015)

Automated 3D Ultrasound Biometry Planes Extraction for First Trimester Fetal Assessment

Hosuk Ryou[1]($\boxtimes$), Mohammad Yaqub[1], Angelo Cavallaro[2],
Fenella Roseman[2], Aris Papageorghiou[2], and J. Alison Noble[1]

[1] Institute of Biomedical Engineering, Department of Engineering Science,
University of Oxford, Oxford, UK
hosuk.ryou@eng.ox.ac.uk
[2] Nuffield Department of Obstetrics and Gynaecology,
University of Oxford, Oxford, UK

Abstract. In this paper, we present a fully automated machine-learning based solution to localize the fetus and extract the best fetal biometry planes for the head and abdomen from $11–13^{+6days}$ week 3D fetal ultrasound (US) images. Our method to localize the whole fetus in the sagittal plane utilizes Structured Random Forests (SRFs) and classical Random Forests (RFs). A transfer learning Convolutional Neural Network (CNNs) is then applied to axial images to localize one of three classes (head, body and non-fetal). Finally, the best fetal head and abdomen planes are automatically extracted based on clinical knowledge of the position of the fetal biometry planes within the head and body. Our hybrid method achieves promising localization of the best biometry fetal planes with 1.6 mm and 3.4 mm for head and abdomen plane localization respectively compared to the best manually chosen biometry planes.

Keywords: 3D ultrasound · First-trimester scan · Random Forests · Convolutional Neural Networks · Fetal plane localization

1 Introduction

Routine first trimester US screening is performed in most developed countries at $11–13^{+6days}$ weeks of fetal gestational age [1]. The aims of this scan are to confirm fetal viability and detect multiple pregnancy; and to screen major abnormalities such as chromosomal defects [2]. Early detection of major fetal abnormalities is important because early termination of pregnancy is associated with lower risks to the mother [3]. Hence, there is interest in investigating whether some of the diagnostic checks performed at the mid-trimester scan can be brought forward to first trimester screening. To allow this, fetal diagnostic planes have to be first detected by the clinician. This task is challenging for clinicians at early gestation. The automation of such task is the focus of this paper.

Electronic supplementary material The online version of this chapter (doi:10.1007/978-3-319-47157-0_24) contains supplementary material, which is available to authorized users.

© Springer International Publishing AG 2016
L. Wang et al. (Eds.): MLMI 2016, LNCS 10019, pp. 196–204, 2016.
DOI: 10.1007/978-3-319-47157-0_24

First trimester screening is traditionally done using 2D US imaging. The advent of 3D fetal US scanning has some potential benefits as it is possible to reconstruct anatomical planes after image acquisition. In addition, while several 2D images have to be obtained to visualize all important fetal anatomical landmarks, several fetal body parts can be imaged at once using one 3D US image which has the potential to reduce examination times and hence improve clinical workflow. For example, Dyson et al. [4] showed that the use of 3D US images provided additional information in 51 % of 103 anomalies when compared with 2D US alone. However in the first trimester, fetal organs are smaller compared to the second and third trimesters. Therefore, to allow for proper assessment of abnormalities, the detection of consistent and accurate biometry fetal planes is needed before performing measurements.

With the overall aim to aid sonographers in first trimester US image interpretation, we present here a method to detect the best biometry fetal head and abdominal planes, which are presented for sonographer guidance [1]. Specifically, we propose fetal localization in the sagittal plane using an object proposal approach and SRFs as a pre-processing step. Having localized the fetal region of interest, we partition it into two parts - head and body - using transfer learning based CNNs [5]. The best biometry planes for the head and abdomen are extracted by utilizing clinical knowledge of the position of fetal biometry planes within the structures. We compare our automatic method with manually selected planes by an experienced clinician.

2 Related Work

There are actually a number of methods proposed for the detection from fetal US data [6–8]. Maraci et al. [6], for example, used dynamic texture analysis and Support Vector Machines (SVM) for classification of each frames from 2D US videos in second trimester. Chen et al. [8] used transferred recurrent neural network to automatically detect the standard plane for head and abdomen. These methods showed promising results, however, their data was taken based on fetal axial planes which means the fetal parts cover most of the image which makes it less challenging to detect the fetus. Most of all, our data does not require time to search for each fetal parts since it is 3D. In addition, the gestational age range was at later trimester which in general makes the fetal US structure clearer. On the other hand, our data is taken based on Crown Rump Length (CRL) protocol and we are focused on first trimester fetal data. Since the fetal volumes are acquired in the sagittal plane to allow all the fetus to fit in the volume, fetal structures typically appear smaller than non-fetal parts.

3 Localization of the Fetus in the Sagittal Plane

In our solution, the first task is to remove the non-fetal parts to simplify the localization of the fetus. Specifically, we localize the bounding box which encloses the fetus in the sagittal plane. We exploit the fact that the boundary between amniotic fluid and the fetus is generally clear. Therefore, a method that exploits these sharp boundaries is developed to facilitate localizing the fetus by guiding the bounding box localization around the fetus. The main issue with relying on fetal edges is the fact that the boundary between the back of the fetus and non-fetal tissue is typically ambiguous. To address this, we propose a method which learns the best bounding boundary box from a set of candidate boxes. The following two subsections describe our proposed method.

3.1 Edge Detection Using Structured Random Forests

Inspired by Zitnick, et al. [9], we propose a method which generates a number of bounding boxes as object proposals based on edge detection using SRFs [10]. SRFs directly predict the local structure of an image patch by using structural information of pixel neighborhoods to focus on certain patterns in the image patch. This produces much cleaner edges which in turn provides better bounding boxes. In this work, we used a 48×48 image patch size to capture more global structure appearance rather than local since small edges are less important for detecting the boundary of the fetus in our application. We used intensity, gradient magnitudes and gradient orientations features to train SRFs.

3.2 Detection of the Fetus Region-of-Interest

Given the edges from an SRF, a score to measure the number of edges enclosed within the region of interest (ROI) compared to the number of edges overlapping the ROI boundary is computed [9]. The larger the score the more enclosed object within the box. Relying on the box with the largest score to identify the best enclosing box around the fetus does not guarantee a proper localization of the fetus. Therefore, a set of candidate boxes are retained and the appearance of the best box which surrounds the fetus is learnt using a RF classifier.

In the RFs classifier [11] which learns the appearance of the best bounding box, we use unary, binary feature from both raw and signed symmetry-mapped images, and also use Haar-based features only from raw images. Signed symmetry-mapped images are pre-processed images that show local phase information such as local maximum and minimum of intensity. They are known to be robust to speckle and the low contrast nature of US images [7]. With this classifier, we classify the boxes into two classes: the box with the whole fetus (positive) and the box without the whole fetus (negative). Within the positive boxes, the top three boxes with the largest class probabilities are chosen. Empirically, using more than three boxes worsen the accuracy because of using more irrelevant boxes. Therefore, we only used the top three boxes in this work. The final bounding box is then found using the following empirical approach to ensure that the final box contains the whole fetus without losing any fetal parts. The average box from the three candidates is computed and the resulting box is considered correctly localized if the Intersection over Union (IoU) ≥ 0.5 and $\frac{Intersection}{Ground-truth} \geq 0.95$ which seemed visually acceptable.

4   Detection of the Best Head and Abdominal Planes

Given the best bounding box placement of the sagittal plane, the US volume is cropped in the axial plane to reduce the search space for the best axial biometry planes. We empirically chose the width of the cropped volume based on the box height as shown in Fig. 1.

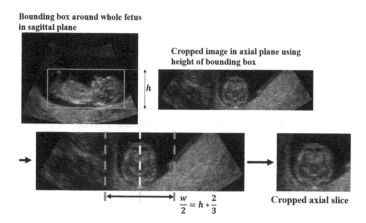

Fig. 1. Based on the box height, the width of the image in axial plane can be calculated as (4/3) times the height centered at the middle of the image. Using these, we obtain final cropped axial slice.

Once the range of axial slices where the fetus exists is detected, we classify the fetal axial slices into three classes: head, body and non-fetal. We then search for the best biometry head plane among head candidates only and the best abdominal biometry plane among abdominal candidates only. In the following two subsections, we describe these two steps in detail.

4.1   Fetal-Partitioning via Transfer Learning CNNs

In this step, we aim to partition the fetal axial slices into three classes: head, body and non-fetal. It is important that the slices are classified into the correct class so that a good partition can be obtained. We address this task as a classification problem using CNNs [12]. CNNs has advantages that it automatically learns the visual feature descriptors that are invariant to the translation. However, medical imaging applications, such as this work, usually use small datasets due to ethics approval constraints or availability of data only from small clinical trials. Hence, there is no guarantee that a CNN will satisfactorily solve the problem. Therefore, in this work, we propose to use transfer learning [5] to transfer learnt-features from a different pre-trained network and then fine-tune the CNN on our dataset to reduce overfitting. Also, it can reduce the time required to build the base networks. In this paper, we use a pre-trained network trained on a second-trimester fetal US data [13]. In addition, the network in [13] initialized its layers from AlexNet [12]. Since we transfer the learnt features from the second trimester fetal US dataset, one may assert that the extracted features should be useful for our US data. Our network consists of 5 convolutional layers and two fully connected layers that have 4096 neurons. We use max pooling layers to non-linearly downsample the feature maps. The output of the last fully connected layer is fed to a Softmax layer (multinomial logistic regression) which is used as a cost function.

For this task, it is also important that the biometry planes for head and abdomen must be within the predicted ranges for the head and body respectively.

4.2   Detection of Best Plane for Fetal Head and Abdomen Biometry

Based on the partitioned regions of the fetal slices, we use a greedy approach to find the best plane for both the head and abdomen. From the training data, we perform a linear regression to predict the distance of the best head plane from the approximate fetal crown as a function of the length of the head. Similarly, we perform another linear regression for the best abdominal plane from the approximate fetal rump as a function of the length of the body.

During testing, as shown in Fig. 2, we first find the set of axial planes which belongs to the head and body. We then get the distribution of each set to estimate whether the head is located on the left or right side of the image. We then exploit the anatomical constraint that if the head is found to be located to the left, random body slices should not appear on the left side of the image. Using this constraint, image slices located on the left which have been previously classified as body are reassigned to the head class. Based on this result, we then apply linear regression to locate the best plane for the head and abdomen.

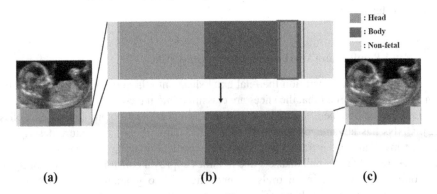

Fig. 2. Exploit the anatomical constraint. (a) Acquire the set of axial planes which belong to the head and body. (b) Misclassified slices (red box) are corrected since the head is on the left according to the partitioning result. (c) The final partitioning result. (Color figure online)

5   Experiments

The volumetric US data used in this work was acquired in the same clinical protocol which is used to image the 2D CRL view [1]. This makes our solution consistent with the current clinical workflow in the standard dating scan. During 3D image acquisition, the whole fetus must be present and the fetus has to be in neutral position [1]. The first trimester fetal volumes were obtained from participating mothers in the INTERGROWTH-21st [14]. Image resolution was 0.33 mm^3. Images were acquired following a standardized protocol which is similar to the acquisition protocol in the current clinical practice. This ensures that the fetus is facing upward and in a neutral position as mentioned in Sect. 3. We acquired total 64 3D US first trimester volume. The axial slices from a volume which belong to the head, body were manually selected by an expert which were then used to train the proposed solution. The expert also specified the best manual biometry plane for the head and abdomen which we used as ground truth to compare with the automatic biometry plane.

6   Results

6.1   Localization of the Fetus in the Sagittal Plane

As shown in Fig. 3(b), the edge strength is strong between the fetus and amniotic fluid, but it is weak between the fetus and non-fetal tissue. As mentioned in Sect. 3.2, a large number of candidate bounding boxes are generated and by excluding the out-of-range boxes, the number of boxes can be reduced significantly, for example, 1000 to 100 for one test data. We achieved a correct localization rate of 84.4 % using the criterion as mentioned in Sect. 3.2.

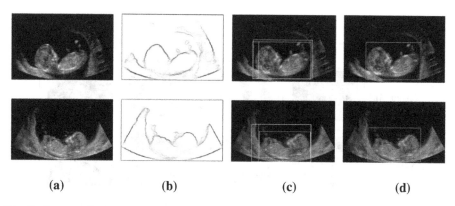

(a)   (b)   (c)   (d)

Fig. 3. Progress for bounding box around the fetus (a) Original image (b) Edge-mapped image (c) 3 bounding boxes based on the detected edges that received top 3 highest class probabilities (d) Final bounding box by averaging 3 boxes.

6.2   Fetal-Partitioning and Extraction of Biometry Planes

We performed 3-fold cross validation and the mean accuracy of correct classification of each slice using CNNs was 76.9 %. Figure 4 shows visual results of the fetal slice partitioning step. From the partitioning result, it was also found that most of the ground truth biometry planes were within the range of the head and the body. The mean distance between the manually and automatically extracted biometry planes is 1.6 ± 0.2 mm for the fetal head and 3.4 ± 0.4 mm for the fetal abdomen. Some typical results are shown in Fig. 5.

For the demonstration of the whole progress along with the results, please refer to the supplementary material of this paper.

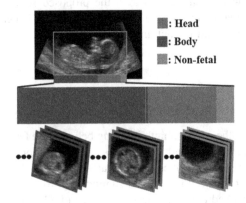

■: Head
■: Body
■: Non-fetal

Fig. 4. The partitioning result. (Color figure online)

	Head		Abdomen	
	Good	**Bad**	**Good**	**Bad**
Manual	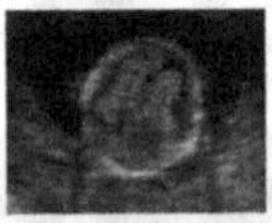	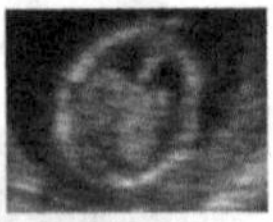	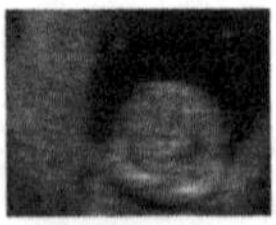	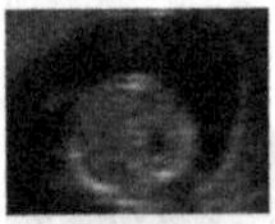
Automatic	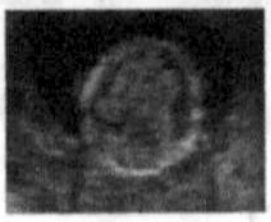	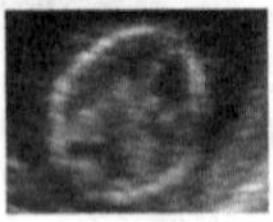	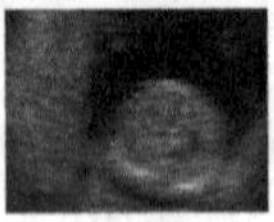	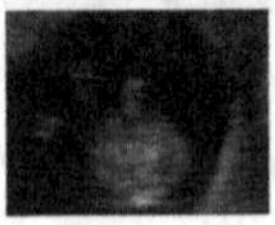
Difference	0.3 mm	2.6 mm	0.3 mm	11.9 mm

Fig. 5. Manually selected and automatically selected best planes for the fetal head and fetal abdomen with distances of difference between them

7 Discussion and Conclusion

We have developed a method for automatic localization of the fetus in a 3D US scan and subsequent detection of the best biometry planes for both the fetal head and fetal abdomen in the axial plane. The localization of the whole fetus in the sagittal plane using the bounding box approach alone helps a clinician better visualize the whole fetus but also measure the CRL. We showed a method which partitions the fetal volume into the fetal head and body using CNNs and extracts the biometry planes for fetal head and abdomen using linear regression with promising results. Extending the current prototype into a clinical tool is within our future vision. The current approach uses multiple machine learning methods to select the best biometry planes. We plan to investigate the use of one CNN framework with multiple tasks to tackle all the steps and compare with the current proposed solution.

References

1. Salomon, L., et al.: ISUOG practice guidelines: performance of first-trimester fetal ultrasound scan. Ultrasound Obstet. Gynecol. **41**(1), 102–113 (2013)
2. Abu-Rustum, R.S., Daou, L., Abu-Rustum, S.E.: Role of first-trimester sonography in the diagnosis of aneuploidy and structural fetal anomalies. J. Ultrasound Med. **29**(10), 1445–1452 (2010)
3. Bartlett, L.A., et al.: Risk factors for legal induced abortion–related mortality in the United States. Obstet. Gynecol. **103**(4), 729–737 (2004)
4. Dyson, R., et al.: Three-dimensional ultrasound in the evaluation of fetal anomalies. Ultrasound Obstet. Gynecol. **16**(4), 321–328 (2000)
5. Chen, H., et al.: Standard plane localization in fetal ultrasound via domain transferred deep neural networks. IEEE J. Biomed. Health Inform. **19**(5), 1627–1636 (2015)
6. Maraci, M.A., Napolitano, R., Papageorghiou, A., Noble, J.: Searching for structures of interest in an ultrasound video sequence. In: Wu, G., Zhang, D., Zhou, L. (eds.) MLMI 2014. LNCS, vol. 8679, pp. 133–140. Springer, Heidelberg (2014)
7. Rahmatullah, B., Papageorghiou, A.T., Noble, J.: Integration of local and global features for anatomical object detection in ultrasound. In: Ayache, N., Delingette, H., Golland, P., Mori, K. (eds.) MICCAI 2012, Part III. LNCS, vol. 7512, pp. 402–409. Springer, Heidelberg (2012)
8. Chen, H., Dou, Q., Ni, D., Cheng, J.-Z., Qin, J., Li, S., Heng, P.-A.: Automatic fetal ultrasound standard plane detection using knowledge transferred recurrent neural networks. In: Navab, N., Hornegger, J., Wells, W.M., Frangi, A.F. (eds.) MICCAI 2015, Part I. LNCS, vol. 9349, pp. 507–514. Springer, Heidelberg (2015). doi:10.1007/978-3-319-24553-9_62
9. Zitnick, C.L., Dollár, P.: Edge boxes: locating object proposals from edges. In: Fleet, D., Pajdla, T., Schiele, B., Tuytelaars, T. (eds.) ECCV 2014, Part V. LNCS, vol. 8693, pp. 391–405. Springer, Heidelberg (2014)
10. Dollár, P., Zitnick, C.: Structured forests for fast edge detection. In: Proceedings of the IEEE International Conference on Computer Vision (2013)
11. Yaqub, M., et al.: Investigation of the role of feature selection and weighted voting in random forests for 3-D volumetric segmentation. IEEE Trans. Med. Imaging **33**(2), 258–271 (2014)

12. Krizhevsky, A., Sutskever, I., Hinton, G.E.: Imagenet classification with deep convolutional neural networks. In: Advances in Neural Information Processing Systems (2012)
13. Gao, Y., Maraci, M.A., Noble, J.A.: Describing ultrasound video content using deep convolutional neural networks. In: 2016 IEEE 13th International Symposium on Biomedical Imaging (ISBI) (2016)
14. Papageorghiou, A.T., et al.: International standards for fetal growth based on serial ultrasound measurements: the Fetal Growth Longitudinal Study of the INTERGROWTH-21st Project. Lancet **384**(9946), 869–879 (2014)

Learning for Graph-Based Sensorless Freehand 3D Ultrasound

Loïc Tetrel[(✉)], Hacène Chebrek, and Catherine Laporte

Department of Electrical Engineering, École de technologie supérieure,
1100 Rue Notre-Dame O, Montréal, QC H3C 1K3, Canada
`loic_tetrel@yahoo.fr`, `catherine.laporte@etsmtl.ca`

Abstract. Sensorless freehand 3D ultrasound (US) uses speckle decorrelation to estimate small rigid motions between pairs of 2D images. Trajectory estimation combines these motion estimates to obtain the position each image relative to the first. This is prone to the accumulation of measurement bias. Whereas previous work concentrated on correcting biases at the source, this paper proposes to reduce error accumulation by carefully choosing the set of measurements used for trajectory estimation. An undirected graph is created with frames as vertices and motion measurements as edges. Using constrained shortest paths in the graph, random trajectories are generated and averaged to obtain trajectory estimate and uncertainty. To improve accuracy, a Gaussian process regressor is trained on tracked US sequences to predict systematic motion measurement error, which is then used to weigh the edges of the graph. Results on speckle phantom imagery show significantly improved trajectory estimates in comparison with the state-of-the-art, promising accurate volumetric reconstruction.

Keywords: Freehand 3D ultrasound · Speckle decorrelation · Sensorless reconstruction · Measurement selection · Gaussian process regression

1 Introduction

Compared to traditional 2D ultrasound (US), 3D US allows a better evaluation of the anatomical structures. A 3D probe can be used to obtain US volumes, but it is expensive and offers a limited field of view. Using freehand 3D US with a conventional 2D probe, the sonographer sweeps the area of interest to acquire a sequence of 2D frames. Volume reconstruction of this sequence requires the six degree of freedom (6DoF) motions of all the frames relative to the first one. During the acquisition, the probe can be tracked by a position sensor, but this imposes extra cost, is cumbersome and requires calibration. Instead, using the information of the images themselves to perform a sensorless registration of the frames [2–4, 8, 17] allows easy and inexpensive transducer tracking.

This is possible because speckle patterns are correlated out-of-plane in nearby images. Under Rayleigh scattering conditions, this phenomenon is entirely predictable from transducer characteristics and can be used to measure elevational

© Springer International Publishing AG 2016
L. Wang et al. (Eds.): MLMI 2016, LNCS 10019, pp. 205–212, 2016.
DOI: 10.1007/978-3-319-47157-0_25

displacement [3]. This approach can be adapted to work outside Rayleigh scattering conditions, allowing measurements in imagery of real tissues [2,6,12]. In-plane displacement can be estimated from the position of the correlation peak. By dividing the image into patches, each with a local 3D displacement estimate, the global 6DoF rigid motion can be estimated by a least squares approach [17].

Freehand motion does not produce pure elevational translations. Unfortunately, other types of motion (particularly rotations), also affect speckle correlation, leading to biased motion estimates [13]. Moreover, elevational translation measurements are limited by speckle correlation range, so we need to combine multiple measurements to estimate each frame's position relative to the first [8]. This results in the accumulation of bias and strongly affects the accuracy of the trajectory estimate. This is the challenge addressed in this paper.

A few papers proposed to correct measurement biases at the source. Correction of the elevational decorrelation curve was proposed to increase accuracy under probe rotation [1,9]. It was also suggested that because the measurement biases are systematic, corrections can be learned from tracked synthetic image sequences to improve the accuracy of sensorless motion estimation [4]. However, we found this approach difficult to generalize to real imagery.

Our approach to the problem is to reduce error accumulation by carefully selecting the measurements used for trajectory estimation. For this purpose, previous work has proposed using maximally spaced images (thereby reducing the number of error accumulation steps) [8], or fusing multiple redundant elevational motion estimates along with measurements of their uncertainty [10]. A hypothesis testing approach was also proposed to eliminate biased measurements arising from inaccurate tissue models used outside Rayleigh scattering conditions [11]. None of these works considered how to choose the *best* motion estimates for trajectory estimate.

We hypothesize that wisely choosing the motions estimated by speckle decorrelation *and* minimizing the number of measurements involved improves probe trajectory estimation. To this end, a graph-based trajectory estimate method, along with a learning-based technique for characterizing measurement error, are proposed in Sect. 2. Experimental results illustrating the benefits of this approach are given in Sect. 3. Section 4 summarizes our contribution.

2   Method

A 2D probe is used to acquire a sequence of N frames $\{f_0, f_1, ... f_N\}$ (Fig. 1a). The estimated position of frame N is denoted $M_N = m_{0N}$, where $m_{ij} \in SE(3)$, $i, j \in \{0, ..., N\}$, is the rigid motion between f_i and f_j (Fig. 1b). To simplify experimental validation, we assume that probe motion is monotonic, that there are no intersection between frames, and that we are under Rayleigh scattering conditions. These assumptions could easily be dropped by using methods proposed in the literature [2,6,8,10,12] without invalidating the methods proposed here.

To reduce the error in $M_{k=1,...,N}$, graph-based trajectory estimation from the m_{ij} is proposed (Fig. 1). We first estimate the motion m_{ij} between all pairs of

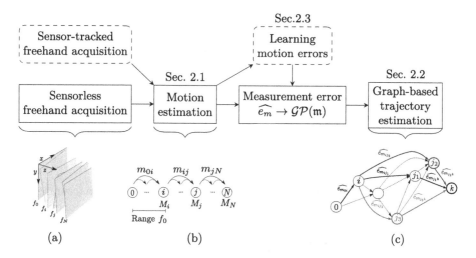

Fig. 1. Block diagram of the method including training (dashed) and testing (solid). (a) Freehand acquisition. (b) Sensorless motion estimation. (c) Reconstruction of frame f_k for $n = 3$ constrained shortest paths through j_1, j_2, j_3.

frames $\{f_i, f_j\}$ using speckle decorrelation (Sect. 2.1). A directed graph is then constructed with frames as vertices and the edges representing the motion estimates between pairs of frames. Using a Gaussian process relating measurement error to the parameters of m_{ij} in a tracked training sequence, it is possible to estimate the error of our sensorless measurements (Sect. 2.3), which we use to weigh the edges of the graph. To retrieve the position M_k of each frame f_k, we generate n random trajectories using a constrained shortest path algorithm and estimate their mean and variance (Sect. 2.2).

2.1   Rigid Motion Estimation

Estimating motion between pairs of frames requires calibrating a probe-specific elevational speckle decorrelation model [17]. Thus, a speckle phantom is scanned at fixed regular elevational intervals. The images are divided into p non-overlapping patches and the normalized cross-correlation between pairs of corresponding patches is measured. Measurements corresponding to identical elevational displacements are averaged, yielding p local empirical speckle decorrelation curves.

For a new pair of frames $\{f_i, f_j\}$, the in-plane motion of each patch is estimated by maximizing correlation and its out-of-plane motion is read off the local speckle decorrelation curve at peak correlation. The rigid motion $m_{i,j}$ is found from these p local 3D translation measurements (Fig. 2) using least squares [18].

2.2   Graph-Based Trajectory Estimation

Given the motion measurements m_{ij} of a sequence of frames, we want to estimate M_k. One possibility is to compose consecutive pairwise transformations:

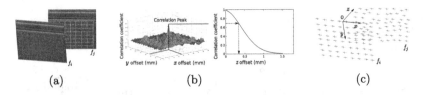

(a)   (b)   (c)

Fig. 2. (a) US image divided in p patches. (b) 3D translation estimate of one patch using speckle decorrelation. (c) Estimation of $m_{i,j}$ by Procrustes alignment.

$$M_k = m_{0,k} = m_{0,1} \circ m_{1,2} \circ \dots \circ m_{k-1,k}. \tag{1}$$

This is error prone because (1) empirical decorrelation curves are inaccurate for very short distances and (2) it accumulates biases over many measurements.

The set of motion measurements can be described by a directed unweighted graph, whose vertices represent the frames and whose edges are available motion estimates between pairs of frames. Then, the estimated position of f_k minimizing the accumulation of biases is Dijkstra's shortest path from vertex 0 to vertex k.

Averaging Multiple Solutions. Assuming that motion measurements are subject to random noise as well as bias, we further reduce error by averaging n positions close to the optimal one. Trajectory i is obtained by randomly selecting a vertex $0 < j_i < k$ and finding the shortest path from vertex 0 to vertex k that uses j_i. To average the n positions of f_k, we use Govindu et al.'s intrinsic averaging [7] with the shortest path to f_k as an initial guess. We also compute the standard deviation for the six rigid motion parameters, which is related to the error of the estimated position M_k.

2.3 Learning to Characterize Measurement Error

We can improve measurement selection by weighting the graph edges by measurement error. A typical error measure for sensorless freehand 3D US trajectory estimation is the mean target registration error (mTRE) [5] with respect to position sensor data. In our context, such data are not available on-line. However, there is a predictable relationship between the motion parameters and the measurement error [4]. Thus, we hypothesize that there exists a function g such that mTRE $= g(m)$, where m is a sensorless motion measurement. Knowing input-output pairs $\{m_{i,j}, \text{mTRE}_{m_{i,j}}\}$ from an accurately tracked sequence, g could, in principle, be learned. However, position sensors are not sufficiently accurate to measure the small motion between two consecutive frames of a typical freehand 3D US acquisition ($\sim 5 \times 10^{-2}$ mm).

Error Measure. The first task is to define an error measure e for a sensorless motion measurement m, knowing the position sensor output. The idea is to create a window bounded by two frames f_l and f_k such that the displacement $d_{\kappa\lambda}$ between the two frames leads to negligible sensor error, i.e., $d_{\kappa\lambda} > 2$ mm. We compute n trajectory estimates $\{\widehat{T_{\kappa\lambda_1}}...\widehat{T_{\kappa\lambda_n}}\}$ from vertex κ to vertex λ using the constrained random positions of Sect. 2.2 and compute their errors

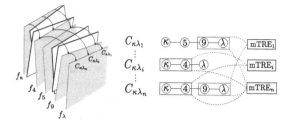

Fig. 3. Assigning mTREs to motions $m_{\kappa,4}$ (blue) and $m_{9,\lambda}$ (red) for window $[\kappa, \lambda]$. (Color figure online)

$\{\mathrm{mTRE}_1...\mathrm{mTRE}_n\}$ with respect to the sensor measurement T_{lk}. The computation of one transformation $\widehat{T_{\kappa\lambda_i}} = m_{\kappa,x} \circ ... \circ m_{y,\lambda}$ biased by mTRE_i involves many pairwise motion measurements. The process is repeated with different windows and the *error* $e_{m_{i,j}}$ of each sensorless motion measurement m_{ij} is defined as the average mTRE of all the window-wise position estimates it was involved in (Fig. 3).

Error Prediction Model. Finding a function $e_m = g(m)$ that relates the estimated motion $m_{i,j}$ to its error $e_{m_{i,j}}$ is a non-linear regression problem which we solve using Gaussian processes $(\mathcal{GP})$ [14]. $\mathcal{GP}$ regression is a Bayesian approach which assumes that $g(m)$ behaves according to $p(g|m_1,...,m_n) = \mathcal{N}(\mathcal{M},\mathcal{K})$, where $\mathcal{M}$ is the mean vector and $\mathcal{K}$ is the covariance function of the motions m. We used a pure quadratic mean function and a squared exponential covariance function to capture the smoothness of e_m. Error on inputs m, outputs e_m and lengthscale l were trained using quasi-newton optimization with the MATLAB Statistics and Machine Learning Toolbox. To have independency between the parameters of the rotation, we mapped the motion from Lie group $SE(3)$ to Lie Algebra $\mathfrak{se}(3)$ with the log function $\mathfrak{m} = \log(\mathrm{m})$ [7].

3   Experiments and Results

3.1   Data Acquisition

Images of a speckle phantom were acquired using an ATL HDI5000 US scanner with a linear 4–7 MHz transducer at a depth of 3 cm. The phantom was first scanned elevationally over 50 mm at regular 0.05 mm intervals by mounting the transducer on a robot arm following a purely translational trajectory, controlled by a step motor with a precision of 5 μm. The images were divided into 8 × 8 patches of size 55 × 32 pixels (Fig. 2a) and the speckle decorrelation curve corresponding to each patch was computed as described in Sect. 2.1.

Nine freehand sequences tracked with a Micron Tracker optical sensor were then acquired with the transducer moving mainly elevationally, with total displacements up to 30 mm. The optically tracked transducer was calibrated temporally and spatially using our adaptation of Rousseau et al.'s plane phantom methods [15,16]. We found experimentally that this setup produces volume measurements within 97 % accuracy.

3.2   Evaluation of Probe Trajectory Estimation

We evaluated five approaches for probe trajectory estimation: (1) the nearest neighbor (NN) approach (Eq. 1); (2) Housden *et al.*'s approach [8] which generates a coarse sequence (CSq) with blocks of three nearly equally spaced frames; (3) the farthest neighbor approach (FN), which takes the first and third frames of each block of CSq, and is better suited to monotonic sequences; (4) the average unweighted graph-based trajectory estimate (GA) of Sect. 2.2; (5) the proposed approach (GMeA) which is GA weighted by measurement error (Sect. 2.3). For GMeA, the $\mathcal{GP}$ was trained using one freehand sequence.

Each approach was tested on the eight other sequences, labeled S1-S8 with $n = 1000$ random positions for GA and GMeA. Table 1 shows the mTRE of the last frame of each sequence (measured at the patch centers) with respect to the optical sensor data, along with the total elevational displacement $|z|$ of the probe. GMeA improves accuracy by 20 % compared to FN. For all methods, error increases with $|z|$. This is expected as longer sequences require more measurements for position estimation and error accumulation cannot be avoided entirely. Some trajectories are clearly estimated less accurately than others (e.g., S2 vs S6), probably due to differences in rotational motion.

Table 1. mTRE of the last frame in S1-S8, as estimated by each method with total elevational displacement $|z|$ for reference and best results in bold.

	S1	S2	S3	S4	S5	S6	S7	S8
total $|z|$	20 mm	21 mm	25 mm	27 mm	36 mm	38 mm	52 mm	56 mm
NN	11.041	11.866	15.492	13.897	10.699	12.790	15.321	18.973
CSq	4.395	3.816	5.820	4.683	6.207	10.531	12.655	13.713
FN	2.036	1.028	3.758	2.412	4.758	10.486	10.578	10.999
GA	**1.781**	0.767	3.488	2.055	3.961	10.160	9.790	10.503
GMeA	1.803	**0.731**	**3.039**	**1.995**	**3.735**	**9.345**	**9.154**	**9.999**

To perform meaningful comparisons over the methods and image sequences, the mTREs of all the frames in each sequence (measured at the patch centers) were normalized by the total probe displacement. A Kolmogorov-Smirnov test showed that the results are not normally distributed. Thus, we performed a Friedman test to evaluate the influence of the methods on each sequence, except NN and CSq which are clearly less accurate than the others (Table 1). A Tukey contrast on the ranked means tested the hypothesis that the approaches GA and GMeA have the same accuracy as FN. Because we worked on minimizing drift, the effect of our methods is stronger towards the end of each sequence. A statistically significant difference between GMeA and FN was found when considering the last 35 frames of each sequence ($p < 0.05$), and for the last 10 frames ($p \ll 0.001$). GA was not found significantly different from FN.

Figure 4 shows detailed results for sequence S4. CSq over-estimates rotations and under-estimates elevational translations because there is confusion between

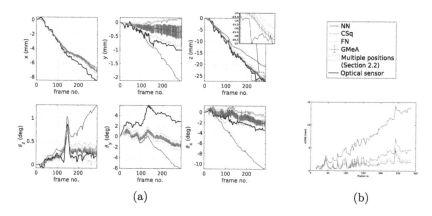

Fig. 4. (a) Freehand trajectories of (CSq, FN and GMeA) for the six degrees of freedom in sequence S4. (b) Error comparison of (NN, CSq, FN, GMeA).

rotation and translation induced decorrelation [9]. The averaging step of GMeA improves the rotational and translational estimates, whereas FN has more difficulty following the optical sensor data. Choosing the best measurements in the graph, as characterized by GMeA, improves the trajectory estimate compared to GA. The standard deviations of the estimated position parameters are a measure of uncertainty for the 3D reconstruction step. They grow with time as there are more plausible motion measurements to choose from. This difficulty is intrinsic to the sensorless approach. Qualitative results shown in Fig. 5 highlight the improved accuracy of volumetric reconstruction with GMeA versus CSq compared to that obtained with the optical sensor.

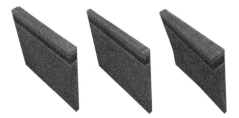

Fig. 5. (Left to right) Volumetric reconstruction of sequence S4 with optical sensor, GMeA and CSq.

4   Conclusion

This paper shows that measurement error can effectively be learned from tracked data and used towards improved sensorless freehand 3D US reconstruction. Our error weighted graph-based method significantly improves over the state-of-the-art. Future work will concentrate on adapting our method to non-Rayleigh scattering conditions.

References

1. Afsham, N., et al.: A generalized correlation-based model for out-of-plane motion estimation in freehand ultrasound. IEEE Trans. Med. Imaging **33**(1), 186–199 (2014)
2. Afsham, N., et al.: Nonlocal means filter-based speckle tracking. IEEE Trans. Ultrason. Ferroelectr. **62**(8), 1501–1515 (2015)
3. Chen, J.F., et al.: Determination of scan-plane motion using speckle decorrelation: theoretical considerations and initial test. Int. J. Imaging Syst. Technol. **8**(1), 38–44 (1997)
4. Conrath, J., Laporte, C.: Towards improving the accuracy of sensorless freehand 3D ultrasound by learning. In: Wang, F., Shen, D., Yan, P., Suzuki, K. (eds.) MLMI 2012. LNCS, vol. 7588, pp. 78–85. Springer, Heidelberg (2012). doi:10.1007/978-3-642-35428-1_10
5. van De Kraats, E.: Standardized evaluation methodology for 2-D-3-D registration. IEEE Trans. Med. Imaging **24**(9), 1177–1189 (2005)
6. Gee, A.H., et al.: Sensorless freehand 3D ultrasound in real tissue: speckle decorrelation without fully developed speckle. Med. Image Anal. **10**(2), 137–149 (2006)
7. Govindu, V.M.: Lie-algebraic averaging for globally consistent motion estimation. In: Proceedings of CVPR, vol. 1, pp. 684–691 (2004)
8. Housden, R.J., et al.: Sensorless reconstruction of unconstrained freehand 3D ultrasound data. Ultrasound Med. Biol. **33**(3), 408–419 (2007)
9. Housden, R., et al.: Rotational motion in sensorless freehand three-dimensional ultrasound. Ultrasonics **48**(5), 412–422 (2008)
10. Laporte, C., Arbel, T.: Combinatorial and probabilistic fusion of noisy correlation measurements for untracked freehand 3-D ultrasound. IEEE Trans. Med. Imaging **27**(7), 984–994 (2008)
11. Laporte, C., Arbel, T.: Measurement selection in untracked freehand 3D ultrasound. In: Jiang, T., Navab, N., Pluim, J.P.W., Viergever, M.A. (eds.) MICCAI 2010. LNCS, vol. 6361, pp. 127–134. Springer, Heidelberg (2010). doi:10.1007/978-3-642-15705-9_16
12. Laporte, C., Arbel, T.: Learning to estimate out-of-plane motion in ultrasound imagery of real tissue. Med. Image Anal. **15**(2), 202–213 (2011)
13. Li, P.C., et al.: Tissue motion and elevational speckle decorrelation in freehand 3D ultrasound. Ultrason. Imaging **24**(1), 1–12 (2002)
14. Rasmussen, C.E.: Gaussian Processes for Machine Learning. MIT Press, Cambridge (2006)
15. Rousseau, F., et al.: Confhusius: a robust and fully automatic calibration method for 3D freehand ultrasound. Med. Image Anal. **9**, 25–38 (2005)
16. Rousseau, F., et al.: A novel temporal calibration method for 3D ultrasound. IEEE Trans. Med. Imaging **25**(8), 1108–1112 (2006)
17. Tuthill, T.A., et al.: Automated three-dimensional US frame positioning computed from elevational speckle decorrelation. Radiology **209**(2), 575–582 (1998)
18. Umeyama, S.: Least-squares estimation of transformation parameters between two point patterns. IEEE Trans. Pattern Anal. **13**(4), 376–380 (1991)

Learning-Based 3T Brain MRI Segmentation with Guidance from 7T MRI Labeling

Renping Yu[1,2], Minghui Deng[3], Pew-Thian Yap[2], Zhihui Wei[1], Li Wang[2], and Dinggang Shen[2(✉)]

[1] School of Computer Science and Engineering,
Nanjing University of Science and Technology, Nanjing, China
[2] Department of Radiology and BRIC, UNC at Chapel Hill, Chapel Hill, NC, USA
dgshen@med.unc.edu
[3] College of Electrical and Information,
Northeast Agricultural University, Harbin, China

Abstract. Brain magnetic resonance image segmentation is one of the most important tasks in medical image analysis and has considerable importance to the effective use of medical imagery in clinical and surgical setting. In particular, the tissue segmentation of white matter (WM), gray matter (GM), and cerebrospinal fluid (CSF) is crucial for brain measurement and disease diagnosis. A variety of studies have shown that the learning-based techniques are efficient and effective in brain tissue segmentation. However, the learning-based segmentation methods depend largely on the availability of good training labels. The commonly used 3T magnetic resonance (MR) images have insufficient image quality and often exhibit poor intensity contrast between WM, GM, and CSF, therefore not able to provide good training labels for learning-based methods. The advances in ultra-high field 7T imaging make it possible to acquire images with an increasingly high level of quality. In this study, we propose an algorithm based on random forest for segmenting 3T MR images by introducing the segmentation information from their corresponding 7T MR images (through semi-automatic labeling). Furthermore, our algorithm iteratively refines the probability maps of WM, GM, and CSF via a cascade of random forest classifiers to improve the tissue segmentation. Experimental results on 10 subjects with both 3T and 7T MR images in a leave-one-out validation, show that the proposed algorithm performs much better than the state-of-the-art segmentation methods.

1 Introduction

Magnetic resonance (MR) imaging is a powerful tool for in vivo diagnosis of brain disorders. Accurate measurement of brain structures in MR image is important for studying both brain development associated with growth and brain alterations associated with disorders. These studies generally require to first segment structural T1-weighted MR images into white matter (WM), gray matter (GM), and cerebrospinal fluid (CSF). Thus MR image segmentation is a key processing

© Springer International Publishing AG 2016
L. Wang et al. (Eds.): MLMI 2016, LNCS 10019, pp. 213–220, 2016.
DOI: 10.1007/978-3-319-47157-0_26

step in medical image analysis, such as morphometry, automatic tissue labeling, tissue volume quantification and image registration, and has considerable importance to the effective use of medical imagery in clinical and surgical setting. Although this diversity of processing applications promotes the development of various automatic segmentation techniques, accurate automated tissue segmentation still remains a difficult task.

So far, many learning-based techniques have been applied for tissue segmentation, including support vector machines (SVM) [1], artificial neural networks (ANN) [2], deep convolutional neural networks (CNNs) [3], and random decision forests [4,5]. The performance of learning-based segmentation methods is largely dependent on the quality of the training dataset. In general, training datasets were most commonly generated by manual labeling of 3T MR images, which typically exhibit insufficient signal-to-noise ratio (SNR) and intensity contrast. The inaccuracy and unreliability of these manual delineations affect image segmentation and subsequent quantitative statistical analysis.

By the end of 2010, more than 20 ultra-high field MR scanners, mainly 7T, have been in operation in the world for human medical imaging [6]. 7T scanners give images with significantly higher intensity contrast, greater SNR [7], and more anatomical details [8]. The utilization of higher field strengths allows the visualization of brain atrophy that is not evident at lower field strength, promoting better understanding of neurological disorders, cerebrovascular accidents, or epileptic syndromes [9].

In this paper, we present an automatic learning-based algorithm for segmentation of 3T brain MR images by introducing the segmentation information obtained from their corresponding 7T MR images. Specifically, to integrate information from multiple sources, we harness the learning-based multi-source integration framework (LINKS) strategy [5], which is based on random forest and has been applied to accurate tissue segmentation of infant brain images. In particular, image segmentation is achieved by automatically learning the contribution of each source through random forest with an auto-context strategy [10,11]. By iteratively training random forest classifiers based on the image appearance features and also the context features of progressively updated tissue probability maps, a sequence of classifiers is trained. Specifically, the first random forest classifier provides the initial tissue probability maps for each training subject. These tissue probability maps are then further used as additional input images to train the next random forest classifier, by combining the high-level multi-class context features from the probability maps with the appearance features from the T1-weighted MR images. Repeating this process, a sequence of random forest classifiers can be obtained. In the application stage, given an unseen image, the learned classifiers are sequentially applied to progressively refine the tissue probability maps for achieving final tissue segmentation.

2   Materials and Methods

10 volunteers (4 males and 6 females) with age of 30 ± 8 years were recruited for this study. All the participants were scanned at both 3T Siemens Trio scanner

and 7T Siemens ultra-high field MR imaging scanner with a circular polarized head coil. The 3T T1-weighted images were obtained with 144 sagittal slices using two sets of parameters: (1) 300 slices, voxel size $0.8594 \times 0.8594 \times 0.999$ mm^3; and (2) 320 slices, voxel size $0.8594 \times 0.999 \times 0.8594$ mm^3. The 7T T1-weighted MR images were acquired with 192 sagittal slices using two sets of parameters: (1) 300 slices, voxel size $0.80 \times 0.80 \times 0.80$ mm^3; and (2) 320 slices, voxel size $0.6 \times 0.6 \times 0.6$ mm^3. The 7T MR images were linearly registered to the spaces of their corresponding 3T MR images.

Standard image preprocessing steps were performed before tissue segmentation, including skull stripping, intensity inhomogeneity correction, histogram matching, and removal of both cerebellum and brain stem by using in-house tools. Specifically, the segmentations of 7T MR images were obtained by first using the publicly available software, FSL [12], to generate a relatively accurate segmentation, and then performing necessary manual corrections by an experienced rater via ITK-SNAP (www.itksnap.org).

2.1 Proposed Algorithm

Brain tissue segmentation is carried out using a cascade of random forest classifiers, which will be trained using *the appearance features* obtained from 3T MR images and the *ground truth segmentation labels* obtained by semi-automatic delineation of corresponding 7T MR images. The main motivation for using segmentation information from 7T MR images is because of their greater contrast and details compared with 3T MR images, as illustrated in Fig. 1. An overview of our proposed algorithm is shown in Fig. 2, in which a series of classifiers are trained with both T1-weighted MR images and tissue probability maps of WM, GM and CSF as input. Specifically, the first classifier is trained by only the appearance features from the T1-weighted MR images. When training the subsequent random forests, the context features of WM, GM, and CSF probability maps, generated in the previous iteration, are used as additional input for training. Note that the context features capture information of voxel neighborhood and thus improve classification robustness. This training process is repeated and finally a series of random forests are constructed with progressively refined probability maps. In the testing stage, each voxel of an unseen T1-weighted MR image goes through each trained random forest sequentially. Each classifier will

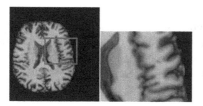
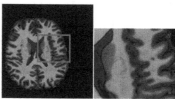

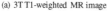
(a) 3T T1-weighted MR image   (b) Corresponding 7T T1-weighted MR image

Fig. 1. Comparison between 3T and 7T T1-weighted MR images.

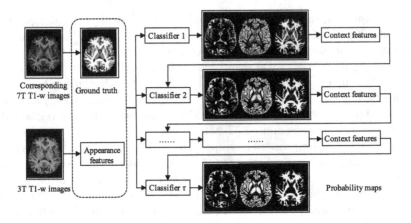

Fig. 2. Method overview. The appearance features from the T1-weighted MR images and the context features from the WM, GM, and CSF probability maps are used for training a sequence of random forest classifiers.

produce a set of GM, WM, and CSF tissue probability maps, which together with the T1-weighted MR image are used as input to the next trained classifier for producing the improved GM, WM, and CSF tissue probability maps.

In our work, we employ the random forest to train the classifiers. The random forest (RF) is an ensemble of decision trees that is based on bagging and random decision forests. Based on the decisions given by all the trees, the class of input feature vector is determined using majority voting. The random forest is able to capture complex data structures and is resistant to both over-fitting (when trees are deep) and under-fitting (when trees are shallow) [13]. Each tree classifier $h(X, \Theta_k)$ is constructed using the feature vectors of a random subset of training voxels X. Each element of the feature vector corresponds to a feature type. At each node of the tree, splitting is based on a small randomly selected group of feature elements. The random generated vector Θ_k determines both the voxel subset and the nodal feature subsets associated with the tree. Its randomness promotes diversity among the tree classifiers [14].

2.2 Appearance and Context Features

In this paper, we use 3D Haar-like features to compute both appearance and context features, due to computational efficiency. Specifically, for each voxel x, its Haar-like features are computed as the local mean intensity of any randomly displaced cubical region (R_1), or the mean intensity difference over any two randomly displaced, asymmetric cubical regions (R_1 and R_2) [5]:

$$f(x, I) = \frac{1}{R_1} \sum_{u \in R_1} I(u) - b \frac{1}{R_2} \sum_{v \in R_2} I(v), \quad R_1 \in R, \quad R_2 \in R \qquad (1)$$

where R is the region centered at voxel x, I is the image under consideration, and parameter $b \in \{0, 1\}$ indicates whether one or two cubical regions are used. Within R, the intensities are normalized to have unit L_2 norm. For each voxel, a large number of features can be extracted.

3   Experiments

In this study, we train a sequence of 10 random forest classifiers, each consisting of 20 forests with maximal depth of 100. A number of 30,000 voxel samples, randomly selected from the brain region of each training subject, were used to train the decision trees in each random forest, with the voxel neighborhood size of $9 \times 9 \times 9$, minimum 8 samples for each leaf node, and 100,000 random Haar-like features for each tree. Example results, shown in Fig. 3, indicate that the tissue probability maps are progressively improved and increasingly consistent with the ground truth, by using the sequential random forest classifiers.

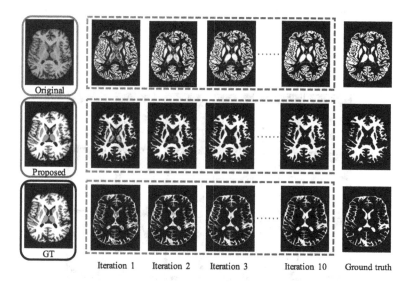

Fig. 3. The first column shows the original image, the segmentation results obtained by the proposed algorithm, and the ground truth segmentation. Subsequent columns show the tissue probability maps of GM, WM, and CSF output by the sequential random forest classifiers. The last column shows the ground-truth tissue probability maps.

3.1   Comparison with Other Methods on 10 Subjects

We compared our method with other segmentation methods provided in the following software packages: FSL and Medical Image Processing, Analysis, and Visualization (MIPAV). The leave-one-out cross-validation based Dice ratios for the 10 training subjects are reported in Table 1. The results indicate that the proposed method outperforms other methods for all three tissue types in most cases. Specifically, for the average Dice ratio of all 10 subjects, our method performs much better than any other comparison methods. For example, compared to the best method, our method improves about 7 % for GM, >3 % for WM, and >12 % for CSF.

Table 1. Comparison of tissue segmentation performance in terms of Dice ratio.

	Dice (%)	Sub.1	Sub.2	Sub.3	Sub.4	Sub.5	Sub.6	Sub.7	Sub.8	Sub.9	Sub.10	Mean (±STD)
GM	**Proposed**	**87.54**	**88.81**	**88.78**	**87.94**	**86.33**	**92.62**	**90.72**	**90.31**	**91.38**	**90.45**	**89.49 ± 1.83**
	FSL	83.39	81.85	81.32	83.09	81.03	81.07	78.75	83.07	82.13	77.57	81.33 ± 1.80
	MIPAV	84.31	81.74	81.66	80.56	81.92	83.89	79.70	84.47	83.43	83.85	82.55 ± 1.58
	SPM	77.39	77.58	79.71	77.75	7953	78.81	79.60	78.01	84.63	70.21	78.32 ± 3.36
WM	**Proposed**	93.80	**94.18**	**94.26**	**93.25**	**93.45**	**95.90**	**95.27**	94.07	**95.62**	95.36	**94.52 ± 0.90**
	FSL	**94.15**	87.96	88.60	89.98	85.17	95.29	90.13	**95.00**	92.76	**95.87**	91.49 ± 3.46
	MIPAV	92.82	87.49	88.69	86.85	86.76	92.32	90.33	94.37	92.02	94.90	90.66 ± 2.91
	SPM	82.08	79.78	81.41	81.25	80.26	83.21	87.30	83.46	84.82	84.22	82.78 ± 2.18
CSF	**Proposed**	**79.85**	**78.18**	**76.34**	**77.09**	**73.29**	**88.11**	**86.15**	**80.50**	**77.58**	**82.62**	**79.97 ± 4.32**
	FSL	64.79	60.46	60.75	63.12	49.70	77.48	69.73	64.94	66.29	70.72	64.80 ± 6.99
	MIPAV	64.69	59.65	59.89	61.51	48.34	75.14	69.67	70.75	63.80	69.59	64.30 ± 7.21
	SPM	67.77	63.32	51.76	69.70	51.90	78.32	73.43	77.83	75.15	61.91	67.11 ± 9.28

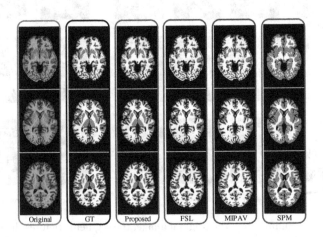

Fig. 4. Comparison of segmentation results by different methods on a typical subject. Each row shows the results on a representative slice.

Qualitative results for visual inspection are also shown in Figs. 4, 5 and 6. From Fig. 4, we can obverse that our method, compared with FSL, MIPAV and SPM, produces results that are significantly consistent with the ground-truth segmentations. WM surfaces generated by the ground truth and different methods are shown in Fig. 5. Figure 6 shows the differences of the label maps with respect to the ground-truth segmentations, indicating that the proposed method produces better segmentation with less false positives and false negatives.

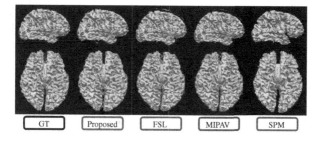

Fig. 5. Comparison of WM surfaces generated by ground truth and different methods.

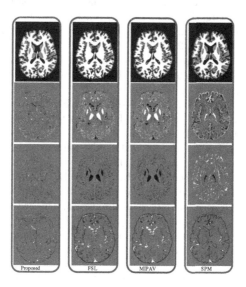

Fig. 6. Label differences with the manual segmentation. The first column shows the segmentation results by different methods. The next three rows show the differences of the GM, WM and CSF label maps with the ground-truth. Black and white denote false negatives and false positives, respectively.

4 Conclusion

In this paper, we presented a method for robust and accurate segmentation of 3T T1-weighted MR images by introducing the segmentation information from their corresponding 7T MR images (with high image quality). The proposed algorithm could combine the T1-weighted MR images with the tentatively estimated tissue probability maps to progressively refine the tissue probability maps by using the sequential random forest classifiers. Comparison results demonstrate the advantage of the proposed method in terms of accuracy.

Acknowledgement. This work was supported by the China Scholarship Council (No. 201506840071) and the Research Fund for the Doctoral Program of Higher Education of China (RFDP) (No. 20133219110029).

References

1. Morra, J.H., Tu, Z., Apostolova, L.G., et al.: Comparison of AdaBoost and support vector machines for detecting Alzheimers disease through automated hippocampal segmentation. IEEE Trans. Med. Imaging **29**, 30 (2010)
2. Pitiot, A., Delingette, H., Thompson, P.M., Ayache, N.: Expert knowledge-guided segmentation system for brain MRI. NeuroImage **23**, 85–96 (2004)
3. Zhang, W., Li, R., Deng, H., Wang, L., Lin, W., Ji, S., Shen, D.: Deep convolutional neural networks for multi-modality isointense infant brain image segmentation. NeuroImage **108**, 214–224 (2015)
4. Mitra, J., Bourgeat, P., Fripp, J., Ghose, S., Rose, S., Salvado, O., Christensen, S.: Lesion segmentation from multimodal MRI using random forest following ischemic stroke. NeuroImage **98**, 324–335 (2014)
5. Wang, L., Gao, Y., Shi, F., Li, G., Gilmore, J.H., Lin, W., Shen, D.: LINKS: learning-based multi-source integration framework for segmentation of infant brain images. NeuroImage **108**, 160–172 (2015)
6. Rauschenberg, J.: 7T higher human safety the path to the clinic adoption. Proc. Intl. Soc. Mag. Reson. Med. **19**, 7 (2011)
7. Hahn, A., Kranz, G.S., Seidel, E.M., Sladky, R., Kraus, C., Küblböck, M., Windischberger, C.: Comparing neural response to painful electrical stimulation with functional MRI at 3 and 7T. NeuroImage **82**, 336–343 (2013)
8. Braun, J., Guo, J., Ltzkendorf, R., Stadler, J., Papazoglou, S., Hirsch, S., Bernarding, J.: High-resolution mechanical imaging of the human brain by three-dimensional multifrequency magnetic resonance elastography at 7T. Neuroimage **90**, 308–314 (2014)
9. MARTIN VAQUERO, P.A.U.L.A., COSTA, S., et al.: Magnetic resonance imaging of the canine brain at 3 and 7T. Vet. Radiol. Ultrasound **52**, 25–32 (2011)
10. Zikic, D., Glocker, B., Konukoglu, E., Criminisi, A., Demiralp, C., et al.: Decision forests for tissue-specific segmentation of high-grade gliomas in multi-channel MR. Med. Image Comput. Comput. Assist. Interv. **15**, 369–376 (2012)
11. Zikic, D., Glocker, B., Criminisi, A.: Encoding atlases by randomized classification forests for efficient multi-atlas label propagation. Med. Image Anal. **18**, 1262–1273 (2014)
12. Smith, S.M., Jenkinson, M., Woolrich, M.W., Beckmann, C.F., Behrens, T.E., Johansen-Berg, H., Niazy, R.K.: Advances in functional and structural MR image analysis and implementation as FSL. Neuroimage **23**, 208–219 (2004)
13. Maiora, J., Ayerdi, B., Grana, M.: Random forest active learning for AAA thrombus segmentation in computed tomography angiography images. Neurocomputing **126**, 71–77 (2014)
14. Pinto, A., Pereira, S., Dinis, H., Silva, C.A., Rasteiro, D.M.: Random decision forests for automatic brain tumor segmentation on multi-modal MRI images. In: IEEE 4th Portuguese BioEngineering Meeting, pp. 1–5 (2015)

Transductive Maximum Margin Classification of ADHD Using Resting State fMRI

Lei Wang[1,2], Danping Li[1,3], Tiancheng He[1], Stephen T.C. Wong[1], and Zhong Xue[1(✉)]

[1] Houston Methodist Research Institute,
Weill Cornell Medicine, Houston, TX 77030, USA
zxue@houstonmethodist.org
[2] School of Electronic Engineering, Xidian University, Xi'an 710071, China
[3] School of Telecommunications Engineering,
Xidian University, Xi'an 710071, China

Abstract. Resting-state functional magnetic resonance imaging (rs-fMRI) provides key neural imaging characteristics for quantitative assessment and better understanding of the mechanisms of attention deficit hyperactivity disorder (ADHD). Recent multivariate analysis studies showed that functional connectivity (FC) could be used to classify ADHD from normal controls at the individual level. However, there may not be sufficient large numbers of labeled training samples for a hand-on classifier especially for disease classification. In this paper, we propose a transductive maximum margin classification (TMMC) method that uses the available unlabeled data in the learning process. On one hand, the maximum margin classification (MMC) criterion is used to maximize the class margin for the labeled data; on the other hand, a smoothness constraint is imposed on both labeled and unlabeled data projection so that similar samples tend to share the same label. To evaluate the performance of TMMC, experiments on a benchmark cohort from the ADHD-200 competition were performed. The results show that TMMC can improve the performance of ADHD classification using rs-fMRI by involving unlabeled samples, even for small number of labeled training data.

Keywords: ADHD classification · rs-fMRI · Maximum margin classification · Transductive learning

1 Introduction

Attention deficit hyperactivity disorder (ADHD) is one of the most common neurobehavioral disorders of childhood. ADHD children often demonstrate age-inappropriate problems such as inattention, impulsivity and hyperactivity, and clinically cognitive, emotional, and motor processes of these children are affected [1]. Clinical diagnosis is based on integration of parent and teacher reports and assessment of ADHD symptoms along a standardized scale [2]. In addition, recent research works showed that ADHD can also be characterized by neuroimaging such as functional MRI. For example, abnormal brain activations were found in task-related experiments on the ventrolateral prefrontal cortex (VLPFC) [3] and the putamen [4]; abnormalities in the default

© Springer International Publishing AG 2016
L. Wang et al. (Eds.): MLMI 2016, LNCS 10019, pp. 221–228, 2016.
DOI: 10.1007/978-3-319-47157-0_27

networks of resting state fMRI (rs-fMRI) were also found in prefrontal cortex, inferior frontal cortex, sensorimotor cortex, anterior cingulated cortex, putamen, temporal cortex, and cerebellum [5, 6]; Castellanos et al. [7] showed functional connectivity (FC) differences in ADHD than controls between anterior cingulate and precuneus/posterior cingulate cortex regions and between precuneus and other default-mode network components.

To quantify FC characteristics from neuroimaging and extract the distinct imaging markers to classify ADHD brains from normal controls, various clustering, classification, and machine learning algorithms can be applied. Univariate between-group statistics might be of less capability to distinguish one group from another than multivariate analysis. Recent multivariate pattern-based machine learning methods for neuroimaging data take into account interactions among different regions and are ideally suited to make predictions for individual subjects based on brain imaging patterns. These multivariate analysis methods are highly desirable to find objective neuroimaging based diagnostic biomarkers to aid traditional diagnostic methods [8]. For example, reliable prediction can be achieved by utilizing these classic machine learning techniques, such as KPCA [9], SVM [10], ELM [11], hyper-networks [12] and others.

However, one major issue with these traditional pattern classification methods is that we might not have sufficient labeled training samples to feed the classifier. A large number of training samples are needed to perform reliable disease detection. In fact, this is a common problem encountered in machine learning community, where labeled data are often scarce or limited, and a large number of unlabeled data are easy to collect in many applications ranging from natural to medical images classification. This has motivated researchers to develop learning methods that can exploit both labeled and unlabeled data for learning the classification. Such a learning paradigm developed over the past decade or so is referred to as semi-supervised learning.

In this paper, we propose a semi-supervised learning method based on the transductive learning [13, 14], called transductive maximum margin classification (TMMC), in which the unlabeled data are employed in the training stage together with the labeled data. This paradigm is useful for finding neuroimaging diagnostic biomarkers, since in general the amount of structural MRI or fMRI data with diagnosis is less than the larger pool of unlabeled imaging data (no matter a patient or a normal control is concerned). Like image retrieval, the imaging features of labeled datasets and the grouping (or clustering) information of unlabeled datasets can be combined together and utilized in the transductive learning. Our rationale is that a classifier that can not only provide large margins among the groups of labeled data but also maintain data-mapping smoothness (i.e., data with similar features are more likely to be classified into the same group) can improve its performance, robustness and reliability compared to the training that only uses the labeled data.

The idea of TMMC stems from recent developments in graph-based transductive learning techniques. Specifically, in TMMC, we apply the maximum margin criteria to ensure large margins among different groups of the labeled training data, and utilize the smoothness constraint on the graph formed by both labeled and unlabeled data so that data close to each other are more likely to share the same label. Using functional connectivity as features, TMMC can be used in a semi-supervised fashion.

In experiments, we evaluate and demonstrate the performance of our learning framework on a benchmark cohort from the well-known ADHD-200 global competition, where many supervised multivariate pattern classification methods had set themselves as standards for automatic diagnosis of ADHD. By comparing with the conventional supervised learning methods the resulting learning model improves classification performance. Moreover, the experiments provide the evidence that the test dataset structure of brain connectivity features can be functionally integrated with the labeled brain connectivity graphs, providing a more reliable neuroimaging based diagnosis of individual subject, from this dataset itself.

2 Method

Traditionally a classifier is trained using labeled training samples, and the model is utilized for testing samples, and for validation the testing samples need to be labeled also. For semi-supervised learning, beside the labeled training samples, unlabeled samples are employed for training. It has been shown that the use of unlabeled data can considerably improve the classification accuracy and reliability. The proposed TMMC estimates the optimal projection of original data onto the feature space by jointly making use of two kinds of information under semi-supervised setting: the discriminative information by maximizing the classification margin of the labeled data (maximum margin criterion); and the smoothness constraints on both labeled and unlabeled data to ensure a smooth projection on the feature space. The contribution of TMMC lies in the integration of these two criteria to form a semi-supervised learning framework for analyzing the FC networks of the neuroimaging data of ADHD.

2.1 Maximum Margin Classification (MMC)

Many classifiers attempt to first solve a projection $\mathbf{A}$ of the input data so that the between-class difference is maximized and within-class difference is minimized. MMC is one of such projections and acts in a similar way as linear discriminant analysis (LDA). By reformulating the trace-ratio problem of the LDA criterion into a trace-subtraction problem, MMC not only retains the benefits of maximum margin theory from the statistical learning community but also has the add-on advantages that the non-singular requirement of the within-class scatter matrix is no more required. Thus it would be easier to combine MMC with other constraints analytically.

Given N rs-fMRI connectivity networks, we denote them as the labeled training sample set, $\mathbf{X}_l = [\mathbf{x}_1, \mathbf{x}_2, \ldots, \mathbf{x}_N] \in \mathrm{R}^{d \times N}$, where $\mathbf{x}_i$ is the vector formed by the connectivity matrix of subject i. Each sample has been labeled as $k_i \in \{1, 2, \ldots, c\}$, with c the number of classes. We also denote n_m as the number of samples for class m. The average of the training samples of class m and that of all the training samples are given by $\mu_m = \frac{1}{n_m} \sum_{i:k_i=m} \mathbf{x}_i$ and $\mu = \frac{1}{n} \sum_{i=1}^{n} \mathbf{x}_i = \frac{1}{n} \sum_{m=1}^{c} n_m \mu_m$, respectively. Using the MMC criterion [15], the optimal projection matrix $\mathbf{A}$ can be obtained as follows,

$$\mathbf{A} = \arg\ \max_{\mathbf{A}}\mathrm{tr}(\mathbf{A}^{\mathrm{T}}\mathbf{S}_b\mathbf{A} - \mathbf{A}^{\mathrm{T}}\mathbf{S}_w\mathbf{A}), \qquad (1)$$

where $\mathbf{S}_b = \sum_{m=1}^{c} n_m (\mu_m - \mu)(\mu_m - \mu)^{\mathrm{T}}$ and $\mathbf{S}_w = \sum_{m=1}^{c} \sum_{i:k_i=m} (\mathbf{x}_i - \mu_m)(\mathbf{x}_i - \mu_m)^{\mathrm{T}}$ are the between-class and the within-class scatter matrices of $\mathbf{X}_l$, respectively.

To balance the two variances a parameter α is introduced, and the optimal projection matrix can be obtained by minimizing the following objective function,

$$J(\mathbf{A}) = \mathrm{tr}\big(\mathbf{A}^{\mathrm{T}}(\alpha\mathbf{S}_w - \mathbf{S}_b)\mathbf{A}\big). \qquad (2)$$

2.2 Smoothness Constraints

The smoothness constraints imply that data with similar features are more likely to share the same label, and hence they should also be close in the projection space. Because no label information is needed for enforcing such constraints, the unlabeled data can be involved in this stage. Thus, given M additional unlabeled connectivity matrices, we concatenate them to the above labeled training data, i.e., $\mathbf{X} = [\mathbf{x}_1, \mathbf{x}_2, \ldots, \mathbf{x}_N, \mathbf{x}_{N+1}, \ldots \mathbf{x}_{N+M}]$. Such smoothness constraints should yield a preference for decision boundaries in low-density regions so that there are fewer points close to each other in different classes. This task can be accomplished by first forming an undirected and weighted graph $\mathbf{G}$ among the sample data, with each vertex as a sample and the edges as the similarity among them. Then, we can determine that the projection should be smooth along the edges of the graph by applying graph Laplacian regularization. Specifically, given graph $\mathbf{G}$ and its Laplacian matrix $\mathbf{L} = \mathbf{D} - \mathbf{W}$, where $\mathbf{D}$ is the degree matrix and $\mathbf{W}$ is the adjacency matrix of the graph, similar to [13, 14], the optimal projection can be obtained by minimizing,

$$T(\mathbf{A}) = \mathbf{tr}(\mathbf{A}^T\mathbf{XMXA}), \qquad (3)$$

where $\mathbf{M} = (\mathbf{I} + \beta\mathbf{L})^{-1}(\beta\mathbf{L})$. β is the coefficient to control the influence of the graph Laplacian to the smoothness of the decision function.

2.3 Transductive-MMC

The MMC criterion ensures that the projection matrix yields a subspace so that labeled data pairs within the same class are close and the data pairs in different classes are far away from each other. On the other hand, using the smoothness constraint, the same projection matrix will result in a subspace so that similar data points, even their labels being unknown, are still close to each other after mapping. Herein, we propose a transductive MMC method to combine the MMC criterion and the smoothness constraints in the semi-supervised learning, by optimizing the objective function,

$$E(\mathbf{A}) = J(\mathbf{A}) + \eta T(\mathbf{A}) = \mathbf{tr}(\mathbf{A}^T[\eta\mathbf{XMX} + (\alpha\mathbf{S}_w - \mathbf{S}_b)]\mathbf{A}), \qquad (4)$$

where $\eta > 0$ is a parameter to control the trade-off between the discriminative strength of labeled data and the global smoothness constraints from both labeled and unlabeled data. The minimization of the above objective function can be achieved by the minimal eigenvalue solution to the generalized eigenvalue problem,

$$[\eta \mathbf{XMX} + (\alpha \mathbf{S}_w - \mathbf{S}_b)]a_k = \lambda_k a_k, k = 1, \ldots, d, \tag{5}$$

where λ_k is the kth smallest eigenvalue of $[\eta \mathbf{XMX} + (\alpha \mathbf{S}_w - \mathbf{S}_b)]$, and $\mathbf{a}_k$ is the corresponding eigenvector. The algorithm of TMMC learning is summarized as follows.

TMMC Algorithm
Input: dataset $\mathbf{X} = [\mathbf{x}_1, \mathbf{x}_2, \ldots, \mathbf{x}_N, \mathbf{x}_{N+1}, \ldots \mathbf{x}_{N+M}]$; parameters α, β, η; subspace dimension d.
Output: Projection matrix $\mathbf{T}_{\text{TMMC}}$

— Step 1. Normalize the dataset matrix $\mathbf{X}$;
— Step 2. Calculate the adjacent matrix $\mathbf{W}$ and Laplacian matrix $\mathbf{L}$;
— Step 3. Calculate matrix $\mathbf{M}$;
— Step 4. Calculate between-class scatter matrix $\mathbf{S}_b$ and within-class scatter matrix $\mathbf{S}_w$ of the labeled data $\mathbf{X}_l$;
— Step 5. Calculate the generalized eigenvalues and eigenvectors using Eq.(5);
— Step 6. Construct $\mathbf{T}_{\text{TMMC}}$ by selecting the eigenvectors corresponding to the d smallest eigenvalues.

In summary, the key idea for the proposed TMMC is to incorporate the smoothness constraint from both labeled and unlabeled data into the traditional maximum margin criterion so that the feature distribution from the large number of unlabeled data can help improve the robustness and accuracy of the classifier guided by the labeled training data. After the projection the k-Nearest Neighbors (KNN) algorithm is used to identify the class label of each testing sample.

3   Results

Dataset. fMRI data were downloaded from the ADHD-200 global competition (http://fcon_1000.projects.nitrc.org/indi/adhd200/). A description of ADHD-200 global competition data acquisition can be found from the same website. Anatomical and rs-fMRI scans were performed at 7 different facilities on children and young adults ages 7 to 21 years, approximately half male. Participants were diagnosed as either typically developing (TD) or ADHD-Hyperactive, ADHD-Inattentive, or ADHD-Combined type. These data and various metadata describing subject phenotypic traits (including diagnosis) were made available through the ADHD-200 Consortium. ADHD-Hyperactive type cases were not used herein because the small number of samples. This leads to a 3-class classification problem. We used all the training data in the experiments (768 subjects). Only the FC data derived from rs-fMRI are used to test the performance and the feasibility of our proposed TMMC.

Data Processing. Preprocessing of rs-fMRI data were performed by the Athena Pipeline, based on the publicly available AFNI and FSL software packages. The pipeline includes registering onto the MNI atlas, slice time correction, the removal of nuisance variance, a bandpass filter between 0.009 Hz and 0.08 Hz, and a 6-mm FWHM Gaussian filter. Then, region-specific average time courses were extracted from each subject's data using the CC200 [16] template atlas, which consists of 190 brain regions-of-interest (ROIs) guided by normalized cut clustering. Functional

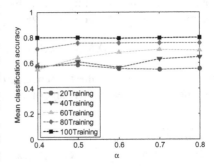

Fig. 1. Robustness of parameter α.

connectivity is measured as the Pearson correlation coefficient of time courses of any two ROIs, resulting in connectivity matrix for each sample. The upper triangular each FC matrix is extracted and concatenated as the input data of TMCC.

Performance Comparison. We compared the classification performance of TMMC with the classic linear dimensionality reduction methods including linear discriminant analysis (LDA), transductive component analysis (TCA) [14], semi-supervised discriminant analysis (SDA) [17]. KNN ($K = 1$) is subsequently used after these projections. On the other hand, support vector machine (SVM) [10] was also included as a reference method, since it is a benchmark maximum margin method.

First, we verified the multiclass classification performance of the proposed TMMC method for three groups: TD, ADHD-C and ADHD-I. We used the 768 subjects for cross-validation. We randomly chose 20, 40, 60, 80, and 100 subjects as the labeled training set and the rest (with no label) as the unlabeled training set and the testing data. We repeated 20 times for each case and calculated the mean and standard deviation of the results. The regularization parameter β and η are tuned from the 2-dimensional grid:$\{0.1, 0.5, 0.9, \ldots, 2.9\}$, while α is fixed as 0.6.

Table 1 shows the classification accuracy for three-class classification. It can be seen that TMMC outperforms other methods, and with increasing number of training samples, the performance is improved. To investigate the robustness of parameter

Table 1. Comparison of classification accuracy performance (%) of the proposed TMMC method and classic classifiers for multiclass classification problem (mean ± standard deviation).

Method	20 training	40 training	60 training	80 training	100 training
LDA	41.7 ± 4.9	42.3 ± 5.6	43.7 ± 2.2	44.1 ± 3.5	48.4 ± 3.5
MMC	44.6 ± 7.4	48.3 ± 4.6	49.8 ± 4.9	51.2 ± 4.5	54.6 ± 3.4
TCA	39.2 ± 3.5	41.0 ± 3.3	40.3 ± 2.9	39.5 ± 2.4	38.0 ± 2.0
SDA	39.2 ± 3.5	45.1 ± 3.6	49.5 ± 9.3	51.6 ± 7.6	55.0 ± 5.3
SVM	41.4 ± 4.1	43.2 ± 3.0	46.0 ± 2.2	46.4 ± 2.6	47.4 ± 2.4
TMMC	**56.8 ± 7.1**	**56.4 ± 5.5**	**68.2 ± 8.9**	**74.6 ± 2.3**	**79.7 ± 9.4**

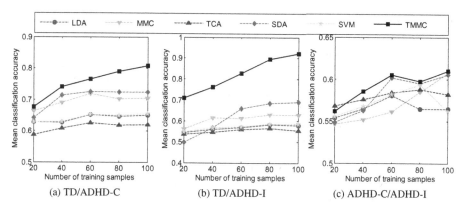

Fig. 2. Comparison of classification performance for different training numbers.

selection, we tested the performance for a range of α for TMCC, as shown in Fig. 1. It can be seen that the performance of TMMC is quite stable for different α.

To further investigate the ability to distinguish different groups, we performed two-class classification: TD/ADHD-C, TD/ADHD-I, and ADHD-C/ADHD-I, using similar cross-validation strategy. The parameters were set as the same. Figure 2 plots the average classification accuracy for different number of training samples. It can be seen that with the increasing training samples, the accuracy of most classifiers is improved. For TD/ADHD-C and TD/ADHD-I, TMMC yields consistently high accuracy over other methods. However, this improvement is not as big for ADHD-C/ADHD-I. This result indicates that TMMC performs a better task to distinguish typical development from the two types of ADHD, and it is still a challenging problem to identify ADHD-C from ADHD-I. Further investigation needs also be performed by considering the batch-effects of the datasets.

4 Conclusion

To tackle the problem of limited number of labeled training samples especially for high-dimensional feature classification, we proposed a transductive maximum margin classifier (TMMC) that applies graphical smoothness constraints among both labeled and unlabeled datasets with the maximum margin classification criterion. TMMC is evaluated by comparing with other algorithms using the functional connectivity matrices of rs-fMRI data to distinguish ADHD from controls and to separate two ADHD groups. TMMC extends the conventional MMC into a semi-supervised framework through a smoothness transductive fashion. Experimental results on the ADHD competition data cohort showed that TMMC outperforms the methods closely related to it. In future works, we will extend our method to multi-view classification in order to utilize multi-modality imaging data for more reliable disease diagnosis.

Acknowledgements. This work was partially supported by National Natural Science Foundation of China (No. 61203137, 61401328), Natural Science Foundation of Shaanxi Province (No. 2014JQ8306, 2015JM6279), the Fundamental Research Funds for the Central Universities (No. K5051301007), and NIH 5-R03-EB018977 (ZX).

References

1. Cortese, S.: The neurobiology and genetics of attention-deficit/hyperactivity disorder (ADHD): what every clinician should know. Eur. J. Paediatr. Neurol. **16**(5), 422–433 (2012)
2. Colby, J.B., Rudie, J.D., Brown, J.A., Douglas, P.K., Cohen, M.S., Shehzad, Z.: Insights into multimodal imaging classification of ADHD. Front. Syst. Neurosci. **6**(59), 1–18 (2012)
3. Teicher, M.H., Anderson, C.M., Polcari, A., Glod, C.A., Maas, L.C., Renshaw, P.F.: Functional deficits in basal ganglia of children with attention-deficit/hyperactivity disorder shown with functional magnetic resonance imaging relaxometry. Nat. Med. **6**(4), 470–473 (2000)
4. Durston, S., Tottenham, N.T., Thomas, K.M., Davidson, M.C., Eigsti, I.M., Yang, Y., Ulug, A.M., Casey, B.J.: Differential patterns of striatal activation in young children with and without ADHD. Biol. Psychiatry **53**(10), 871–878 (2003)
5. Cao, Q., Zang, Y., Sun, L., Sui, M., Long, X., Zou, Q., Wang, Y.: Abnormal neural activity in children with attention deficit hyperactivity disorder: a resting-state functional magnetic resonance imaging study. NeuroReport **17**(10), 1033–1036 (2006)
6. Zang, Y.F., He, Y., Zhu, C.Z., Cao, Q.J., Sui, M.Q., Liang, M., Tian, L.X., Jiang, T.Z., Wang, Y.F.: Altered baseline brain activity in children with ADHD revealed by resting-state functional MRI. Brain Dev. **29**(2), 83–91 (2007)
7. Castellanos, F.X., Margulies, D.S., Kelly, C., Uddin, L.Q., Ghaffari, M., Kirsch, A., Shaw, D., Shehzad, Z., Di Martino, A., Biswal, B., Sonuga-Barke, E.J., Rotrosen, J., Adler, L.A., Milham, M.P.: Cingulate-precuneus interactions: a new locus of dysfunction in adult attention-deficit/hyperactivity disorder. Biol. Psychiatry **63**(3), 332–337 (2008)
8. Lim, L., Marquand, A., Cubillo, A.A., Smith, A.B., Chantiluke, K., Simmons, A., Mehta, M., Rubia, K.: Disorder-specific predictive classification of adolescents with attention deficit hyperactivity disorder (ADHD) relative to autism using structural magnetic resonance imaging. PLoS ONE **8**(5), e63660 (2013)
9. Sidhu, G.S., Asgarian, N., Greiner, R., Brown, M.R.: Kernel principal component analysis for dimensionality reduction in fMRI-based diagnosis of ADHD. Front. Syst. Neurosci. **6**(74), 1–16 (2012)
10. Cheng, W., Ji, X., Zhang, J., Feng, J.: Individual classification of ADHD patients by integrating multiscale neuroimaging markers and advanced pattern recognition techniques. Front. Syst. Neurosci. **6**(58), 1–11 (2012)
11. Peng, X., Lin, P., Zhang, T., Wang, J.: Extreme learning machine-based classification of ADHD using brain structural MRI data. PLoS ONE **8**(11), e79476 (2013)
12. Jie, B., Wee, C.Y., Shen, D., Zhang, D.: Hyper-connectivity of functional networks for brain disease diagnosis. Med. Image Anal. **32**(1), 84–100 (2016)
13. Liu, W., Chang, S.-F.: Robust multi-class transductive learning with graphs. In: CVPR, pp. 381–388. IEEE (2009)
14. Liu, W., Tao, D., Liu, J.: Transductive component analysis. In: ICDM, pp. 433–442. IEEE (2008)
15. Li, H., Jiang, T., Zhang, K.: Efficient and robust feature extraction by maximum margin criterion. IEEE Trans. Neural Netw. **17**(1), 157–165 (2006)
16. Craddock, R.C., James, G.A., Holtzheimer, P.E., Hu, X.P., Mayberg, H.S.: A whole brain fMRI atlas generated via spatially constrained spectral clustering. Hum. Brain Mapp. **33**(8), 1914–1928 (2012)
17. Cai, D., He, X., Han, J.: Semi-supervised discriminant analysis. In: ICCV, pp. 1–7. IEEE (2007)

Automatic Hippocampal Subfield Segmentation from 3T Multi-modality Images

Zhengwang Wu, Yaozong Gao, Feng Shi, Valerie Jewells,
and Dinggang Shen[✉]

Department of Radiology and BRIC, UNC at Chapel Hill, Chapel Hill, NC, USA
dgshen@med.unc.edu

Abstract. Hippocampal subfields play important and divergent roles in both memory formation and early diagnosis of many neurological diseases, but automatic subfield segmentation is less explored due to its small size and poor image contrast. In this paper, we propose an automatic learning-based hippocampal subfields segmentation framework using multi-modality 3T MR images, including T1 MRI and resting-state fMRI (rs-fMRI). To do this, we first acquire both 3T and 7T T1 MRIs for each training subject, and then the 7T T1 MRI are linearly registered onto the 3T T1 MRI. Six hippocampal subfields are manually labeled on the aligned 7T T1 MRI, which has the 7T image contrast but sits in the 3T T1 space. Next, corresponding appearance and relationship features from both 3T T1 MRI and rs-fMRI are extracted to train a structured random forest as a multi-label classifier to conduct the segmentation. Finally, the subfield segmentation is further refined iteratively by additional context features and updated relationship features. To our knowledge, this is the first work that addresses the challenging automatic hippocampal subfields segmentation using 3T routine T1 MRI and rs-fMRI. The quantitative comparison between our results and manual ground truth demonstrates the effectiveness of our method. Besides, we also find that (a) multi-modality features significantly improved subfield segmentation performance due to the complementary information among modalities; (b) automatic segmentation results using 3T multi-modality images are partially comparable to those on 7T T1 MRI.

1 Introduction

Hippocampal subfields play important and divergent roles in both memory formation and early diagnosis of many neurological diseases. However, due to the small size and poor image contrast, it is less explored. Previously, either manual or automatic hippocampal subfields segmentation depends on ultra-high resolution or 7T/9.4T MR images [1–3], which are not universally available. Hence, it is desirable to develop hippocampal subfields segmentation methods using universal scanners (such as 3T scanner). However, few authors [4] have tried to

D. Shen—This work was supported by the National Institute of Health grants 1R01 EB006733

© Springer International Publishing AG 2016
L. Wang et al. (Eds.): MLMI 2016, LNCS 10019, pp. 229–236, 2016.
DOI: 10.1007/978-3-319-47157-0_28

segment hippocampal subfields using 3T routine T1 MRI and the result is not satisfactory due to low spatial resolution and poor tissue contrast.

Recently, many researches have revealed various connectivity patterns between the hippocampus and other brain regions in fMRI, where different subfields serve for different functions during the brain activities [5,6]. This implies that there might be some distinct connectivity patterns among different hippocampal subfields, which motivated us to use the rs-fMRI to assist the hippocampal subfields segmentation to achieve better performance with 3T scanners.

In this paper, multi-modality images, including 3T T1 MRI and 3T resting-state fMRI (rs-fMRI), are used together to segment hippocampal subfields in a learning based strategy. In order to get the hippocampal subfields for learning on 3T T1 MRI, both 7T T1 and 3T T1 MRI for each training subject are acquired and the 7T T1 MRI is linearly registered (using Flirt [7]) onto the 3T T1 MRI of the same subject. Six hippocampal subfields (the subiculum (Sub), CA1, CA2, CA3, CA4, and the dentate gyrus (DG), see Fig. 1 (a)) are manually labeled on the aligned 7T T1 MRI, which has the 7T contrast but sits in 3T space. In the next step, corresponding appearance and relationship features from both 3T T1 MRI and 3T rs-fMRI are extracted to train a structured random forest as a multi-label classifier to conduct the segmentation. Finally, the subfields segmentation result is further refined iteratively by additional context features and updated relationship features. To our knowledge, this is the first work that addresses the challenging automatic hippocampal subfields segmentation using 3T routine T1 MRI and rs-fMRI. The quantitative comparison between our results and manual labels demonstrates that the proposed method is quite effective. In addition, we also get two promising conclusions, (a) multi-modality features provide complementary information and significantly improve subfields segmentation performance compared to the use of a single modality, and (b) through the proposed method, a comparable segmentation performance is achieved with 3T multi-modality MRI comparing to that using 7T T1 MRI.

2   Motivation and Main Framework

The main challenge of subfields segmentation on 3T routine T1 MRI is the ambiguous subfield boundary caused by low contrast and resolution, as shown in Fig. 1(a-2). To compensate such ambiguity, the relationship features from rs-fMRI are adopted to assist the appearance features from T1 MRI for hippocampal subfields segmentation. Figure 1(b-1) gives an illustration, where patch 1 (belonging to CA2) and patch 2 (belonging to DG) are quite similar in the T1 MRI. It's hard to distinguish them if only using appearance features from T1 MRI. However, if the relationship features (e.g., functional connectivity pattern $\{c_1, \ldots, c_{36}\}$) between each patch and the reference regions are obtained from the rs-fMRI (here, 36 is the number of reference regions in our study), then we can potentially distinguish these appearance-similar patches through the differences of their relationship features, as shown in Fig. 1(b-2).

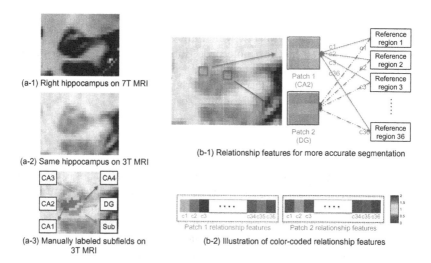

(a-1) Right hippocampus on 7T MRI

(a-2) Same hippocampus on 3T MRI

(a-3) Manually labeled subfields on 3T MRI

(b-1) Relationship features for more accurate segmentation

(b-2) Illustration of color-coded relationship features

Fig. 1. (a) Hippocampal subfields demonstration in 7T and 3T MRI, as well as their manual segmentations. (b) Main idea of using relationship features for subfields segmentation.

The main workflow of our method is shown in Fig. 2. For a training subject, its appearance features from T1 MRI and relationship features from rs-fMRI are used to train a structured random forest [8] as a multi-label classifier to conduct the segmentation, and then an auto-context model [9] is adopted to refine the classifier iteratively. In the next iteration, the additional context features and the updated relationship features are firstly calculated based on current segmentation probability maps, and then both of them as well as the appearance features are combined to train a new classifier. This procedure will be repeated iteratively to refine the classifier. When a testing subject comes, similarly, the classifier at iteration **0** uses the appearance features and relationship features to generate the segmentation probability maps; then, the context features and the updated relationship features can be obtained for the iteration **1**. This procedure is also done iteratively until reaching the maximum iteration, where the final segmentation probability maps are used to generate the final segmentation.

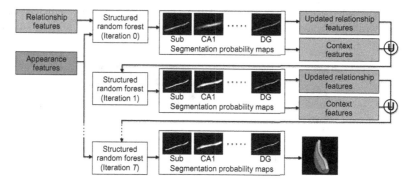

Fig. 2. The segmentation refinement procedure via the auto-context model.

In our framework, the appearance features are the 3D Haar features [10] and gradient based texture features [11], which are calculated from the 3T T1 MRI and will not be updated in the whole procedure; the context features are also the 3D Haar features but they are calculated from the segmentation probability maps. The key part is the calculation and updating of the relationship features, which is explained in detail in the following section.

3   Relationship Feature Calculation and Updating

In the preprocessing, the rs-fMRI is linearly registered onto the T1 MRI space [7] for extracting corresponding appearance and relationship features. After that, *first*, the reference regions are constructed, and the connectivity pattern is obtained through the Pearson correlation of fMRI signals between the local patch and each reference region; *second*, this connectivity pattern is enhanced and explored to formulate the final relationship features.

Reference Region Construction and Connectivity Pattern Computation. Since rs-fMRI is from the BOLD signal, a rational assumption is that the BOLD signals are highly correlated inside each subfield, but less correlated across different subfields. So ideally we can choose each subfield as the reference when calculating the connectivity pattern. This is easy for the training images, but is infeasible for testing images since subfields are not segmented yet.

To address this problem, we use a multi-atlas based segmentation [12] to do a rough segmentation, and then obtain the segmentation probability map (See Fig. 3) for each subfield, denoted as $P_{[t]}^{Sub}$, $P_{[t]}^{CA1}$, $P_{[t]}^{CA2}$, $P_{[t]}^{CA3}$, $P_{[t]}^{CA4}$ and $P_{[t]}^{DG}$, where t denotes iteration in our framework. Note, when $t = 0$, the probability maps are the roughly segmented results by [12]; when $t \geq 1$, they are the segmentation results by the classifier in each iteration.

By applying a threshold to the probability map, the segmentation of each subfield can be obtained (see Fig. 3). However, it's not appropriate to directly use subfield region as the reference region, because averaging the BOLD signals in the whole subfield might be over-smoothing. To address this issue, we further divide each subfield region into 6 subregions. The advantages of the subdivision include: (a) each subregion is smaller than the whole subfield, which reduces the negative impact caused by over-smoothing; (b) since the segmented subfield

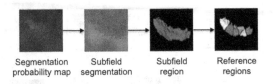

Segmentation   Subfield   Subfield   Reference
probability map   segmentation   region   regions

Fig. 3. Demonstration of constructing reference regions from the segmentation probability map of one subfield.

might contain mis-segmented voxels from the neighboring subfields, the BOLD signals from divided subregions of this subfield might be more accurate. Also, since the classifier in this paper is structured random forest, it will automatically select the most discriminative features among all subregions to guide the classification.

To make the division of each subfield consistent across different subjects, the division is firstly carried out on one atlas image (or training image), and then the centroid of each subregion is obtained. For a new image, the atlas image is first non-rigidly registered onto it, which provides a deformation field that brings the centroid of each subregion to the new image. Finally, the subfield can be divided by assigning the label of each voxel with that of the closest centroid.

We use these subregions as the reference regions, and denote the average BOLD signal in each reference region as $\mathbf{b}_k^R$, $k = 1, \ldots, 36$, where 36 is the number of reference regions since each of 6 subfields is divided into 6 subregions.

For any voxel i, denoting its mean BOLD signal in the local patch as $\mathbf{b}(i)$, its connectivity to the k-th reference region $c_k(i), k = 1, \ldots, 36$, is the Pearson correlation coefficient between $\mathbf{b}(i)$ and $\mathbf{b}_k^R$. Then, for any voxel i, its connectivity pattern to all reference regions is $\mathbf{c}(i) = \{c_k(i), k = 1, \ldots, 36\}$, where $\{c_k(i), 1 \leq k \leq 6\}$ is connectivity pattern from subfield 'Sub', and $\{c_k(i), 7 \leq k \leq 12\}$ is the connectivity pattern from subfield 'CA1', and etc.

Connectivity Pattern to Relationship Features. For two voxels i and j, i.e., i belonging to CA1 and j belonging to CA2, their corresponding connectivity patterns are $\mathbf{c}(i)$ and $\mathbf{c}(j)$. Because each subfield is relatively small, the difference between $\mathbf{c}(i)$ and $\mathbf{c}(j)$ might be subtle, which is less beneficial for classification. Thus, we employ the segmentation probability maps to amplify the difference.

For any voxel i, the probability map values $P_{[t]}^{\mathcal{S}}(i)$ indicate its probabilities belonging to subfield $\mathcal{S}$, where $\mathcal{S} \in \{$Sub, CA1, CA2, CA3, CA4, DG$\}$. They can be used to weight the connectivity pattern to obtain the weighted connectivity pattern, i.e., $\mathbf{r}(i) = \{r_k(i) | k = 1, \ldots, 36\}$, where $r_k(i) = P_{[t]}^{\mathcal{S}}(i) * c_k(i)$. For $1 \leq k \leq 6$, $P_{[t]}^{\mathcal{S}}$ is $P_{[t]}^{Sub}$; For $7 \leq k \leq 12$, $P_{[t]}^{\mathcal{S}}$ is $P_{[t]}^{CA1}$, and etc. Through the above formula, the connectivity pattern is weighted according to current predicted segmentation probability maps and thus become more discriminative. For each voxel, a 36 dimensional weighted connectivity pattern can be obtained. So, for the whole image, 36 weighted connectivity maps can be obtained. Then, the 3D Haar features can be extracted from those weighted connectivity maps to explore more patterns. Finally these Haar features form our relationship features.

In our study, 100 Haar features are extracted for each voxel from its local patch in each of the 36 weighted connectivity maps. Thus, totally $36*100 = 3600$ relationship features are used for each voxel.

Updating the Relationship Features. At each iteration of the refinement, the segmentation probability maps are updated according to the prediction of the current classifier, which will be used to update the reference regions. Then, the new relationship features can be updated according to the new reference regions and new segmentation probability maps. In such a way, the relationship features can be updated at each iteration.

4   Experiments

Materials. Each subject has 7T T1 MRI, 3T T1 MRI and 3T rs-fMRI data. The 3T scanner (Siemens Trio scanner) of T1 parameters were TR = 1900 ms, TE = 2.16 ms, TI=900ms and with isotropic 1 mm resolution. Rs-fMRI scans were performed using a gradient-echo EPI sequence and the parameters were as follows: TR = 2000 ms, TE = 32 ms, FA = 80, matrix = 6464, resolution = 3.75*3.75*4 mm^3. A total of 150 volumes were obtained by 5 mins. The 7T scanner (Siemens Magnetom) of T1 parameters were TR = 6000 ms, TE = 2.95 ms, TI = 800/2700 ms and with isotropic 0.65 mm resolution. 6 hippocampal subfields for 8 subjects (with ages of 30±8 years) are manually labeled. Then, the leave-one-out strategy is adopted to evaluate the performance of the proposed method.

Segmentation Performance Analysis. A typical hippocampal subfield segmentation result is demonstrated in Fig. 4 by overlapping our result on 3T MRI. By comparing with manual segmentation results, it can be seen that our method can effectively segment hippocampal subfields.

The quantitative analysis is reported in Table 1. Each entry shows mean ± standard deviation of Dice ratios in a leave-one-out cross validation (only mean value is reported for J. Pipitone's work [4], where they also used 3 T structural MRI, but treated CA2 and CA3 (or CA4 and DG) as one subfield). From the table, it can be seen that the segmentation results using combined T1 MRI and rs-fMRI at 3 T are consistently better than those using only one single modality. The consistently increased mean value and decreased standard deviation indicate that multi-modality data provides complementary information, which is beneficial for subfield segmentation.

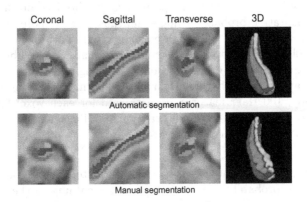

Fig. 4. Subfield segmentation results demonstration for one subject.

Table 1. Segmentation performance using different image modalities. Bolded numbers indicate the best performance using 3T MRI scanner.

	Sub	CA1	CA2	CA3	CA4	DG
3T T1	0.63±0.15	0.64±0.17	0.63±0.14	0.65±0.11	0.66±0.15	0.53±0.13
3 T rs-fMRI	0.61±0.13	0.65±0.11	0.62±0.07	0.61±0.08	0.64±0.08	0.46±0.15
3T T1 + rs-fMRI	**0.68±0.05**	**0.68±0.10**	**0.66±0.06**	**0.67±0.06**	**0.69±0.05**	**0.57±0.10**
7T T1	0.75±0.04	0.68±0.09	0.68±0.04	0.68±0.06	0.72±0.04	0.65±0.09
J. Pipitone [4]	0.58	0.56	0.41		0.68	

Besides, our result is also compared to the result of using 7T T1 MRI with the same appearance features as the 3T T1 MRI. The comparison result is also reported in Table 1. Comparing the fourth and fifth rows in the table, it can be seen that by using the complementary features from 3T T1 MRI and 3 T rs-fMRI, the segmentation results (CA1 - CA4) are comparable to those obtained using 7T T1 MRI. However, for the subiculum (Sub) and dentate gyrus (DG), more discriminative appearance features from 7T T1 MRI seem beneficial, and the results using 3T MRI are inferior. However, in most clinical settings, considering 7 T scanners are not available, our approach has the practical advantage.

Segmentation Refinement Evaluation. The segmentation results using different numbers of iterative refinement are reported in Fig. 5 (with the mean Dice ratio). From the figure, it can be seen that the iterative segmentation refinement is quite effective, especially in iteration **1** and **2**. The reason is, at each step, the previous segmentation result provides tentative label predictions of the neighboring voxels, which can be used to learn the relationship among neighboring predictions in the random forest. This information refines voxel-wise segmentations that are performed independently. In our case, after iteration **2**, the segmentation results become stable. So two iterations are used in this paper.

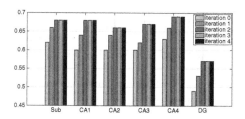

Fig. 5. Subfield segmentation results (mean Dice ratio) at different iterations.

5   Conclusion

In this paper, we utilize multi-modality images, i.e., 3T T1 MRI and 3 T rs-fMRI, to segment hippocampal subfields. This automatic segmentation algorithm uses a structured random forest as the multi-label classifier, followed by iterative segmentation refinement. To the best of our knowledge, this is the first work that investigates hippocampal subfield segmentation using the 3 T routine T1 MRI and rs-fMRI. The quantitative comparison between our results and the manually labeled subfields showed that our method is effective. Through these experimental results, we have reached two promising conclusions, (a) multi-modality features can provide complementary information which significantly improves the subfield segmentation compared to the single modality; (b) the segmentation results using 3 T scanner are comparable to those obtained using 7 T scanner. This shows a clear clinical advantage of our hippocampal subfield segmentation method using 3 T multi-modality MRI, considering that the 7 T scanner is currently not available in clinical assessment.

References

1. Van Leemput, K., Bakkour, A., et al.: Automated segmentation of hippocampal subfields from ultra-high resolution in vivo MRI. Hippocampus **19**, 549–557 (2009)
2. Yushkevich, P.A., Pluta, J.B., et al.: Automated volumetry and regional thickness analysis of hippocampal subfields and medial temporal cortical structures in mild cognitive impairment. Hum. Brain Mapp. **36**, 258–287 (2015)
3. Iglesias, J.E., Augustinack, J.C., Nguyen, K., Player, C.M., Player, A., Wright, M., Roy, N., Frosch, M.P., McKee, A.C., Wald, L.L., et al.: A computational atlas of the hippocampal formation using ex vivo, ultra-high resolution MRI: application to adaptive segmentation of in vivo mri. NeuroImage **115**, 117–137 (2015)
4. Pipitone, J., Park, M.T.M., et al.: Multi-atlas segmentation of the whole hippocampus and subfields using multiple automatically generated templates. Neuroimage **101**, 494–512 (2014)
5. Stokes, J., Kyle, C., et al.: Complementary roles of human hippocampal subfields in differentiation and integration of spatial context. J. Cogn. Neurosci. **27**, 546–559 (2015)
6. Blessing, E.M., Beissner, F., et al.: A data-driven approach to mapping cortical and subcortical intrinsic functional connectivity along the longitudinal hippocampal axis. Hum. Brain Mapp. **37**, 462–476 (2016)
7. Jenkinson, M., Bannister, P., et al.: Improved optimization for the robust and accurate linear registration and motion correction of brain images. Neuroimage **17**, 825–841 (2002)
8. Huynh, T., Gao, Y., et al.: Estimating CT image from MRI data using structured random forest and auto-context model. IEEE T-MI **35**, 174–183 (2016)
9. Tu, Z., Bai, X.: Auto-context and its application to high-level vision tasks and 3D brain image segmentation. IEEE T-PAMI **32**, 1744–1757 (2010)
10. Hao, Y., Wang, T., et al.: Local label learning (LLL) for subcortical structure segmentation: application to hippocampus segmentation. Hum. Brain Mapp. **35**, 2674–2697 (2014)
11. Cui, X., Liu, Y.e.a.: 3D HAAR-like features for pedestrian detection. In: ICME-2007, pp. 1263–1266. IEEE (2007)
12. Wang, H., Suh, J.W., et al.: Multi-atlas segmentation with joint label fusion. IEEE T-PAMI **35**, 611–623 (2013)

Regression Guided Deformable Models for Segmentation of Multiple Brain ROIs

Zhengwang Wu, Sang Hyun Park, Yanrong Guo, Yaozong Gao,
and Dinggang Shen[✉]

Department of Radiology and BRIC, UNC at Chapel Hill, Chapel Hill, NC, USA
dgshen@med.unc.edu

Abstract. This paper proposes a novel method of using regression-guided deformable models for brain regions of interest (ROIs) segmentation. Different from conventional deformable segmentation, which often deforms shape model locally and thus sensitive to initialization, we propose to learn a regressor to explicitly guide the shape deformation, thus eventually improves the performance of ROI segmentation. The regressor is learned via two steps, (1) a joint classification and regression random forest (CRRF) and (2) an auto-context model. The CRRF predicts each voxel's deformation to the nearest point on the ROI boundary as well as each voxel's class label (e.g., ROI *versus* background). The auto-context model further refines all voxel's deformations (i.e., deformation field) and class labels (i.e., label maps) by considering the neighboring structures. Compared to the conventional random forest regressor, the proposed regressor provides more accurate deformation field estimation and thus more robust in guiding deformation of the shape model. Validated in segmentation of 14 midbrain ROIs from the IXI dataset, our method outperforms the state-of-art multi-atlas label fusion and classification methods, and also significantly reduces the computation cost.

1 Introduction

Segmenting the brain into distinct ROIs is the foundation work for establishing relationships (functional network construction) between different brain ROIs. Recently, more and more discoveries reveal the importance of analyzing brain functional networks for understanding human brain, emotion and behaviors [1]. Therefore, better brain ROI segmentation is highly demanded.

Previously, many automatic methods have been proposed for brain ROI segmentation. One popular approach is the *multi-atlas label fusion based segmentation* [2]. In this approach, atlases with pre-segmented ROI labels are registered onto the target image. The aligned labels are then fused to derive the final segmentation of target image. However, it suffers from high-computational cost, due to nonlinear registration and local correspondence searching. To compromise for the computational cost, the number of used atlases is generally small,

---

D. Shen—This work was supported by the National Institute of Health grants 1R01 EB006733.

L. Wang et al. (Eds.): MLMI 2016, LNCS 10019, pp. 237–245, 2016.
DOI: 10.1007/978-3-319-47157-0_29

e.g., 20 atlases. For example, this approach often selects a subset of the most relevant atlases, which unfortunately loses some potentially useful information in other unselected atlases. On the other hand, the *classification-based approach* has also been proposed. Without relying on nonlinear registration, this approach is very efficient. However, its performance is limited since it overlooks the spatial information of brain ROIs. Moreover, classification based approach may produce weird ROI shapes and unsmooth boundaries, since the labeling of neighboring voxels is independent and no shape constraint is imposed. To address this limitation, Ma et al. [3] combined these two approaches into a single framework by extracting additional features from aligned atlases to train ROI classifiers. However, similar to the multi-atlas based approach, the efficiency is still a big concern due to the need of nonlinear registration.

In this paper, we propose a novel deformable model to segment brain ROIs. Different from conventional methods, which search local boundaries to deform the shape model, we explicitly learn a regressor to guide the shape deformation inspired by, which firstly addressed the regressor guided deformable segmentation. The difference between our work and [4] is that we introduced the context features to refine learned regressor. Specifically, we propose a joint **c**lassification and **r**egression **r**andom **f**orest (CRRF) regressor, which predicts both the deformation and ROI label of each voxel. Experimental results show that the incorporation of ROI classification into deformation estimation framework could significantly improve the deformation estimation in CRRF. To further impose the structured information during voxel-wise deformation prediction, an auto-context model is also adopted. It iteratively refines the estimated deformation fields by employing the neighboring predictions as new features to refine the training of the regressor. Compared with existing methods, our method has three advantages: (1) it is registration-free and thus very efficient; (2) it does not suffer from initialization problem as in the conventional deformable models; (3) it can impose both global-shape and local-smoothness constraints during the deformable ROI segmentation. We applied our method to IXI data set for segmenting 14 midbrain ROIs. The quantitative comparison between our results and manual segmentations proved the effectiveness, and also demonstrated its outstanding performance over several state-of-the-art methods.

2   Method

2.1   Main Framework

The main framework of our method is illustrated in Fig. 1. For each ROI, a shape model (represented as a triangle mesh in the 3D space [5]) is initialized to the image center and then iteratively deformed to the target ROI boundary under the guidance of the estimated deformation field (DF). Here, the DF is efficiently estimated by a CRRF and refined in the auto-context model, which will be detailed in Sect. 2.2. Section 2.3 presents how the estimated DF guides the shape model's deformation to the target ROI iteratively. In this paper, a multi-resolution strategy is also adopted to increase both the robustness and efficiency

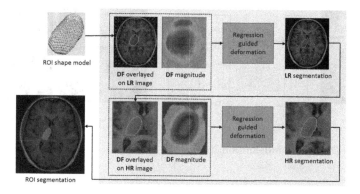

Fig. 1. Main framework of our proposed method. DF denotes deformable field. **LR** and **HR** denote low resolution and high resolution, respectively.

of our proposed method. Specifically, the coarse-level DF is first estimated in the down-sampled image space. It is used to roughly guide the shape model onto the ROI boundary. Then, the fine-level DF is estimated only in a local region surrounding the ROI for voxel-level refinement, thus improving both the efficiency of segmentation in the fine resolution, as well as the robustness of segmentation by using the coarse-level DF to guide the deformation.

Based on the above framework, each brain ROI can be independently segmented by the proposed deformable model. This can be done in a parallel way, which could greatly improve the segmentation efficiency. However, it potentially brings the issue of overlapping among different ROIs. To address this issue, a merging step is further adopted to combine all segmented ROIs into a single multi-label segmentation, which is detailed in Sect. 2.4.

2.2   Deformation Field Estimation

This section is organized as follows. First, we summarize overall pipeline of deformation field estimation, including the definition of deformation at each voxel and also the sampling strategy used in the training stage. Then, we present a joint classification and regression random forest (CRRF) for estimating both the deformation and ROI label of each voxel. Finally, we elaborate how to combine CRRF with auto-context for iteratively refining the deformation field.

Overall Pipeline. The deformation at each voxel is defined as a 3D displacement from this voxel to the nearest voxel on the ROI boundary, as illustrated in Fig. 2. It is given in the training images, but unknown for a testing image. In the *training stage*, we uniformly sample a set of voxels from training images. For each voxel, we compute its deformation and extract its ROI label, and then use them as the ground-truth prediction targets. The appearance features for each voxel are the 3D Haar-like features [6] extracted from the local patch. The choice of Haar-like features is due to its computational efficiency by using the integral

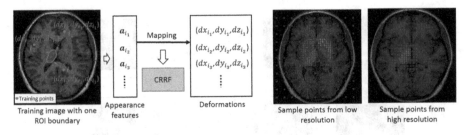

Fig. 2. Deformation definition.　　　　Fig. 3. Two sampling strategies.

image. Given features and prediction targets, we can use them to train a CRRF for each brain ROI. In the *testing stage*, each voxel of the testing image will be visited. Specifically, the appearance features of each visited voxel are extracted from the local patch and then fed into the learned CRRF to estimate the deformation at this voxel towards a brain ROI. Through this voxel-wise estimation, a deformable field can be finally obtained for each brain ROI under segmentation. To iteratively refine the deformation field by auto-context, additional 3D Haar features are extracted from the intermediate deformation field. Since they encode the neighboring prediction information, the combination of these features with original appearance features could lead to the structured refinement of the deformation field. This refinement step can be iteratively conducted for updating the deformation field.

Sampling/Training Strategy. Figure 3 illustrates the sampling strategies used in the low and high resolutions. In the low resolution, the training voxels are uniformly sampled all over the whole image, and a single CRRF is trained to jointly predict the deformations of a voxel to all ROIs. In the high resolution, the training voxels are randomly sampled near each ROI, and CRRF is trained separately for each ROI. The joint CRRF training can encode the spatial relationship between ROIs, thus improving the robustness of localization in the low resolution. In the high resolution, the specificity of the CRRF can be improved by sampling around the individual ROIs for training ROI-specific CRRFs.

Joint Classification and Regression Random Forest (CRRF). To adapt random forest for joint classification and regression, the objective function of random forest at each node is modified as follows:

$$\arg\max_{f,\tau} \frac{1}{Z_V}\left(V - \sum_{q\in\{L,R\}} \frac{N^q}{N}V^q\right) + \frac{1}{Z_E}\left(E - \sum_{q\in\{L,R\}} \frac{N^q}{N}E^q\right)$$

where f and τ are the pair of feature and threshold of one node to be optimized. V, E, N denote the average variance, entropy and the number of training samples at this node. The superscript $q \in \{L, R\}$ indicates the measurement computed after splitting this node into left(L) and right(R) child nodes. Z_V and Z_E are the average variance and entropy at the root node, respectively. The first term in the above formula is for the deformation regression, and the second term is

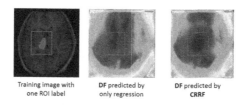

Fig. 4. Qualitative comparison between deformation fields (DFs) estimated by conventional regression forest (middle) and our CRRF (right).

for the ROI classification. With the above modification, a single random forest can be utilized to simultaneously predict the deformation and ROI label of a voxel. Similar to the theory of multi-task learning, we find that the joint classification and regression random forest produces better deformation field than the conventional regression forest, as illustrated in Fig. 4.

Iterative Auto-Context Refinement. With CRRF, the deformation at each voxel can be predicted from the local appearance. However, independent voxel-wise estimation neglects the relationship among deformations of neighboring voxels. Thus, the estimated deformation field is often noisy and unsmooth. To overcome it, an auto-context model [7] is adopted to iteratively refine the deformation field. In auto-context model, a sequence of CRRF is trained iteratively, as schematically illustrated in Fig. 5. In iteration **0**, the CRRF is trained with only appearance features. Once the first CRRF is obtained, it can be used to estimate a tentative deformation field as well as a ROI probability map. In iteration **1**, additional 3D Haar features are extracted from both the tentative deformation field and ROI probability map. These features are context features, because they encode both the neighboring deformation and ROI label information. By combing context features with appearance features, a second CRRF can be trained to refine both the deformation field and ROI probability map. This procedure can be repeatedly conducted until the maximum iteration T is reached.

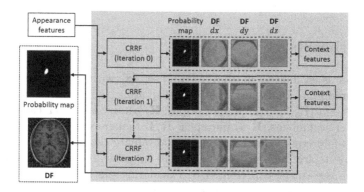

Fig. 5. Illustration of iterative auto-context refinement.

2.3   Regression Guided Deformable Segmentation

The mean ROI shape model is first initialized at the image center. Then, based on the estimated deformation field $\mathbf{D}$, we propose a hierarchical strategy to deform the shape model under the guidance of the estimated deformable field. Denote the vertex set of the shape model as $\mathcal{V} = \{\mathbf{p}_1, \cdots, \mathbf{p}_m, \cdots, \mathbf{p}_{|\mathcal{V}|}\}$, where $\mathbf{p}_m$ is the m-th vertex and $|\mathcal{V}|$ is the total number of vertices. Let $\mathbf{D}_{\mathbf{p}_m}$ denote the estimated deformation for vertex $\mathbf{p}_m$ in the image domain. The whole deform procedure is conducted in the following 3 steps, *First*, a translation vector $\mathbf{\Delta}$ is estimated as the average deformation of all vertices, i.e., $\mathbf{\Delta} = \sum_{m=1}^{|\mathcal{V}|} \mathbf{D}_{\mathbf{p}_m} / |\mathcal{V}|$, which brings the deformable model into the correct position of ROI. *Second*, a rotation matrix $\mathbf{R}$ is estimated between the deformed shape model $\hat{\mathcal{V}}$ and the original shape model $\mathcal{V}$, which brings the deformable model to the correct orientation, i.e., $\arg\min_{\mathbf{R}} ||\hat{\mathcal{V}} - \mathbf{R}\mathcal{V}||_2^2$, s.t., $\mathbf{R}\mathbf{R}^T = 1$, where $\hat{\mathcal{V}} = \{\mathbf{p}_1 + \rho\mathbf{D}_{\mathbf{p}_1}, \cdots, \mathbf{p}_m + \rho\mathbf{D}_{\mathbf{p}_m}, \cdots, \mathbf{p}_{|\mathcal{V}|} + \rho\mathbf{D}_{\mathbf{p}_{|\mathcal{V}|}}\}$, and ρ is the step size. Similarly, an affine transformation matrix can be also estimated to correct the scaling and shearing parameters of the deformable model. *Finally*, once the pose of deformable model is well estimated, the deformable model can be freely deformed locally under the deformation field. To maintain the mesh quality, the deformable model is further smoothed and re-meshed after each iteration of free-form deformation. With an explicit deformation field, the proposed deformable model is able to improve both the robustness to initialization and the flexibility of deformation.

2.4   ROI Merging

Once all ROIs are independently segmented by the proposed regression-guided deformable models, the final step is to address the potential overlapping issue by fusing all the individual ROI segmentations together. To merge all ROI segmentations, we utilize the ROI probability maps from CRRF. Note that each ROI probability map tells the probability of a voxel belonging to the ROI. Thus, for a voxel in the overlapping region, its ROI label can be determined by the one with the maximum probability value across all ROIs.

3   Experiments

Our method is evaluated in the IXI dataset [8] with 30 subjects. In this study, 14 midbrain ROIs are used for evaluating the segmentation performance, i.e., Right(**R**)/Left(**L**) hippocampus, **R**/**L** amygdala, **R**/**L** caudate, **R**/**L** nucleus(nuc.) accumbens, **R**/**L** putamen, **R**/**L** thalamus and **R**/**L** globus pallidus. The 3-fold cross validation is used to evaluate the performance. At each fold, 20 subjects are used for training and 10 subjects are used for testing. The quantitative assessment is presented by calculating the Dice ratio between the automatic segmentations and manual ROI segmentations. Five state-of-the-art segmentation methods are compared with our method, including, (a) majority voting (MV) [9]; (b) local weighted voting (LWV) [10]; (c) patch based label fusion (PLF) [11]; (d) sparse patch based label fusion (SPLF) [12]; (e) random forest classification (RFC) [3].

Table 1. Comparison with other methods. Bolded numbers indicate the best performance.

Method	MV	LWV	PLF	SPLF	RFC	Ours
R. Hippocampus	0.71	0.76	0.81	0.80	0.70	**0.83**
L. Hippocampus	0.70	0.73	0.78	0.79	0.72	**0.81**
R. Amygdala	0.71	0.74	0.77	0.75	0.71	**0.78**
L. Amygdala	0.73	0.73	0.79	0.76	0.73	**0.80**
R. Caudate	0.80	0.82	0.86	0.83	0.73	**0.89**
L. Caudate	0.80	0.83	0.86	0.83	0.82	**0.90**
R. nuc. accumbens	0.58	0.60	0.64	0.68	0.63	**0.72**
L. nuc. accumbens	0.57	0.60	0.64	0.68	0.60	**0.71**
R. Putamen	0.81	0.83	0.86	0.83	0.83	**0.88**
L. Putamen	0.80	0.83	0.86	0.83	0.79	**0.88**
R. Thalamus	0.84	0.85	0.88	0.84	0.88	**0.91**
L. Thalamus	0.84	0.86	0.88	0.84	0.85	**0.90**
R. Globus pallidus	0.76	0.77	0.80	0.79	0.77	**0.82**
L. Globus pallidus	0.72	0.75	0.78	0.78	0.72	**0.83**

All comparison results are reported in Table 1. It can be seen that our method consistently achieves the best performance for all 14 ROIs (with the mean Dice ratio of 0.83). Compared to the results of multi-atlas based methods (columns 2–5), our method has improved the Dice ratio by 0.07 on average. This indicates the effectiveness of our method. Furthermore, the computational time of our method (about 3 min) for segmenting all 14 ROIs is also much less than those of multi-atlas based methods (about 10–15 minutes on average, with the same number of atlases as used as training images in our method). Column 6 shows the segmentation results using random forest classification, with both the same multi-resolution training strategies and the same auto-context refinement. Although this simple random forest classification method can run as fast as our method, its performance is generally limited because it overlooks the spatial information of ROIs and also does not enforce the shape constraints of the ROIs during the segmentation. Our method obtains higher average dice ratio by 0.08 than the simple random forest classification.

Typical segmentation result using our proposed method is also demonstrated in Fig. 6. It can be seen, compared to the manual labels, our results are smoother. This is understandable, since manual ROI labeling need to validate at 3 cross-sectional views during manual delineation, the smoothness is thus difficult to

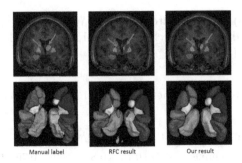

Fig. 6. Qualitative segmentation comparison obtained by RFC and our method.

maintain. For the RFC method, since each voxel is independently segmented, there are some mis-classifications, as shown in Fig. 6. Clearly, the ROIs segmented by our method are more coherent and do not contain the isolated voxels.

4   Conclusion

In this paper, we have proposed learning a regressor to explicitly predict the deformation field for guiding the deformable segmentation of multiple brain ROIs. Specifically, a joint classification and regression random forest (CRRF) is developed to estimate both the deformation and label of each voxel. Compared to the conventional regression forest, CRRF provides better deformation estimations. To tackle the limitation of independent voxel-wise estimation, an auto-context model is further adopted to iteratively refine the estimated deformation field by considering the neighboring prediction results. Validated on the 14 midbrain ROIs of IXI dataset, our method outperforms other five multi-atlas based label fusion and classification approaches.

References

1. Satterthwaite, T.D., Davatzikos, C.: Towards an individualized delineation of functional neuroanatomy. Neuron **87**, 471–473 (2015)
2. Aljabar, P., Heckemann, R.A., et al.: Multi-atlas based segmentation of brain images: atlas selection and its effect on accuracy. Neuroimage **46**, 726–738 (2009)
3. Ma, G., Gao, Y., Wu, G., Wu, L., Shen, D.: Atlas-guided multi-channel forest learning for human brain labeling. In: Menze, B., Langs, G., Montillo, A., Kelm, M., Müller, H., Zhang, S., Cai, W.T., Metaxas, D. (eds.) MCV 2014. LNCS, vol. 8848, pp. 97–104. Springer, Heidelberg (2014). Revised Selected Papers
4. Glocker, B., Pauly, O., Konukoglu, E., Criminisi, A.: Joint classification-regression forests for spatially structured multi-object segmentation. In: Fitzgibbon, A., Lazebnik, S., Perona, P., Sato, Y., Schmid, C. (eds.) ECCV 2012, Part IV. LNCS, vol. 7575, pp. 870–881. Springer, Heidelberg (2012)
5. Cootes, T.F., Taylor, C.J., et al.: Active shape models-their training and application. Comput. Vis. Image Underst. **61**, 38–59 (1995)

6. Cui, X., Liu, Y.e.a.: 3D HAAR-like features for pedestrian detection. In: ICME-2007, pp. 1263–1266. IEEE (2007)
7. Tu, Z., Bai, X.: Auto-context and its application to high-level vision tasks and 3D brain image segmentation. IEEE T-PAMI **32**, 1744–1757 (2010)
8. Brain Development Org: IXIDataSet. http://www.brain-development.org
9. Wang, H., Suh, J.W., Das, S.R., Pluta, J.B., Craige, C., Yushkevich, P.A.: Multi-atlas segmentation with joint label fusion. IEEE T-PAMI **35**, 611–623 (2013)
10. Artaechevarria, X., Munoz, A., et al.: Combination strategies in multi-atlas image segmentation: application to brain MR data. IEEE T-MI **28**, 1266–1277 (2009)
11. Coupé, P., Manjón, J.V., et al.: Patch-based segmentation using expert priors: application to hippocampus and ventricle segmentation. NeuroImage **54**, 940–954 (2011)
12. Wu, G., Wang, Q., Zhang, D., Shen, D.: Robust patch-based multi-atlas labeling by joint sparsity regularization. In: MICCAI Workshop STMI (2012)

Functional Connectivity Network Fusion with Dynamic Thresholding for MCI Diagnosis

Xi Yang, Yan Jin, Xiaobo Chen, Han Zhang, Gang Li, and Dinggang Shen[✉]

Department of Radiology and Biomedical Research Imaging Center,
University of North Carolina at Chapel Hill, Chapel Hill, NC, USA
dgshen@med.unc.edu

Abstract. The resting-state functional MRI (rs-fMRI) has been demonstrated as a valuable neuroimaging tool to identify mild cognitive impairment (MCI) patients. Previous studies showed network breakdown in MCI patients with thresholded rs-fMRI connectivity networks. Recently, machine learning techniques have assisted MCI diagnosis by integrating information from multiple networks constructed with a range of thresholds. However, due to the difficulty of searching optimal thresholds, they are often predetermined and uniformly applied to the entire network. Here, we propose an element-wise thresholding strategy to dynamically construct multiple functional networks, i.e., using possibly different thresholds for different elements in the connectivity matrix. These dynamically generated networks are then integrated with a network fusion scheme to capture their common and complementary information. Finally, the features extracted from the fused network are fed into support vector machine (SVM) for MCI diagnosis. Compared to the previous methods, our proposed framework can greatly improve MCI classification performance.

1 Introduction

Alzheimer's disease (AD) is an irreversible neurodegenerative disease resulting in progressive decline of memory and cognitive function. Mild cognitive impairment (MCI) is an intermediate stage between normal aging and AD. It is often misdiagnosed due to lacking of obvious clinical symptoms. Therefore, if MCI patients can be accurately diagnosed before the clinical onset of AD, treatments can be given in time to slow down the AD progress.

Recently, a variety of imaging modalities have been used for AD studies, such as structural MRI [1,2], diffusion MRI [3,4], and resting-state functional MRI (rs-fMRI) [5]. Different from structural and diffusion MRI that reveals brain morphological changes, rs-fMRI can examine both functional integration and segregation of brain networks that are undermined by MCI [6]. In previous studies, functional connectivity (FC) networks for characterizing pairwise correlation

D. Shen—This work was supported by the National Institute of Health grants 1R01 AG042599 and 1R01 AG041721.

L. Wang et al. (Eds.): MLMI 2016, LNCS 10019, pp. 246–253, 2016.
DOI: 10.1007/978-3-319-47157-0_30

between different brain regions were constructed with rs-fMRI data and revealed the disrupted network topological properties in MCI [7].

Machine learning techniques are able to utilize features extracted from FC networks to identify MCI patients with a relatively high accuracy. Specifically, first, for reducing both the noise and unreliable connections, FC networks were often thresholded based on the connectivity strength, i.e., the FCs larger than a specific value were preserved and others were set to zero. Then, with a set of different threshold values, different topological views of the same original network can be derived to provide complementary information for enhancing the diagnosis. For example, Jie *et al.* [5] extracted features from multiple complementary thresholded networks and integrated them using multi-kernel learning for classification. Nevertheless, this method has two main drawbacks. (1) In terms of the thresholding strategy, they simply used a range of predetermined thresholds which might not be optimal. Thus, the classification performance often fluctuated greatly with a small change of threshold value, especially when the derived networks are very sparse. More importantly, all connections in the FC network are thresholded by the same *unified* threshold, which may be not reasonable since noise level in different brain regions could vary significantly. (2) In terms of the fusion strategy, searching for an optimal combination of the kernels, each designed for a derived network, becomes a daunting task, especially when the number of networks is large.

In this paper, we propose a novel classification framework with a dynamic thresholding strategy and then a network fusion scheme to address the above drawbacks. Specifically, for each subject, instead of thresholding all connections in its network by a set of predetermined values (i.e., network-wise thresholding), we propose to threshold each connection in the network (i.e., each element in the connectivity matrix) by a different threshold value (i.e., element-wise thresholding), which is randomly sampled from a distribution learned from all subject data. With this "element-wise" thresholding strategy, multiple FC networks can be dynamically constructed. To effectively integrate various information contained in these networks, we further adopt a novel network fusion method [8] to integrate these dynamic networks for capturing their common and complementary information. During the network fusion process, each thresholded network is iteratively updated under the interaction of two networks: a sparse network carrying the important strongest connectivity information of its own and the average of the other networks. Through such a fusion scheme, the full spectrum of complementary information can be integrated, without optimizing the weights of the kernels as in multi-kernel learning. After obtaining the fused network for each subject, we extract the local clustering coefficients (graph topological properties) of the network as features. Feature selection is then performed with the Least Absolute Shrinkage and Selection Operator (LASSO) [9] and the selected features are finally fed into support vector machine (SVM) for MCI classification. The performance of our proposed framework is evaluated with the Alzheimer's Disease Neuroimaging Initiative Phase-2 (ADNI-2) database.

2   Method

The overview of our method is illustrated in Fig. 1. The whole procedure can
be divided into six steps: network construction, dynamic thresholding, network
fusion, feature extraction, feature selection, and classification. Each step will be
described in details below.

2.1   Data Preprocessing and Network Construction

The dataset was downloaded from the ADNI-2 database (http://adni.loni.usc.
edu/), which contained 30 normal controls (13M/17F; age: 74.3 ± 5.7) and 29
MCI subjects (16M/13F; age: 73.6 ± 4.8). Each subject was scanned with a 3.0T
Philips Achieva scanner with the same protocol: a matrix size of $64 \times 64 \times 48$ and
an isotropic voxel size of 3.3 mm. Among the 140 collected rs-fMRI volumes, the
first 10 volumes were discarded to ensure the magnetization equilibrium, and the
remaining volumes were processed by SPM8 (http://www.fil.ion.ucl.ac.uk/spm/
software/spm8). The data was slice-timing corrected, head motion corrected,
normalized to the standard space, and parcellated into 116 regions of interest
(ROIs) with the Automated Anatomical Labeling (AAL) atlas [10]. Then the
mean rs-fMRI time series at each ROI was computed.

An original FC network can be represented by 116 nodes (i.e., 116 ROIs) and
the edges connecting them (i.e., connections between each pair of 116 ROIs). The
connection strength is computed by Pearson's correlation between two mean
time series between a pair of ROIs. Here, we only considered the magnitudes
of correlation coefficients. Thus, we use their absolute values, i.e., the resultant
connection strengths range from 0 to 1.

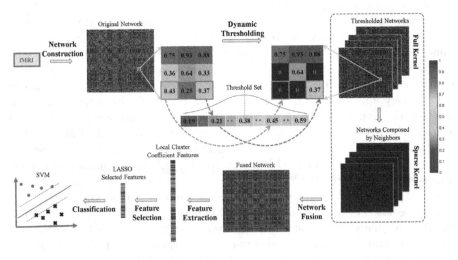

Fig. 1. Overview of connectivity network fusion with dynamic thresholding.

2.2 Dynamical Network Thresholding

The original FC network is usually dense and noisy. To better remove noise and also locate more biologically meaningful features for classification, the network needs to be sparse by proper thresholding. Previous methods for network-wise thresholding typically set up a set of *unified* thresholds for the entire network. However, for one thing, it is extremely difficult to find an optimal set of predetermined thresholds with brutal force; for another, it is not reasonable to use a uniform threshold for all connections, since correlation coefficients are often affected by different levels of noise.

Instead of using a unified threshold for the entire network, we used a dynamic threshold for each connection in the network. As the previous study had indicated that network sparsity between 25 % and 75 % was appropriate for MCI diagnosis [5], we recorded the thresholds corresponding to the 25 % and the 75 % network sparsity, respectively. Then, we generated the thresholds with a step size $\triangle$ between these two estimated thresholds. After finding thresholds across all subjects, we modeled the distribution of all these thresholds with a Gaussian function $N(\mu, \sigma)$, where μ was the mean of all the thresholds, and σ was the standard deviation. The rationale of using a Gaussian distribution was that the optimal threshold most likely appeared in the center of the Gaussian distribution based on previous studies [5] and the observation of our data. Then, for each connection element, we randomly sampled a value from the estimated Gaussian distribution and then used it to threshold this connection element in the original FC network. By implementing this element-specific thresholding for all elements, we obtained a new dynamically-thresholded network. For each subject, we repeated this for N times and constructed a set of dynamically-thresholded networks $\{W_i^j\}$, where $j = 1, ..., N$ for the subject i. An illustration of this procedure is shown in the Dynamic Thresholding step in Fig. 1.

Compared to the one-size-fits-all network-wise method [5], this element-wise dynamic strategy *not only* reduced the influence of threshold selection to the classification result, *but also* treated each connection separately. Besides, we obtained more different topological views of the original FC network for each subject.

2.3 Network Fusion

The dynamically-thresholded networks extracted in Sect. 2.2 provided complementary information for MCI classification. To leverage their common and complementary information, we adopted a recently developed Similarity Network Fusion (SNF) algorithm to fuse these networks [8].

To use SNF for our application, for each network W_i^j of subject i, two kernel matrices were constructed: (1) a *full kernel matrix*, which was the network itself; (2) a *sparse kernel matrix*, which encoded the sparse yet strong connection information. Let N_u denote a set of k-nearest neighbors (the top k strongest connections) of the node u (including u itself) in W_i^j, then the *sparse kernel* S_i^j could be represented as:

$$S_i^j(u,v) = \begin{cases} W_i^j(u,v) & v \in N_u \\ 0 & otherwise \end{cases} \tag{1}$$

where the connection between nodes v and u existed only if v was within the k-nearest neighbors of u. Based on these two kernel matrices, each network could be iteratively updated as follows:

$$(W_i^j)^{(m+1)} = S_i^j \times \frac{\sum_{c\neq j}(W_i^c)^{(m)}}{N-1} \times (S_i^j)^T, c = 1, ..., N \tag{2}$$

where $(W_i^c)^{(m)}$ denotes the network W_i^c for subject i at the m-th iteration and $(W_i^j)^{(m+1)}$ is the updated W_i^j after $m+1$ iterations.

By interacting with other thresholded networks, W_i^j can integrate the information provided by other topological views of the original network. Meanwhile, the *sparse kernel matrix* S_i^j guides the iterative process through the strongest connections of W_i^j and thus can suppress the noise effectively. From the perspective of matrix multiplication, Eq. (2) implies that the connection of any two nodes in W_i^j also relies on the connections of their neighbors among other thresholded networks. In other words, if the respective neighbors of two nodes are strongly connected in other thresholded networks, their connection can be strengthened after the updates even though it may be weak itself and vice versa.

After the iterative process converged, we averaged the N networks to obtain our final fused dynamically dynamically-thresholded network for subject i:

$$W_i = \frac{\sum_j W_i^j}{N}, j = 1, ..., N \tag{3}$$

Comparing to those thresholded networks W_i^j, the benefits of W_i are two-fold. First, it doesn't rely on any individual threshold as in W_i^j, and thus is less affected by noise; Second, it incorporates all the common and complementary information from all N networks $(W_i^j, j = 1, ..., N)$ after SNF, so it can better represent the underlying ground truth of FC.

2.4   Classification

With the fused network W_i for each subject i, the local weighted clustering coefficients (LWCCs) x_i [11] were extracted as features. LWCCs are a the commonly used connectivity measures that compute the degree to which nodes in a graph tend to cluster together. Mathematically, for a subject i, let $x_i = [x_i^1, ..., x_i^L]^T \in \mathbb{R}_{L \times 1}$, where L is the number of ROIs. Let d_l be the number of edges the node l connects and $W_i(p,q)$ be the edge strength between any two nodes p and q in W_i, then x_i^l can be computed as $(l = 1, ..., L)$:

$$x_i^l = \frac{2\sum_{p,q}[W_i(l,p)W_i(p,q)W_i(q,l)]^{1/3}}{d_l(d_l-1)} \tag{4}$$

Once the features were extracted, the LASSO feature selection scheme [9] was applied to select the most relevant features for MCI classification by minimizing the following objective function:

$$\min_{a,b} \frac{1}{2} \sum_{i=1}^{N} (y_i - a^T x_i - b)^2 + \gamma \|a\|_1 \qquad (5)$$

where a denoted the weight coefficient vector and $\|a\|_1$ is the l_1-norm of a. The regularization parameter γ balanced between the fitting error and the sparsity of solution; y_i and b were the class label of subject; x_i and intercept, respectively. The corresponding features of non-zero components of a were selected and fed into SVM classifier for MCI classification.

3 Experimental Results

3.1 Experimental Setup

In our experiment, the step size for threshold selection is $\triangle = 0.01$ and the number of dynamically-thresholded networks is $N = 50$ (Sect. 2.2). In network fusion (Sect. 2.3), $k = 26$ was set for the k-nearest neighbors of S_i^j, and the stopping criterion for iteration was $\|(W_i^j)^{(m+1)} - (W_i^j)^{(m)}\| \leq 0.01$. The SLEP (http://www.yelab.net/software/SLEP/) was used for feature selection with LASSO, while the LIBSVM (https://www.csie.ntu.edu.tw/~cjlin/libsvm/) was utilized for SVM classification (Sect. 2.4).

To evaluate our proposed framework, dynamic thresholding with network fusion (**DTN**), we compared it with four other methods: the original Pearson's correlation FC network (**PCN**), the network-wise thresholding with network fusion (**NTN**), the mean dynamic element-wise thresholding without fusion (**MTN**), and the traditional network-wise thresholding with multi-kernel learning (**MKL**). In PCN, we fed the original FC network directly to SVM for classification. In NTN, we generated 50 networks with the traditional network-wise thresholding and then fused them with our network fusion scheme. In MTN, we averaged over the 50 dynamic element-wise thresholded networks without network fusion for SVM classification. In MKL, 5 networks were randomly selected with network-wise thresholding and then fed into multi-kernel classification [5].

The classification performance was evaluated by the classical measures including accuracy (ACC), sensitivity (SEN), specificity (SPE), and area under the receiver operating characteristic curve (AUC). For all methods, the classification performance were evaluated through leave-one-out cross-validation.

3.2 Classification Performance

The classification results are reported in Table 1. Figure 2 plots the receiver operating characteristic (ROC) curves of all the methods. Our proposed framework outperforms all 4 comparison methods.

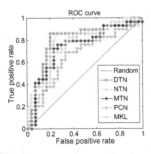

Fig. 2. ROC curves of different methods.

Table 1. Classification performances of all methods in percentage.

Method	ACC	AUC	SEN	SPE
PCN	67.8	65.9	69.0	66.7
MKL	72.9	76.9	79.3	66.7
MTN	74.6	72.2	65.5	80.0
NTN	79.7	72.9	79.3	70.0
DTN	83.1	80.5	86.2	80.0

Both MTN and NTN show better performance than PCN, which confirms that the two key steps, dynamic thresholding and network fusion, are both beneficial. Compared to MTN and NTN, the proposed framework DTN further improves the performance, which proves the effectiveness using the combination of both techniques. DTN achieves better performance than NTN because the dynamic element-wise thresholding, a more reasonable threshold selection scheme, which treats each connection individually and reduces the limitation of random threshold selection for the entire network. DTN outperforms MTN because the network fusion scheme can reveal the underlying topology closer to the ground truth than just simply averaging those networks. The fact that DTN acts better than MKL demonstrates that our method overcomes the drawbacks of the previous methods, and is indeed a better algorithm.

To further gain the insights of our algorithm, we randomly selected three normal controls and MCI patients from our dataset, respectively. Figure 3 illustrates their original FC networks and the dynamically-thresholded networks after fusion. Compared to the original networks, our fused networks show more block-like structures with more clear layouts. Besides, the original networks look similar between normal controls and MCI patients, while our fused networks show significant difference between the two groups. The MCI network connections seem to be much weaker, and this is consistent with the well-accepted FC breakdown concept in MCI.

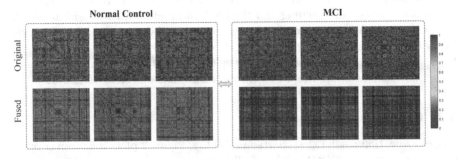

Fig. 3. Original networks and fused networks of three randomly selected normal controls (left) and MCI patients (right) respectively.

4   Conclusion

In this paper, we have proposed a novel classification framework for MCI identification with the FC networks constructed from rs-fMRI data. Unlike the previous network-wise thresholding algorithm that used a fixed value for the entire network, we developed an element-wise dynamic thresholding strategy to reduce the impact of threshold selection. The SNF fusion scheme further enhanced the FC structure by incorporating the complementary information contained in multiple dynamically-thresholded networks. The experimental results demonstrate the superior performance of our framework over other comparison methods, indicating that our method can be potentially used as a practical tool for rs-fMRI based studies.

References

1. Wang, T., et al.: Abnormal changes of brain cortical anatomy and the association with plasma microRNA107 level in amnestic mild cognitive impairment. Front. Aging Neurosci. **8**, 112 (2016)
2. Huang, L., et al.: Longitudinal clinical score prediction in Alzheimer's disease with soft-split sparse regression based random forest. Neurobiol. Aging **46**, 180–191 (2016)
3. Wang, T., et al.: Multilevel deficiency of white matter connectivity networks in Alzheimer's disease: a diffusion MRI study with DTI and HARDI models. Neural Plast. **2016**, 2947136 (2016)
4. Jin, Y., et al.: Automated multi-atlas labeling of the fornix and its integrity in Alzheimer's disease. In: Proceedings of IEEE International Symposium on Biomedical Imaging, pp. 140–143(2015)
5. Jie, B., et al.: Integration of network topological and connectivity properties for neuroimaging classification. IEEE Trans. Biomed. Eng. **61**, 576–589 (2014)
6. Sperling, R.: Potential of functional MRI as a biomarker in early Alzheimer's disease. Neurobiol. Aging **32**(Suppl1), S37–S43 (2011)
7. Toussaint, P.J., et al.: Characteristics of the default mode functional connectivity in normal ageing and Alzheimer's disease using resting state fMRI with a combined approach of entropy-based and graph theoretical measurements. Neuroimage **101**, 778–786 (2014)
8. Wang, B., et al.: Similarity network fusion for aggregating data types on a genomic scale. Nat. Methods **11**, 333–337 (2014)
9. Tibshirani, R.: Regression shrinkage and selection via the lasso. J. Roy. Stat. Soc. Ser. B Methodol. **58**, 267–288 (1996)
10. Tzourio-Mazoyer, N., Landeau, B., et al.: Automated anatomical labeling of activations in SPM using a macroscopic anatomical parcellation of the MNI MRI single-subject brain. Neuroimage **15**, 273–289 (2002)
11. Rubinov, M., Sporns, O.: Complex network measures of brain connectivity: uses and interpretations. Neuroimage **52**, 1059–1069 (2010)

Sparse Coding Based Skin Lesion Segmentation Using Dynamic Rule-Based Refinement

Behzad Bozorgtabar$^{(\boxtimes)}$, Mani Abedini, and Rahil Garnavi

IBM Research - Australia, Carlton, Australia
{sydb,mabedini,rahilgar}@au1.ibm.com

Abstract. This paper proposes an unsupervised skin lesion segmentation method for dermoscopy images by exploiting the contextual information of skin image at the superpixel level. In particular, a Laplacian sparse coding is presented to evaluate the probabilities of the skin image pixels to delineate lesion border. Moreover, a new rule-based smoothing strategy is proposed as the lesion segmentation refinement procedure. Finally, a multi-scale superpixel segmentation of the skin image is provided to handle size variation of the lesion in order to improve the accuracy of the detected border. Experiments conducted on two datasets show the superiority of our proposed method over several state-of-the-art skin segmentation methods.

Keywords: Superpixel-based segmentation · Laplacian sparse coding · Dynamic rule-based refinement

1 Introduction

Malignant melanoma is one of the most common and the deadliest type of skin cancer [17]. Skin lesion segmentation is the first and a crucial step towards developing an automated diagnostic system for melanoma.

In this paper, we propose an unsupervised multi-scale lesion segmentation method, where a Laplacian sparse coding is proposed to measure the probabilities of image superpixels belonging to the lesion. Moreover, the structural information of the lesion pixel and the mutual relationship between the neighbouring superpixels is integrated into our framework to improve the segmentation accuracy. In particular, a new rule-based segmentation refinement is proposed, which enables our method to relate low-level image features to expert domain knowledge. The experimental results have demonstrated that our approach outperforms several state-of-the-art methods in this domain.

2 Related Work

Lesion border detection is a challenging task due to variety of the lesion shapes, colour, textures and presence of artefacts such as hair and fiducial markers. To address these difficulties in the segmentation task, several techniques have

© Springer International Publishing AG 2016
L. Wang et al. (Eds.): MLMI 2016, LNCS 10019, pp. 254–261, 2016.
DOI: 10.1007/978-3-319-47157-0_31

been recently proposed, which can be categorised into main three groups include *threshold-based, active-contour-based* and *region growing* methods.

Thresholding-based methods [4,13] achieved good lesion segmentation results, when there is good contrast between the lesion and the surrounding skin. Alcon et al. [3] proposed a thresholding scheme for the *Macroscopic Pigmented Skin Lesion* images and have proved that Otsu's method may oversegment the skin lesion area. Garnavi et al. [8] applied a hybrid of global thresholding to detect an initial boundary of the lesion, and then employed an adaptive histogram thresholding on optimized colour channels of X (from the *CIE XYZ* colour space) to refine the border.

In *Active-Contour* based techniques, an input skin image is initially smoothed by filtering algorithms such as adaptive anisotropic diffusion filtering. *Gradient Vector Flow* [7] and *Adaptive Snake* [12] are among popular edge-based segmentation methods.

Regarding *region based growing* methods, *Level-Set Active Contours* [9] and *Statistical Region Growing* [6] are the most frequent methods in the literature. Celebi et al. [6] presented a computationally efficient statistical region merging algorithm for dermoscopic images. However, such an approach has difficulties dealing with macroscopic images with complex textures (e.g. multiple lesions) or large variations in colours.

More recently, object saliency-based detection approaches [2,10] have been proposed, which aim to locate region of interest (e.g. skin lesion) that capture human attention within images. These methods show promising segmentation performance. There are also successful segmentation methods by aggregating of the superpixels either using different visual features or superpixels' scales. Mithun et al. [5] proposed a symmetric *Kullback-Leibler* (KL) divergence based clustering method to segment multiple levels of depigmentation in Vitiligo images.

3   System Overview

In this paper, we propose an unsupervised lesion segmentation method which has the following novelties:

- A superpixel-based skin lesion segmentation is proposed, where different confidence maps are generated at multiple superpixels scales. The term '*confidence*' refers to the probability of a superpixel belonging to the lesion. We use sparse feature representation to model the confidence (probability) values of the superpixels. These confidence maps are complementary to each other and are combined through a new multi-scale fusion technique to further improve the lesion border detection performance (see Fig. 1).
- In this paper, a Laplacian multi-task sparse representation is presented, where the similarity of each superpixel to the background seeds (dictionary of the background skin image patches), as well as the pairwise relationship between neighbouring superpixels are exploited jointly, by imposing the graph structure. This graph structure incorporates the colour similarities and spatial smoothness constraints of the superpixels.

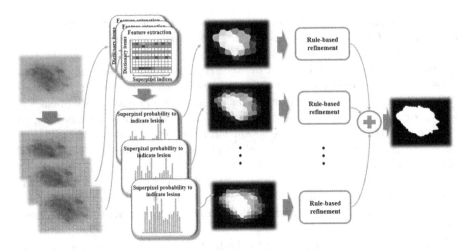

Fig. 1. Illustration of the proposed skin lesion segmentation framework. The first column shows an input skin image and its associated over-segmented image with a set of superpixels. The middle columns display the multi-scale superpixels' probabilities and the confidence maps (generated by the proposed Laplacian multi-task sparse representation). The rightmost image shows the final segmentation result constructed by multi-scale confidence maps fusion.

– More importantly, a new *rule* based lesion segmentation refinement is proposed, where each superpixel confidence score will be updated based on colour properties of the neighbouring superpixels (see Sect. 3.2).

3.1   Single-Scale Lesion Confidence Map

An input skin image is over-segmented at S scales. At any scale, an image is partitioned into N superpixels using the *Simple Linear Iterative Clustering* (SLIC) algorithm [1], whose features (*CIE LAB* colour features and *spatial* location) are denoted in a matrix form as: $Y^s = [y_1^s, \ldots, y_N^s] \in R^{m \times N}$[1], where y_i^s is the ith vectorised superpixel features at scale s.

Laplacian Multi-task Sparse Representation. We formulate the global contrast between the superpixels within the lesion and the surrounding skin area as a Laplacian multi-task sparse learning problem. The proposed sparse feature representation not only encodes the dissimilarity of each superpixel with respect to the background skin, but also considers the pairwise similarities between neighbouring superpixels. In doing so, we build a dictionary representing the background skin. We choose background seeds (templates) in our sparse feature representation framework from the superpixels located on corners of the image

---

[1] m is the feature dimension.

(to avoid inclusion of any lesion). The background templates $B^s = [b_1^s, \ldots, b_K^s] \in R^{m \times K}$ are constructed using the *K-mean* clustering, which can represent the superpixels under a variety of appearance changes by its templates $\{b_i^s\}_{i=1}^{K}$ (b_i is the ith *dictionary* item at scale s). Given these background templates, the sparse representation of the superpixels can be jointly learned based the following optimisation problem:

$$\arg \min_X \|Y - BX\|_F^2 + \frac{\lambda_1}{2} Tr\left(XLX^T\right) + \lambda_2 \|X\|_{2,1} \tag{1}$$

where $\|X\|_{2,1} = \sum_{i=1}^{K} \|X\|_2$, λ_1 and λ_2 are the regularization parameters. We drop Y^s, B^s and X^s to avoid clutters in the equations. L is known as the Laplacian matrix, is symmetric and positive definiteness. Our proposed optimisation problem has the following terms:

1. *Global Contrast*: The probability of the ith superpixel at scale s belonging to the skin lesion is determined by its reconstruction error $\varepsilon_i^s = \|y_i^s - B^s x_i^s\|$ over the background templates B^s, where x_i^s is the corresponding sparse representation.
2. *Mixed Sparsity Norm* $\|X\|_{2,1}$: The clustered boundary templates B represent the possible appearance variations of superpixels such as colour variations, but only a few number of these templates is needed to reliably represent each superpixel. It should be noted that l_1 norm can also be used, but our experiments show that the mixed norm $\|X\|_{2,1}$ is more efficient than l_1 norm especially when the number of clusters increases and it encourages the feature representation matrix to be *row* sparse.
3. *Graph Regularizer Term* $Tr\left(XLX^T\right)$: The mutual relationship between the superpixels is imposed with a graph structure $G = (V, E, W)$, where the superpixels are represented by the graph vertices V and the edges E between superpixels specify their correlation (feature similarity) with their corresponding weights W. In fact, a symmetric weight w_{ij} is the feature similarity measure between the ith superpixel y_i and the jth superpixel $y_j{}^2$. Considering $d_i = \sum_{i=1}^{N} w_{ij}$ as the sum of elements in the ith row of W, $D = diag\{d_1, d_2, \cdots, d_N\}$ is known as the graph degree matrix. As the last part of the formula, by denoting $L = D - W$ as the Laplacian of the graph, we represent the graph regularizer term as $\sum_{ij} \|x_i - x_j\|_2^2 w_{ij} = Tr\left(XLX^T\right)$, which model the pairwise correlations among the superpixels.

The proposed minimisation problem in Eq. 1 for learning the sparse feature representation is rendered as a non smooth convex (unconstrained) optimisation problem, in which, we used an *Accelerated Proximal Gradient* (APG) method [19] for solving this optimisation problem.

The confidence score of the ith superpixel at scale s belonging to the lesion is formulated as a probability value in the form of exponential function of the reconstruction error ε_i^s and is calculated as:

---

^{2} $w_{ij} = exp\left(-\frac{\|y_i, y_j\|}{\sigma^2}\right)$ s.t. $j \in NB(i)$.

$$P_i^s = \frac{1}{exp\left(-\frac{\varepsilon_i^s}{\sigma}\right) + \alpha} \tag{2}$$

where α and σ are the balance weights.

3.2   Dynamic Rule-Based Refinement

To elevate the segmentation accuracy and to further refine the confidence map, a dynamic *rule-based* strategy is devised, where the confidence score of each super-pixel is updated based on its identified neighbours within the graph structure. More specifically, if a certain superpixel is completely dissimilar to its neighbours (e.g. based on colour features), its updated confidence value will be only based on its current value, otherwise, the similar nearby superpixels have a great influence on the superpixel's updated score. In order to balance these two factors, we build a updating matrix $C = diag\{c_1, c_2, \cdots, c_N\}$ whose i^{th} element is $c_i = \frac{1}{max(w_{ij})}$. Finally, the updating rule is defined as:

$$P^{t+1} = C.P^t + (I - C).W^*.P^t \tag{3}$$

where I is the identity matrix and $W^* = W.D^{-1}$ is a normalised version of a symmetric weight matrix W. The updating process starts with the initial P^t when $t = 0$ from Eq. 1, and after a few iterations, the confidence map can reach its steady state.

3.3   Multi-scale Fusion

Since the accuracy of the border detection is sensitive to the number of super-pixels, a multi-scale superpixel segmentation is presented. The lesion confidence maps produced at multiple scales are combined with different weights to construct a strong confidence map, which is then binarised using the *otsu* threshold to obtain the final segmentation result. The weights are determined by measuring the feature similarities between each image pixel z and the corresponding superpixels at different scales that pixel belongs to. Denoting $r(z)$ as the feature representation of pixel z (*CIE LAB* and *spatial* features) and $\bar{y}_z^s$ as the *mean* feature value of the superpixel containing the pixel z at scale s, we compute the overall lesion confidence map as follows:

$$F(z) = \frac{1}{\gamma} \sum_{s=1}^{S} I^s(z) \times P^s(z) \tag{4}$$

where γ is the normalisation parameter and for each pixel, there are S values $\{P^s(z)\}, s = 1, 2, \cdots, S$ of the superpixels containing the pixel at different scales. The scale influence weight $I^s(z)$ for the pixel z is calculated based on its feature distance to $\bar{y}_z^s$ as:

$$I^s(z) = (\|r(z) - \bar{y}_z^s\| + \beta)^{-1} \tag{5}$$

We observed that, this weighted summation performs better than a simple combination of the confidence maps at different scales. Constant β is used to avoid being divided by zero[3].

4   Experimental Results

4.1   Datasets

PH[2] *dataset:* This dataset has been acquired at *Dermatology Service of Hospital Pedro Hispano, Matosinhos, Portugal* [11] with Tuebinger Mole Analyzer system. It provides 200 dermoscopic images with a resolution of 768×560 pixels. The lesions are manually annotated by the expert dermatologists.

ISBI 2016 *challenge dataset:* This dataset contains 900 dermoscopic images[4]. The skin images sizes vary from 1022×767 to 4288×2848 pixels and the ground truth is provided by experts. This dataset contains 727 *benign* and 173 *melanoma* dermoscopic images.

4.2   Performance Measure and Parameters Setting

To measure the performance of the proposed method, we adopt different metrics: *Area Under Curve* (AUC), *Average Precision* (AP), *Dice Similarity Coefficient* (DSC) and *Jaccard Coefficient* (JC), which quantify the spatial overlap between the ground truth and the obtained segmentation binary mask. For example, DSC is defined as the area $\frac{2A_S \cap A_G}{A_S + A_G}$, where A_S and A_G denote the segmentation result and the ground truth, respectively.

The parameters λ_1 and λ_2 in Eq. 1 are empirically set to 0.04 and 0.4, and the maximum number of iteration for the optimisation problem in Eq. 1 and updating process in Eq. 3 is set to 15 and 5, respectively. The number of clusters K and scales S is both set to 3 by cross-validation. The sparse feature representation of the features (*CIE LAB* colour and *spatial* location) are computed separately, and then are multiplied to obtain the final features. The balance weights, α and σ in Eq. 2 are set to 0.1 and 8, respectively. The normalisation factor γ in Eq. 4 is computed by summation of scale weights I^s. The parameter settings are the same for the two different datasets and are found experimentally. The segmentation performance is not very sensitive to these parameters.

We have compared the performance of the proposed lesion segmentation method with several state-of-the-art methods; namely, *AT* [16], *ISO* [14], *Yen thresholing* [15], *LSAC* [9] and *SRG* [6]. We also compare our method with new superpixel-based saliency detection approaches [10,18] that cluster superpixels to different image regions (foreground and background). The results are shown in Tables 1 and 2.

---

[3] The parameter β is set to 0.2.

[4] https://challenge.kitware.com/challenge/n/ISBI_2016_3A_Skin_Lesion_Analysis_Tow ards_Melanoma_Detection.

Table 1. Comparative study between the proposed method and other state-of-the-art methods tested on 'ISBI 2016' dataset.

Methods	AP	JC	DC	AUC
Adaptive thresholding [16]	0.80	0.45	0.56	0.72
ISO [14]	0.77	0.56	0.68	0.82
Yen thresholing [15]	0.77	0.58	0.67	0.81
Level set active contours [9]	0.79	0.46	0.58	0.70
Statistical region growing [6]	0.76	0.43	0.55	0.73
Bootstrap learning [18]	0.75	0.57	0.72	0.78
Contexual hypergraph [10]	0.78	0.60	0.75	0.83
Proposed method $\#SP = 100$	0.79	0.63	0.77	0.83
Proposed method $\#SP = 200$	0.80	0.64	0.78	**0.94**
Proposed method $\#SP = 300$	0.82	0.65	0.78	0.90
Proposed method- fusion	**0.86**	**0.67**	**0.80**	0.91

Table 2. Comparative study between the proposed method and other state-of-the-art methods tested on 'PH^2' dataset.

Methods	AP	JC	DC	AUC
Adaptive thresholding [16]	0.87	0.72	0.80	0.81
ISO [14]	0.62	0.33	0.44	0.84
Yen thresholing [15]	0.67	0.45	0.55	0.87
Level set active contours [9]	0.86	**0.76**	0.83	0.77
Statistical region growing [6]	0.89	0.43	0.61	0.79
Bootstrap learning [18]	0.85	0.60	0.75	0.72
Contexual hypergraph [10]	0.87	0.63	0.77	0.75
Proposed method $\#SP = 100$	**0.91**	0.74	0.85	0.93
Proposed method $\#SP = 200$	0.87	0.75	0.85	0.95
Proposed method $\#SP = 300$	0.79	0.72	0.83	0.92
Proposed method- fusion	0.86	**0.76**	**0.86**	**0.96**

Our method achieves the highest overlap accuracy metric (also lowest *False Positives* (FP) and *False Negatives* (FN)) compared to the other state-of-the-arts with the significant margin ($> 6\%$) in JC metric on *ISBI 2016* challenge dataset.

5 Conclusion

In this paper, we have presented an unsupervised method for skin lesion segmentation that builds upon the sparse coding technique. In addition, the main contribution is a new skin lesion segmentation refinement (smoothness), where the superpixels' confidence scores evolve in time steps according to a set of rules based on the confidence score of each superpixel and its neighbouring superpixels. Experimental results show that our method outperforms the other state-of-the-art methods in most of the metrics with significant margins.

References

1. Achanta, R., Shaji, A., Smith, K., Lucchi, A., Fua, P., Susstrunk, S.: Slic superpixels compared to state-of-the-art superpixel methods. IEEE Trans. Pattern Anal. Mach. Intell. **34**(11), 2274–2282 (2012)
2. Ahn, E., Bi, L., Jung, Y.H., Kim, J., Li, C., Fulham, M., Feng, D.D.: Automated saliency-based lesion segmentation in dermoscopic images. In: 2015 37th Annual International Conference of the IEEE Engineering in Medicine and Biology Society (EMBC), pp. 3009–3012. IEEE (2015)
3. Alcón, J.F., Ciuhu, C., Ten Kate, W., Heinrich, A., Uzunbajakava, N., Krekels, G., Siem, D., De Haan, G.: Automatic imaging system with decision support for inspection of pigmented skin lesions and melanoma diagnosis. IEEE J. Sel. Top. Sig. Process. **3**(1), 14–25 (2009)
4. Cavalcanti, P.G., Yari, Y., Scharcanski, J.: Pigmented skin lesion segmentation on macroscopic images. In: 2010 25th International Conference of Image and Vision Computing New Zealand (IVCNZ), pp. 1–7. IEEE (2010)

5. Das Gupta, M., Srinivasa, S., Antony, M., et al.: KL divergence based agglomerative clustering for automated vitiligo grading. In: Proceedings of the IEEE Conference on Computer Vision and Pattern Recognition, pp. 2700–2709 (2015)
6. Emre Celebi, M., Kingravi, H.A., Iyatomi, H., Alp Aslandogan, Y., Stoecker, W.V., Moss, R.H., Malters, J.M., Grichnik, J.M., Marghoob, A.A., Rabinovitz, H.S., et al.: Border detection in dermoscopy images using statistical region merging. Skin Res. Technol. 14(3), 347–353 (2008)
7. Erkol, B., Moss, R.H., Joe Stanley, R., Stoecker, W.V., Hvatum, E.: Automatic lesion boundary detection in dermoscopy images using gradient vector flow snakes. Skin Res. Technol. 11(1), 17–26 (2005)
8. Garnavi, R., Aldeen, M., Celebi, M.E., Varigos, G., Finch, S.: Border detection in dermoscopy images using hybrid thresholding on optimized color channels. Comput. Med. Imaging Graph. 35(2), 105–115 (2011)
9. Li, C., Kao, C.Y., Gore, J.C., Ding, Z.: Minimization of region-scalable fitting energy for image segmentation. IEEE Trans. Image Process. 17(10), 1940–1949 (2008)
10. Li, X., Li, Y., Shen, C., Dick, A., Van Den Hengel, A.: Contextual hypergraph modeling for salient object detection. In: Proceedings of the IEEE International Conference on Computer Vision, pp. 3328–3335 (2013)
11. Mendonça, T., Ferreira, P.M., Marques, J.S., Marcal, A.R., Rozeira, J.: PH 2-A dermoscopic image database for research and benchmarking. In: 2013 35th Annual International Conference of the IEEE Engineering in Medicine and Biology Society (EMBC), pp. 5437–5440. IEEE (2013)
12. Nascimento, J.C., Marques, J.S.: Adaptive snakes using the EM algorithm. IEEE Trans. Image Process. 14(11), 1678–1686 (2005)
13. Otsu, N.: A threshold selection method from gray-level histograms. Automatica 11(285–296), 23–27 (1975)
14. Ridler, T., Calvard, S.: Picture thresholding using an iterative selection method. IEEE Trans. Syst. Man Cybern. 8(8), 630–632 (1978)
15. Sezgin, M., et al.: Survey over image thresholding techniques and quantitative performance evaluation. J. Electron. Imaging 13(1), 146–168 (2004)
16. Silveira, M., Nascimento, J.C., Marques, J.S., Marçal, A.R., Mendonça, T., Yamauchi, S., Maeda, J., Rozeira, J.: Comparison of segmentation methods for melanoma diagnosis in dermoscopy images. IEEE J. Sel. Topics Sig. Process. 3(1), 35–45 (2009)
17. Society, A.C.: Cancer Facts & Figures 2015. American Cancer Society, Atlanta (2015)
18. Tong, N., Lu, H., Ruan, X., Yang, M.H.: Salient object detection via bootstrap learning. In: Proceedings of the IEEE Conference on Computer Vision and Pattern Recognition, pp. 1884–1892 (2015)
19. Tseng, P.: On accelerated proximal gradient methods for convex-concave optimization. submitted to SIAM J. J. Optim (2008)

Structure Fusion for Automatic Segmentation of Left Atrial Aneurysm Based on Deep Residual Networks

Liansheng Wang[1], Shusheng Li[1], Yiping Chen[1], Jiankun Lin[2],
and Changhua Liu[2(✉)]

[1] Department of Computer Science, School of Information Science and Engineering,
Xiamen University, Xiamen, China
[2] Department of Medical Imaging, The 174th Hospital of PLA
(The Chenggong Hospital Affiliated to Xiamen University), Xiamen, China
liuxingc@126.com

Abstract. Robust and accurate segmentation of the left atrial aneurysm serves as an essential role in the clinical practice. However, automatic segmentation is an extremely challenging task because of the huge shape variabilities of the aneurysm and its complex surroundings. In this paper, we propose a novel framework based on deep residual networks (DRN) for automatic segmentation of the left atrial aneurysm in CT images. Our proposed approach is able to make full use of structure information and adopts extremely deep architectures to learn more discriminative features, which enables more efficient and accurate segmentation. The main procedures of our proposed method are as follows: in the first step, a large-scale of pre-processed images are divided into patches as training units which then are used to train a classification model by DRN; in the second step, based on the trained DRN model, the left atrial aneurysm is segmented with a novel structured fusion algorithm. The proposed method for the first time achieves a fully automatic segmentation of left atrial aneurysm. With sufficient training datasets and test datasets, experimental results show that the proposed framework outperforms the state-of-the-art methods in terms of accuracy and relative error. The proposed method has also a high correlation to the ground truth, which demonstrates it is a promising techniques to left atrial aneurysm segmentation and other clinical applications.

1 Introduction

The left atrial aneurysm is a severe heart disease, which can produce compression symptoms with diverticulum oppressing neighboring atrium and ventricle leading to arrhythmias, embolic manifestations and heart failure [1]. Early diagnosis and therapy plan for left atrial aneurysm are very important. In clinical practice, the volume of the aneurysm is widely used to assess the severity of the aneurysm and track its progression. Currently, the volume is estimated and approximated using the diameters of the aneurysm manually obtained by clinical doctors. More specifically, the manual slice-by-slice segmentation by clinical

© Springer International Publishing AG 2016
L. Wang et al. (Eds.): MLMI 2016, LNCS 10019, pp. 262–270, 2016.
DOI: 10.1007/978-3-319-47157-0_32

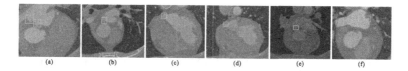

Fig. 1. Original CT images for left atrial aneurysm in different patients. The red boxes denote the left atrial aneurysms in different shapes, sizes and locations. (Color figure online)

doctors from original CT images can provide more accurate results. These manual methods, however, are subjective, inaccurate, non-reproducible and heavily labor-intensive. It is therefore highly desired to automatically segment the left atrial aneurysm, which unwontedly has long been neglected due to the particular challenges caused by the complexity of the aneurysm. The automatical and robust segmentation results can be applied to estimate atrial aneurysm volumes more accurately and other clinical applications, such as quantifying the aneurysm phenotype.

Although several approaches have been proposed to deal with different kinds of cases on CT or MRI images in recent years, conventional segmentation methods rely on the assumption that shape contours are supported by relatively clear edges and region homogeneity. In medical images, edges are not always visible consistently along the entire contour due to low intensity contrast, and region homogeneity is violated by complex image textures and appearances. As can be seen in Fig. 1, the atrial aneurysm tightly attaches to the atrial wall and they have low intensity contrast, which easily leads to the wall segmented as the atrial aneurysm or complete failure to identify the aneurysm in some extreme datasets.

Segmentation, to some extend, can be considered as a classification problem. Recently, convolutional neural network (CNN) is becoming a promising classification method which achieves a high accuracy of classification in many fields, especially in big data analysis. A well trained deep CNN presents high accuracy and efficiency outperforming the traditional models of machine learning. CNNs also have been introduced to medical image processing and shown higher performance [2,3]. However, in our case, CNN is difficult to train an ideal model that segment atrial aneurysm accurately due to the complex characteristics of the aneurysm images. The great challenges of atrial aneurysm segmentation stem from the following aspects. **(1)** The aneurysm tightly attaches to the left atrial wall which makes it difficult to be extracted from the conglutinated tissue (in Fig. 1); in some CT slices the aneurysm is fuzzy and cannot be easily distinguished from the background. **(2)** The atrial aneurysm is surrounded by other anatomical structures that have similar intensity, which leads to low intensity contrast; human can hardly tell the difference between the left atrial aneurysm and the atrial wall. **(3)** In contrast to organs, e.g., cardiac ventricles, the atrial aneurysm largely varies in location, size and shape across different patients; the size of the atrial aneurysm sometimes is very small, the same scale to blood vessels, hence little difference on segmentation will greatly influence the results.

Recent study [4] has shown that exploiting "very deep" models with a depth of sixteen [4] to thirty [5] can achieve significant success and outstanding performance on the challenging ImageNet dataset. However, as the network depth increases, accuracy becomes saturated and then degrades rapidly. In [6], deep residual networks, in which the depth can reach to 152 layers, addresses the degradation problem but still having lower complexity and shows great advantage over existing state-of-the-art models and methods by winning the 1st places in many competitions. The success of deep residual networks relies on a residual mapping as shown in Fig. 2. The original mapping is replaced by $F(x) + x$, i.e., residual mapping which includes *identity* mapping and $F(x)$ mapping, since optimizing the residual mapping is easier [6]. As a consequence, the extremely deep residual nets are designed to learn preferable and informative features which are more robust to different clinical datasets.

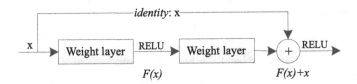

Fig. 2. Residual mapping.

In this paper, we propose a new framework based on deep residual networks to accomplish the segmentation of left atrial aneurysms. To overcome the great image appearance variations and the huge shape variabilities of the aneurysm, we build more powerful models to train the extremely deep network with the depth increasing to 152 layers, which can learn much more complicated and hierarchical discriminative features than conventional CNN. Besides, instead of traditional classification model, we apply a trained DRN model to calculate the probability that whether pixels belong to aneurysm or not. Based on these probabilities and a novel structure fusion algorithm, the left atrial aneurysm is segmented. With sufficient training and testing datasets, experimental results demonstrate that our proposed framework achieves good results, which outperforms state-of-the-art methods. The proposed method also achieves high correlation with the ground truth, which is significant in clinical use.

The contributions of our framework reside in: (1) It is the first automatical and accurate segmentation of left atrial aneurysm, which enables more accurate and efficient volume estimation and other significantly clinical applications; (2) During generating result image, structure fusion is creatively incorporated to the category of each pixel, which can take advantage of the information of each pixel's neighborhood and further improve the accuracy of segmentation. This can also be extensively applied to related applications; (3) A large scale of clinical datasets of the left atrial aneurysm is the first time collected and used in our study.

2   Method

In this section, the details of the method will be introduced. The proposed framework is illustrated in Fig. 3.

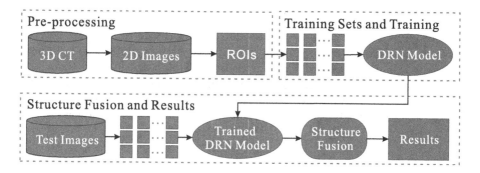

Fig. 3. The workflow of our method.

(1) **Pre-processing:** The training datasets consist of 3D original CT image sequences and corresponding labeled images (shown in Fig. 4(c)). Firstly, we extract a series of single 2D images which contain the left atrial aneurysm in Fig. 4(a). In order to reduce the computational cost and improve the accuracy, Region of Interest (ROI) is extracted manually from the original 2D images to avoid processing the whole image as shown in Fig. 4(b).

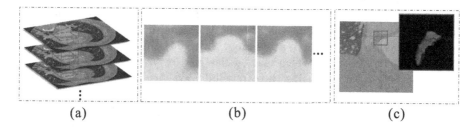

| (a) | (b) | (c) |

Fig. 4. ROI and volume rendering of the aneurysm. (a) Original 2D images, red boxes representing ROI. (b) ROIs extracted from (a). (c) Labeled images with its volume rendering result. (Color figure online)

(2) **Generate Training/Test Sets:** With the help of the ground truth manually labelled by clinical doctors in advance, we divide training units into three categories: the left atrial aneurysm, the atrial wall and the background. Because the feature of atrial aneurysm is easily mixed with the other two categories of features in ROIs, ROIs can not be directly used as training units. To highlight the feature of left atrial aneurysm, we select small patches as training units. In

the processing of the input dataset, the ROIs are divided into a large number of small patches of 7×7 with stride 1×1. For each patch, its category is determined by the major pixels in the patch corresponding to the ground truth. In our study, we focus on a complex segmentation task, and the aneurysm is very small. Therefore, the patches and ROIs may be small compared to traditional classification problem.

(3) **Training:** A 152-layer residual net is constructed to train the model. The input of DRN is a 7×7 tensor and output is a 1×3 vector. The first layer is the entrance of the DRN pipeline and prepares the inputs which have been pre-processed. It fetches the classification units from training sets and puts them into the next layer. Finally, a Softmax layer is connected to the last fully-connected layer. The Softmax layer takes the previous 1×3 vector as input to calculate the loss and the probability P. The probability P is calculated as follows:

$$P\left(Y_i|\chi\right) = \frac{e^{\chi_i}}{\sum_j e^{\chi_j}} \tag{1}$$

where χ is the input vector and $Y \in \{0, 1, 2\}$; $Y_i = 0$ represents the standard output vector of the left atrial aneurysm; $Y_i = 1$ represents the standard output vector of the atrial wall; and $Y_i = 2$ represents the standard output vector of the background.

The Softmax layer is also used to compute the logistic loss of its inputs using predicted labels and actuals labels from ground truth, then backward to the network. The loss function L is defined in Eq. 2:

$$L(y, \chi) = -\log \sum_j e^{\chi_j} - \chi_y \tag{2}$$

The loss function is used to correct the network's weight while training.

(4) **Structure Fusion and Segmentation:** After training, DRN generates a classification model. Prior to the classification, the input test image will be well prepared with the same pre-processing. Therefore, the input test images are divided into 7×7 patches, which will be classified by trained DRN model one by one. Each test patch obtains three possibility values, i.e., possibility vector (denoted as $v = (l, w, b)$), for three categories from the trained model.

Instead of directly choosing the maximal possibility value from v to decide the category of each pixel, structure fusion exploits information of each pixel's neighborhood to determine the category, which makes full use of structure information and further improves the accuracy of final result. The possibility values from v construct three possibility maps as illustrated in Fig. 5(c), i.e., P_l (the left atrial aneurysm), P_w (the atrial wall) and P_b (the background) representing possibility of three category for the indexed pixel in the test images, respectively. In order to take advantage of structure information, these three possibility maps are updated and convoluted with a pre-defined 7×7 weight matrix shown in Fig. 5(d). Each possibility values in the three updated possibility maps can be defined as $x_l \in P_l$, $x_w \in P_w$ and $x_b \in P_b$. Finally, for each corresponding possibility value, $max(x_l, x_w, x_b)$ is calculated as final possibility to determine the

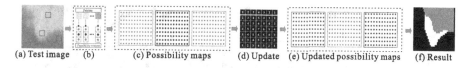

(a) Test image   (b)   (c) Possibility maps   (d) Update (e) Updated possibility maps   (f) Result

Fig. 5. The procedure of segmentation with trained DRN model and structure fusion. (a) Test image. (b) The process of generating possibility vectors with trained DRN model. (c) Three possibility maps for three categories. (d) The convolution weight matrix. (e) Three possibility maps updated by (d). (f) The segmentation result.

category of each pixel. This procedure fuses the three updated possibility maps and generates the segmentation result for the corresponding test images.

3   Experiments and Results

Datasets and Implemetation Details: The data sets were collected from our cooperation hospital, which include 229 patients during the period of 2011 to 2013 diagnosed as left atrial aneurysms by 320-slice dynamic volume CT. Of all there were 160 male patients and 69 female patients. The average age of patients was 59 ± 12, ranging from 21 to 85. For clinical presentation of all patients, 229 patients suffered from palpitations, 85 patients felt the pain in the precordium, 68 patients suffered chest tightness, 76 patients had unstable angina, 34 patients with diabetes and 62 patients combined with hypertension.

In our experiments, we use 155 datasets for training and 74 datasets for testing. We totally get $150,000$ training units and $75,000$ testing units extracted by a 7×7 window. And the classification model will be trained in the defined CNN network using these patches. The final model is trained approximately $330,000$ iterations.

Comparison and Quantitative Analysis: In the study, our method is compared to three current state-of-the-art methods, i.e., the Automatic Feature Learning based on Deep Learning (ALADDIN) [7], the Deep Voting Model (DVM) [8] and ALEXNET [9]. The experimental results are shown in Fig. 6. It is demonstrated that our results are better compared to ALADDIN, DVM and ALEXNET, in which their results are over segmentation because large regions of atrial wall are labelled as aneurysm. It is suggested that our model with structure fusion has more optimal ability to identify the edges between the aneurysm and the atrial wall than ALADDIN, DVM and ALEXNET.

In the clinical diagnosis, the area of the aneurysm is an important criteria which can be an evaluation protocol. The area is calculated by counting the number of pixels in our study. As shown in Fig. 7(a), it is demonstrated that the results of our method is more closer to the ground truth compared to ALADDIN, DVM and ALEXNET. It indicates that our extremely deep network has optimal results for training and our segmentation method is more robust than ALADDIN, DVM and ALEXNET. Figure 7(b) shows the results for the test cases and it is demonstrated that our method outperforms ALADDIN, DVM and ALEXNET in relative error rate with respect to different subjects. This confirms that our method

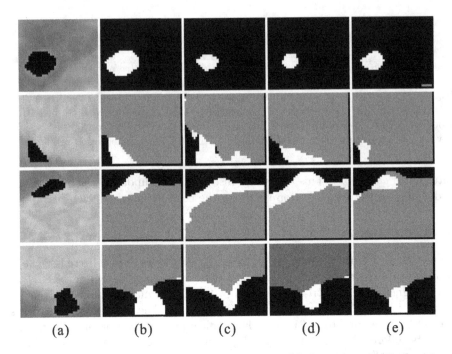

(a)   (b)   (c)   (d)   (e)

Fig. 6. The segmentation comparison of four methods. (a) Ground truth (black regions denotes the aneurysm). (b) Our method. (c) ALADDIN. (d) DVM. (e) ALEXNET. White regions denotes the aneurysm in the results segmented by four methods.

can learn more complicated and discriminative features to overcome the significant challenges including background noise, huge shape variabilities, and low intensity contrast between the aneurysm and atrial wall.

According to the Fig. 7(a), the correlation coefficient is also calculated between predicted area and ground truth's area to further quantitatively evaluate the four methods. The correlation coefficient ($Correl$) measures the correlation between the areas obtained by different methods and manual segmentation. The range of $Correl$ is [0,1], where 1 denotes a perfect fit. For more comprehensive evaluation metrics, precision rate (P), recall rate (R) and F_1 score are used and defined as: $P = \frac{TP}{TP+FP}$, $R = \frac{TP}{TP+FN}$, and $F_1 = \frac{2 \times P \times R}{P+R}$, where TP is the number of true positive, FP is the number of false positive and FN is the number of false negative. The left atrial aneurysm is defined as positive while the other two categories (atrial wall and background) are regarded as negative. As shown in Table 1, our method is superior to the state-of-the-art methods in terms of correlation coefficient, precision rate, recall rate and F_1 score. Therefore, the proposed method can achieve better segmentation and is more stable. Moreover, with high correlation to the ground truth, our method is significant in clinical practice.

Figure 8 illustrates the best segmentation results by our proposed method with lowest errors for atrial aneurysm. This means the result of the automatic segmentation by our method is visually close to the manual one. Although the

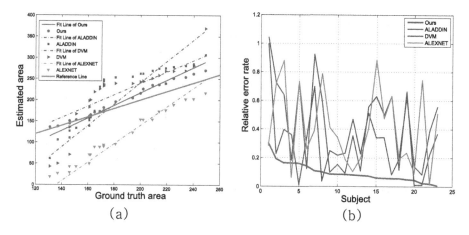

(a)   (b)

Fig. 7. Comparison between the proposed method and other methods. (a) Correlations between the four methods and ground truth in terms of area. (b) Relative error rate for four methods in different subjects.

Table 1. The comparison in average values of false drop rate, precision rate and F_1 score over all test cases for four methods.

Method	Ours	ALADDIN	DVM	ALEXNET
$Correl$	**0.924**	0.711	0.760	0.611
P	**0.828**	0.782	0.674	0.809
R	**0.850**	0.620	0.718	0.657
F_1	**0.839**	0.692	0.695	0.725

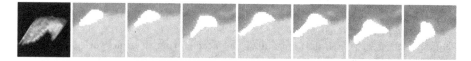

Fig. 8. The best segmentation results by the proposed method. The first image is the volume rendering of the segmented atrial aneurysm. Other images are corresponding original slices with segmented regions in white color.

aneurysm tightly attaches to atrial wall and low intensity contrast between them, the proposed method can provide the high accurate results, which is significant and reliable in clinical use.

4 Conclusion

In this study, we propose a new framework based on deep residual networks to accomplish the automatic segmentation of the left atrial aneurysm. Specifically, a novel structure fusion algorithm is proposed to capture the structure information exhibiting in each pixel's neighborhood, which further produces much more accurate segmentation results. Our proposed method for the first time automatically segment the atrial aneurysm and experiments show that the proposed method achieves highly accurate segmentation results compared to ground truth. In addition, the comparative experiments demonstrate the superior performance of our method over existing state-of-the-art methods. We believe that the framework will serve an effective role in the clinical diagnosis of the atrial aneurysm.

Acknowledgement. This work was supported by National Natural Science Foundation of China (Grant No. 61301010, 61327001, 61271336), the Natural Science Foundation of Fujian Province (Grant No. 2014J05080), Research Fund for the Doctoral Program of Higher Education (20130121120045) and by the Fundamental Research Funds for the Central Universities (Grant No. 2013SH005, 20720150110).

References

1. Reddy, S., Ashwal, A., Padmakumar, R., Reddy, R., Rao, S.: An interesting and rare case of dextrocardia: asymptomatic left atrial aneurysm in an adult. Eur. J. Cardiovasc. Med. **3**(1), 464–465 (2015)
2. Roth, H.R., Lu, L., Seff, A., Cherry, K.M., Hoffman, J., Wang, S., Liu, J., Turkbey, E., Summers, R.M.: A new 2.5 D representation for lymph node detection using random sets of deep convolutional neural network observations. In: Golland, P., Hata, N., Barillot, C., Hornegger, J., Howe, R. (eds.) MICCAI 2014. LNCS, vol. 8673, pp. 520–527. Springer, Heidelberg (2014)
3. Cireşan, D.C., Giusti, A., Gambardella, L.M., Schmidhuber, J.: Mitosis detection in breast cancer histology images with deep neural networks. In: Mori, K., Sakuma, I., Sato, Y., Barillot, C., Navab, N. (eds.) MICCAI 2013. LNCS, vol. 8150, pp. 411–418. Springer, Heidelberg (2013). doi:10.1007/978-3-642-40763-5_51
4. Simonyan, K., Zisserman, A.: Very deep convolutional networks for large-scale image recognition. In: ICLR 2015 (2015)
5. Ioffe, S., Szegedy, C.: Batch normalization: accelerating deep network training by reducing internal covariate shift. In: Proceedings of the 32nd International Conference on Machine Learning, pp. 448–456 (2015)
6. He, K., Zhang, X., Ren, S., Sun, J.: Deep residual learning for image recognition. arXiv preprint arXiv:1512.03385 (2015)
7. Chen, X., Xu, Y., Yan, S., Wong, D.W.K., Wong, T.Y., Liu, J.: Automatic feature learning for glaucoma detection based on deep learning. In: Navab, N., Hornegger, J., Wells, W.M., Frangi, A.F. (eds.) MICCAI 2015. LNCS, vol. 9351, pp. 669–677. Springer, Heidelberg (2015). doi:10.1007/978-3-319-24574-4_80
8. Xie, Y., Kong, X., Xing, F., Liu, F., Su, H., Yang, L.: Deep voting: a robust approach toward nucleus localization in microscopy images. In: Navab, N., Hornegger, J., Wells, W.M., Frangi, A.F. (eds.) MICCAI 2015. LNCS, vol. 9351, pp. 374–382. Springer, Heidelberg (2015)
9. Krizhevsky, A., Sutskever, I., Hinton, G.E.: Imagenet classification with deep convolutional neural networks. In: Advances in Neural Information Processing Systems, pp. 1097–1105 (2012)

Tumor Lesion Segmentation from 3D PET Using a Machine Learning Driven Active Surface

Payam Ahmadvand[1]($\boxtimes$), Nóirín Duggan[1], François Bénard[2,3], and Ghassan Hamarneh[1]

[1] Medical Image Analysis Lab, Simon Fraser University, Burnaby, BC, Canada
{pahmadva,nduggan,hamarneh}@sfu.ca
[2] BC Cancer Agency, Vancouver, BC, Canada
fbenard@bccrc.ca
[3] Department of Radiology, University of British Columbia, Vancouver, BC, Canada

Abstract. One of the key challenges facing wider adoption of positron emission tomography (PET) as an imaging biomarker of disease is the development of reproducible quantitative image interpretation tools. Quantifying changes in tumor tissue, due to disease progression or treatment regimen, often requires accurate and reproducible delineation of lesions. Lesion segmentation is necessary for measuring tumor proliferation/shrinkage and radiotracer-uptake to quantify tumor metabolism. In this paper, we develop a fully automatic method for lesion delineation, which does not require user-initialization or parameter-tweaking, to segment novel PET images. To achieve this, we train a machine learning system on anatomically and physiologically meaningful imaging cues, to distinguish normal organ activity from tumorous lesion activity. The inferred lesion likelihoods are then used to guide a convex segmentation model, guaranteeing reproducible results. We evaluate our approach on datasets from The Cancer Imaging Archive trained on data from the Quantitative Imaging Network challenge that were delineated by multiple users. Our method not only produces more accurate segmentation than state-of-the art segmentation results, but does so without any user interaction.

1 Introduction

Positron emission tomography (PET) is a medical imaging modality that captures functional processes (e.g. metabolism) in the body. Quantitative analysis of tumor tissues in PET is a crucial step towards precise dosimetry and radiation therapy treatment planning. A critical challenge towards quantitative imaging is the ability to distinguish normal activity in the heart, brain and kidneys from abnormal activity due to the presence of malignant lesions. The aim of this paper is to outline a method for automatic localization and segmentation of lesions.

While popular methods for PET segmentation continue to include variants of thresholding [20], more recently sophisticated approaches based on Bayesian-based classification [13], belief function theory [18] and possibility theory [8] have

© Springer International Publishing AG 2016
L. Wang et al. (Eds.): MLMI 2016, LNCS 10019, pp. 271–278, 2016.
DOI: 10.1007/978-3-319-47157-0_33

been proposed. Graph based methods based on the random walker algorithm as well as the maximum-flow method have also been reported [7,14,22]. Table 1 summarizes recent methods for PET and PET-CT segmentation according to whether they handle normal activity, are reproducible[1], the level of user interaction required, as well as the number of parameters which need to be set and whether they utilize CT. The reader is also referred to [11] for a recent survey.

In this paper, we propose a new fully automatic approach to lesion delineation in PET that in contrast with previous works in Table 1, is the only method that is (i) fully automatic (i.e. does not require user-initialization or parameter-tweaking when segmenting novel images); (ii) does not require registered CT scans; and (iii) is able to distinguish between radiotracer activity levels in normal tissue vs. the target tumorous lesions. We focus on 18F-FDG, which is by far the dominant radiotracer used in oncological PET imaging studies. This radiotracer provides unique challenges due to physiological uptake in structures such as the brain, kidneys, and other normal organs. Our method is a hybrid machine learning - active surface formulation, which utilizes physiologically meaningful cues (metabolic activity, anatomical position and regional appearance statistics) and a convex optimization guaranteeing reproducible results.

Table 1. Methods proposed for PET/PET-CT segmentation

Method	Technique	Handles * Normal Activity	Reprod-ucible⁺	User Interaction	Param-eters†	Modality
Song [22] (2013)	Graph based	✗	✗	Seed points and radii for each tumor	7	PET/CT
Ju [14] (2015)	Graph based	✗	✗	Seed points	15	PET/CT
Foster [10] (2014)	Affinity Propagation clust.	✗	◇	Manual correction of registration	7	PET/CT
Lelandais [18] (2012)	Belief-theory with FCM	✗	○	User defined ROI	1	PET/CT
Hatt [13] (2010)	Bayesian based class.	✗	○	User defined ROI	1	PET
Dewalle-Vignion [8] (2011)	Maximum of Intensity Propagations	✗	○	ROI*N‡	1	PET
Abdoli [1] (2013)	Active contours	**	✗	Initial curve	3	PET
Layer [17] (2015)	EM-based GMM	✗	✗	ROI & Seed points	5	PET
Bagci [2] (2013)	Graph based	✗	✗	-	5	PET/CT
Bi [3] (2014)	SVM class.	✓	✗	-	5	PET/CT
Cui [7] (2015)	Graph based	✓	✗	-	3	PET/CT
Lapuyade-Lahorgue [16] (2015)	Fuzzy C-means clust.	✓	✗	-	5	PET
Zeng [24] (2013)	Active surface modeling	✓	✗	-	8	PET
Yu [23] (2009)	kNN class.	✓	✓	-	3	PET/CT
Our Method	Machine Learning & Convex seg.	✓	✓	-	0	PET

*Handles normal activity automatically *i.e.* without user seed points ⁺Accuracy dependent on parameter choice, which includes size of ROI. †Parameters which were empirically set rather than learned. ○Sensitivity to ROI selection not tested. ‡N is the number of projection directions which was set at 3 in [8]. **Discussion of initial curve placement not included. ◇Method is reproducible on the condition that a registered CT is provided and that the method is applied to lung data only.

---

[1] A method is described as non-reproducible when its results are dependent on image-specific parameter tuning/initialization or other user interaction.

2   Method

At a high level, our method consists of the following steps: Firstly, given our emphasis on head-and-neck (H&N) cancer, the bladder is detected and cropped out by removing all transverse slices inferior to the bladder. To reduce inter-subject image variability, the intensity of all volumes is normalized to zero mean and unit variance. In a one-time training stage, seeds from lesions, background, and regions of normal activity are selected manually, along with the associated class labels. The random forest is trained on features extracted from these labeled seed points. For each novel image, a probability map is then generated based on the output of the classifier, which predicts the label likelihood of each voxel. Finally, an active surface is initialized automatically and is optimized to evolve a regularized volume segmentation delineating only the boundaries of tumor lesions.

2.1   Machine Learning: Features and Classification

Most automatic feature learning methods ignore expert domain knowledge and, to avoid overfitting, require a large number of datasets, which are difficult to acquire in many medical imaging domains. We therefore resorted to designing specific features based on the following problem-specific imaging cues:

Radiotracer Uptake (5 Features): The first group of features is based on the standardized uptake value (SUV), which plays an important role in locating tumors. SUV is computed as the ratio of the image-derived radioactivity concentration to the whole body concentration of the injected radioactivity. The activity value of each voxel along with max, min, mean and standard deviation of SUV in a window size $3 \times 3 \times 3$ around each voxel are added to the features vector to encode activity information.

Spatially-Normalized Anatomical Position (1 Feature): Using the approximate position of tumors as a feature is useful since in each type of nonmetastatic cancer, lesions are located in a specific organ (e.g. H&N in our dataset). However, position coordinates must first be described within a standardized frame-of-reference over all the images. The field-of-view of PET images usually spans from the brain to the middle of the femur; however, this is not always the case. To deal with this variability in scans and obtain a common frame of reference across all images, it is necessary to first ensure anatomical correspondence. The most superior point of the bladder, which is a high-uptake organ, is used as the first anatomical landmark. The second landmark used is the most superior part of the image (i.e. top of the brain). Each image is then spatially normalized along the axial direction based on these two landmarks to obtain a new normalized axial position feature with values ranging between 0 (most inferior) to 1 (most superior). No normalization was needed within the transverse plane itself.

PET Image Texture (8 Features): First, four standard 3-D Haar-like features (edge, line, rectangle, and center-surround) are used to capture the general texture pattern of a $10 \times 10 \times 10$ region around each voxel in an image [12]. Second, the following four texture statistics are calculated for each transverse plane: cluster prominence [21], homogeneity [21], difference variance, and inverse difference normalized (INN) [6]. These were found to be particularly useful for distinguishing normal brain from H&N lesion activity along the anteroposterior dimension. The four feature values for a given plane were assigned to each voxel in that plane.

Radiotracer Activity Homogeneity (2 Features): Tumor homogeneity is a measure of the uniformity of tumor pixel intensities [15]. The tumor homogeneity is on a vector of all activity values of 3D neighbors centered around a given voxel. We used two homogeneity features at two scales, using window sizes $3 \times 3 \times 3$ and $4 \times 4 \times 4$, i.e. $n=27$ and 64, respectively.

Classification. In total, the feature vector assigned to each voxel was of length 16. For training, labeled samples (i.e. feature vectors at seed pixels) were collected from the lesion, body, air background, kidneys, heart, and brain regions. These can be considered as six distinguishable classes; however, we consider the heart and kidneys as one class since they are close to each other in terms of location and far from H&N lesions. Having the brain as a separate class was needed to facilitate discrimination between H&N lesions since the brain and lesions are in close proximity. The values of each feature are normalized to zero mean and unit variance over the training samples. A random forest classifier is used to predict the label probability on a voxel-by-voxel basis. The parameters of the classifier were trained using leave-one-image-out cross-validation on the training set. Having more than 50 decision trees did not increase the classification accuracy, and the value for the number of variables randomly sampled at each split was set to the square root of the number of features, as it was automatically set and found to be robust. Although training on thousands of samples using random forests is fast (0.15 s), predicting the labels of millions of voxels using a MATLAB implementation was time-consuming (up to 20 h per volume). Instead, we used a fast C implementation [19], with parallel processing distributed on 4 CPU cores (one slice per core). This resulted in a reduction in prediction time by a factor of 50 to reach the average running time of ~15 min. Figure 1 shows sample probability maps generated by our trained random forest.

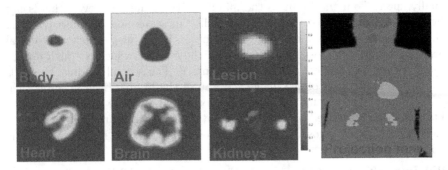

Fig. 1. Example of class probabilities. Images on the left: probability maps over different classes in the transverse plane (different scales used for clarity). Right: maximum probability projection.

2.2   Convex Segmentation with Learned Likelihoods

To produce a final segmentation of the lesion tissue, the posterior model produced by the random forest classifier is included as a data (likelihood) term into the convex segmentation formulation of Bresson et al. [4]:

$$E(u) = \int_{\Omega} |\nabla u(x)|\, dx + \int_{\Omega} u(x)(P_{obj}(x) - P_{bg}(x) + C_A)dx \qquad (1)$$

where $u(x)$ in [0,1] is the segmentation label field, Ω is the image domain, the first term is the boundary regularization term, and the second is the data term. P_{obj} is the probability of a lesion and $P_{bg} = 1 - P_{obj}$ (i.e. P_{bg} groups together the likelihood probabilities of all non-lesion classes), and C_A is a constant that penalizes the area of the segmentation surface and is used to constrain the size of small unconnected components (e.g. small lymph nodes). The contour is automatically initialized as a "box-shell" around the border of the 3D volume. Given the convex formulation, the algorithm converges to the same global solution with any initialization. One hundred (100) segmentation update iterations were enough for convergence for all our experiments.

3   Results

Experimental Setup: We evaluated our approach on the H&N cancer collection provided by The Cancer Imaging Archive (TCIA) [5,9]. Ten images from this collection were selected by the Quantitative Imaging Network (QIN) team for the QIN H&N challenge, in which all lesions and lymph nodes with high activity were delineated by experts. We chose these 10 images for training and tested on 15 new images with one or two lesions in each image from the same collection. The training data came from Siemens Biograph Duo scanner. The reconstruction parameters were 2 iterations/ 8 subsets (iterative reconstruction algorithm: OSEM) with a 5 mm smoothing Gaussian filter and voxel size $0.354 \times 0.354 \times 3.37$ mm. For testing, data from the original scanner as well as additional data from Siemens Biograph 40 scanner was used (also with OSEM reconstruction algorithm, parameters 4 iterations, 8 subsets) with a 7 mm smoothing Gaussian filter and voxel size $0.339 \times 0.339 \times 5$ mm. Six manual segmentations (three users, two trials each) are provided by TCIA for all 25 images. Training seed voxels were collected from the lesions, background, and regions of normal activity, for a total of 1108 seeds. The seed voxels and the manual segmentations of the training data (only) were used to tune hyperparameters and select features; these hyper-parameters were fixed across all test images.

Quantitative Segmentation Results: Our segmentation method was validated against manual segmentations using the Dice similarity coefficient (DSC), Jaccard index, false positive (FP), and false negative (FN) rates. These results are presented in Table 2. Different combinations of classes for training the classifier prior to segmentation were evaluated (Rows 1–5). Note that Row 6 of Table 2 reports the result of the performance of our method without the final

Table 2. Segmentation results. (Row 1–6) variants of our proposed method evaluated on different combinations of classes, with each class surrounded by parentheses (e.g. 2 classes in row 1); (Row 7) competing method; (Row 8) average segmentation agreement for 3 users.

Method	DSC	Jaccard	FP	FN
1 [Air + Body + Kidney + Heart + Brain] [Lesion]	0.71	0.57	0.66	0.03
2 [Air + Body] [Kidney + Heart + Brain] [Lesion]	0.71	0.56	0.60	0.04
3 [Air] [Body] [Kidney + Heart + Brain] [Lesion]	0.73	0.59	0.41	0.05
4 [Air + Body] [Kidney + Heart] [Brain] [Lesion]	0.72	0.57	0.57	0.04
5 [Air] [Body] [Kidney + Heart] [Brain] [Lesion]	0.74	0.60	0.46	0.04
6 [Air] [Body] [Kidney + Heart] [Brain] [Lesion] w/o segmentation	0.71	0.56	0.70	0.03
7 Foster et al. (2014) [10]	0.71	0.58	1.18	0.05
8 Average pairwise agreement between 3 expert segmentations	0.80	0.67	0.27	0.17

segmentation step (i.e. a voxel is assigned to the class with highest random forest probability). Note also that DSC, Jaccard, FP, and FN are the average values obtained from comparing the automatic segmentation with the 6 manual delineations (3 users, 2 delineations each). We compared our method with the state-of-the-art work of Foster et al. [10] using their publicly available PET-only segmentation software (Row 7). In Table 2 we observe that our proposed method, with five different classes and convex segmentation, outperforms [10]. Not only did our method achieve higher DSC and Jaccard and lower FP and FN, but our method is also fully automatic and reproducible. On the other hand, the software of Foster et al. required selecting a 3D region of interest around the lesions and tweaking parameters until the best performing result is obtained, an extra burden that took an experienced user (knowledgeable in PET imaging and understands the meaning of the underlying parameters) on average 5 min per image. Row 8 is the average agreement computed over all scans between manual segmentations produced by the three expert users where each combination of users was included i.e. (user1, user2), (user1, user3) etc.

Segmentation Agreement: We evaluated the inter- and intra-user agreement in lesion delineation and compared it to results from our automated method and those obtained from expert users. We found that user2 has the highest intra-user variability with an average DSC of 0.844, and that user3 agreed the least with the two other users with an average DSC of 0.787. Our fully automated method had an average DSC agreement of 0.741 with other users, i.e. our method falls short by only 4 % from performing as well as expert user3.

Quantitative Segmentation Results: Fig. 2 shows examples of segmentation results from four cases. In the third case, our method segmented a lesion that was missed in the manual segmentation. In the fourth case, a small segmentation leakage into the inferior part of brain is observed.

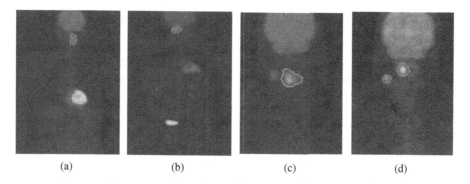

(a)   (b)   (c)   (d)

Fig. 2. Qualitative segmentation results. The PET image is rendered using maximum intensity projection. Our proposed segmentation is shown as red contours, while an example manual segmentation is shown in green. Note in (c) that our method captures a valid lesion missed by the user. In (d), we see an example of segmentation leakage into the inferior part of the brain.

4   Conclusion

We present the first work that fully automates the segmentation of lesions relying solely on PET. Our method is able to isolate abnormal lesion activity from the background and from other tissue regions of normal radiotracer uptake. Our method is a convex segmentation technique that is guided by learned likelihood terms. The learning is based on a classification model trained on anatomically and physiologically meaningful cues. The use of convex formulation together with a trained classifier to learn all parameters precludes the need for human interaction (i.e. initialization and parameter tuning) and results in fully reproducible results on new test images (obtained from a different scanner with different reconstruction parameters). Our approach outperforms a recently published state-of-the-art method for this application and differed in average Dice similarity coefficient DSC by just 4% compared with an expert user. In future work, the approach will be extended to other radiotracers of interest in oncology. It will also be extended to incorporate anatomical information from CT, when available.

Acknowledgements. Funding provided by the Canadian Institutes of Health Research (OQI-137993).

References

1. Abdoli, M., et al.: Contourlet-based active contour model for PET image segmentation. Med. Phys. **40**(8), 082507: 1–082507: 12 (2013)
2. Bagci, U., et al.: Joint segmentation of anatomical and functional images: applications in quantification of lesions from PET, PET-CT, MRI-PET, and MRI-PET-CT images. Med. Image Anal. **17**(8), 929–945 (2013)
3. Bi, L., Kim, J., Feng, D., Fulham, M.: Multi-stage thresholded region classification for whole-body PET-CT lymphoma studies. In: Golland, P., Hata, N., Barillot, C., Hornegger, J., Howe, R. (eds.) MICCAI 2014. LNCS, vol. 8673, pp. 569–576. Springer, Heidelberg (2014). doi:10.1007/978-3-319-10404-1_71

4. Bresson, X., et al.: Fast global minimization of the active contour/snake model. J. Math. Imaging Vis. **28**(2), 151–167 (2007)
5. Clark, K., et al.: The cancer imaging archive (TCIA): maintaining and operating a public information repository. J. Digit. Imaging **26**(6), 1045–1057 (2013)
6. Clausi, D.A.: An analysis of co-occurrence texture statistics as a function of grey level quantization. Can. J. Remote Sens. **28**(1), 45–62 (2002)
7. Cui, H., et al.: Primary lung tumor segmentation from PET-CT volumes with spatial-topological constraint. Int. J. Comput. Assist. Radiol. Surg. **11**(1), 19–29 (2015)
8. Dewalle-Vignion, A., et al.: A new method for volume segmentation of PET images, based on possibility theory. IEEE Trans. Med. Imag. **30**(2), 409–423 (2011)
9. Fedorov, A., et al.: DICOM for quantitative imaging biomarker development: a standards based approach to sharing clinical data and structured PET/CT analysis results in head and neck cancer research. PeerJ **4**, e2057 (2016)
10. Foster, B., et al.: Segmentation of PET images for computer-aided functional quantification of tuberculosis in small animal models. IEEE Trans. Biomed. Eng. **61**(3), 711–724 (2014)
11. Foster, B., et al.: A review on segmentation of positron emission tomography images. Comput. Biol. Med. **50**, 76–96 (2014)
12. Haralick, R.M., et al.: Textural features for image classification. IEEE Trans. Syst. Man Cybern. **6**, 610–621 (1973)
13. Hatt, M., et al.: Accurate automatic delineation of heterogeneous functional volumes in positron emission tomography for oncology applications. Int. J. Radiat. Oncol. Biol. Phys. **77**(1), 301–308 (2010)
14. Ju, W., et al.: Random walk and graph cut for co-segmentation of lung tumor on PET-CT images. IEEE Trans. Image Process. **24**(12), 5854–5867 (2015)
15. Kumar, A., et al.: A graph-based approach for the retrieval of multi-modality medical images. Med. Image Anal. **18**(2), 330–342 (2014)
16. Lapuyade-Lahorgue, J., et al.: Speqtacle: an automated generalized fuzzy c-means algorithm for tumor delineation in PET. Med. Phys. **42**(10), 5720–5734 (2015)
17. Layer, T., et al.: PET image segmentation using a Gaussian mixture model and Markov random fields. EJNMMI Phys. **2**(1), 1–15 (2015)
18. Lelandais, B., Gardin, I., Mouchard, L., Vera, P., Ruan, S.: Segmentation of biological target volumes on multi-tracer PET images based on information fusion for achieving dose painting in radiotherapy. In: Ayache, N., Delingette, H., Golland, P., Mori, K. (eds.) MICCAI 2012. LNCS, vol. 7510, pp. 545–552. Springer, Heidelberg (2012). doi:10.1007/978-3-642-33415-3_67
19. Liaw, A., et al.: Classification and regression by randomForest. R News **2**(3), 18–22 (2002)
20. Nestle, U., et al.: Comparison of different methods for delineation of 18F-FDG PET-positive tissue for target volume definition in radiotherapy of patients with non-small cell lung cancer. J. Nucl. Med. **46**(8), 1342–1348 (2005)
21. Soh, L.K., et al.: Texture analysis of SAR sea ice imagery using gray level co-occurrence matrices. IEEE Trans. Geosci. Remote Sens. **37**(2), 780–795 (1999)
22. Song, Q., et al.: Optimal co-segmentation of tumor in PET-CT images with context information. IEEE Trans. Med. Imag. **32**(9), 1685–1697 (2013)
23. Yu, H., et al.: Automated radiation targeting in head-and-neck cancer using region-based texture analysis of PET and CT images. Int. J. Radiat. Oncol. Biol. Phys. **75**(2), 618–625 (2009)
24. Zeng, Z., et al.: Unsupervised tumour segmentation in PET using local and global intensity-fitting active surface and alpha matting. Comput. Biol. Med. **43**(10), 1530–1544 (2013)

Iterative Dual LDA: A Novel Classification Algorithm for Resting State fMRI

Zobair Arya[1](✉), Ludovica Griffanti[1], Clare E. Mackay[2], and Mark Jenkinson[1]

[1] FMRIB, University of Oxford, Oxford, UK
zarya@fmrib.ox.ac.uk
[2] Department of Psychiatry, University of Oxford, Oxford, UK

Abstract. Resting-state functional MRI (rfMRI) provides valuable information about functional changes in the brain and is a strong candidate for biomarkers in neurodegenerative diseases. However, commonly used analysis techniques for rfMRI have undesirable features when used for classification. In this paper, we propose a novel supervised learning algorithm based on Linear Discriminant Analysis (LDA) that does not require any decomposition or parcellation of the data and does not need the user to apply any prior knowledge of potential discriminatory networks. Our algorithm extends LDA to obtain a pair of discriminatory spatial maps, and we use computationally efficient methods and regularisation to cope with the large data size, high-dimensionality and low-sample-size typical of rfMRI. The algorithm performs well on simulated rfMRI data, and better than an Independent Component Analysis (ICA)-based discrimination method on a real Parkinson's disease rfMRI dataset.

1 Introduction

Neuroimaging biomarkers provide a non-invasive method of obtaining valuable information about structural and functional changes in the brain. A neuroimaging modality that is growing in prominence in clinical research is resting-state functional Magnetic Resonance Imaging (rfMRI) [3].

The aim of rfMRI is to identify regions of the brain that show functional connectivity under rest conditions. It has been estimated that spontaneous neural activity during rest uses over 80 % of the brain's energy, suggesting rfMRI has great potential to discern the progress of diseases such as neurodegeneration [6].

One of the more popular methods for analysing rfMRI data is Independent Component Analysis (ICA). ICA aims to find a set of statistically independent spatial-maps along with their associated time-courses from the rfMRI data. The goal is to express the measured rfMRI signal as a linear combination of source signals. These sources can, for example, be different brain networks, motion artefacts or physiological noise [2].

Recently, a study by Szewczyk-Krolikowski et al. used rfMRI and ICA to compare Parkinson's disease (PD) patients to healthy controls [8]. They showed that the basal ganglia network in the PD group had reduced functional connectivity with a wide range of areas. A post-hoc discrimination method was then employed, with the aim of differentiating healthy controls from PD patients.

© Springer International Publishing AG 2016
L. Wang et al. (Eds.): MLMI 2016, LNCS 10019, pp. 279–286, 2016.
DOI: 10.1007/978-3-319-47157-0_34

ICA can be a powerful exploratory tool but it has non-ideal characteristics for use in a discriminatory framework. The main disadvantages are that the number of independent components is arbitrarily set beforehand and the user has to subjectively choose the component for discrimination, without knowing how well it will discriminate. It is possible to do a statistical test, such as Dual Regression [1], beforehand but such tests may show that more than one component contains useful information, which then complicates its use in creating a discriminant. The challenges with reproducibility of results derived from rfMRI and ICA have been demonstrated in detail by Griffanti et al. in [5].

In this paper, we present a novel algorithm, which is an extension of Linear Discriminant Analysis (LDA), for classifying rfMRI data. Our algorithm employs a supervised learning approach. We apply the algorithm to both simulated and real rfMRI datasets, assessing its performance by leave-one-out cross validation. The advantage of our algorithm is that the whole rfMRI dataset can be fed in without any parcellation or decomposition, and it does not need require the user to make any choices regarding which regions or resting-state networks to use.

Linear Discriminant Analysis

Since our algorithm is based on LDA, we give a short explanation of standard LDA in this section. LDA, when applied to two classes, aims to project a vector of features onto a line, such that the projected between-group mean difference divided by the sum of the projected within group variances is maximised [4]. Let's consider n_1 and n_2 training samples belonging to class 1 and class 2 respectively, with each sample having a set of features $\mathbf{x}_s$, $s = 1, \ldots, (n_1 + n_2)$. Then LDA seeks to maximise the following objective function with respect to $\mathbf{w}$:

$$J_{\text{LDA}} = \frac{\left(\mathbf{w}^T \left(\boldsymbol{\mu}_1 - \boldsymbol{\mu}_2\right)\right)^2}{\sum_{s \in C_1} \left(\mathbf{w}^T \left(\mathbf{x}_s - \boldsymbol{\mu}_1\right)\right)^2 + \sum_{s \in C_2} \left(\mathbf{w}^T \left(\mathbf{x}_s - \boldsymbol{\mu}_2\right)\right)^2 + \lambda} \tag{1}$$

where $\boldsymbol{\mu}_p$ is the set of mean features in class C_p ($C_1 = $ class 1 and $C_2 = $ class 2), λ is a regularisation term and $\mathbf{w}^T \mathbf{w} = 1$. This can be rewritten as:

$$J_{\text{LDA}} = \frac{\mathbf{w}^T \mathbf{S}_B \mathbf{w}}{\mathbf{w}^T \left(\mathbf{S}_W + \lambda \mathbf{I}\right) \mathbf{w}} \tag{2}$$

Here $\mathbf{S}_B = \left(\boldsymbol{\mu}_1 - \boldsymbol{\mu}_2\right) \left(\boldsymbol{\mu}_1 - \boldsymbol{\mu}_2\right)^T$, $\mathbf{S}_W$ is the sum of each class's covariance matrix and $\mathbf{I}$ is the identity matrix (same size as $\mathbf{S}_W$). This has an analytical solution:

$$\mathbf{w}^* = \left(\mathbf{S}_W + \lambda \mathbf{I}\right)^{-1} \left(\boldsymbol{\mu}_1 - \boldsymbol{\mu}_2\right) \tag{3}$$

When there are many more features associated with each sample than there are samples themselves (as is typical in MRI data), $\mathbf{S}_W$ contains a substantial null space and its inverse is ill-posed. To overcome this, a constant λ term is added to the diagonal elements of $\mathbf{S}_W$ for regularisation. This is represented by the $\lambda \mathbf{I}$ term in (3) and the λ term in (1).

For discrimination, $\mathbf{w}^*$ is used to project a test sample down to a scalar value and a number of different strategies can then be employed for classifying this sample based on the scalar value.

2   Methods

2.1   Proposed Algorithm

Consider rfMRI data that has been de-meaned and variance normalised across time for each voxel, belonging to a subject s, and stored in an $n_v \times n_t$ matrix $\mathbf{X}_s$, where n_v = number of voxels and n_t = number of time-points.

   The similarity between two rfMRI time-courses belonging to two different brain regions can be assumed to be a measure of how connected the two regions are. This is due to the fact that if two regions, e.g. region A and region B, are communicating with each other, then a certain amount of region A's intrinsic activity will be encoded in region B's time-course and vice versa.

   If we define vectors $\mathbf{w}$ and $\mathbf{v}$, both of size $n_v \times 1$ and magnitude 1, as a vector of weights corresponding to the spatial maps of regions A and B, then an expression for this similarity metric for subject s can be:

$$y_s = \left(\mathbf{w}^T\mathbf{X}_s\right)\left(\mathbf{v}^T\mathbf{X}_s\right)^T = \mathbf{w}^T\mathbf{X}_s\mathbf{X}_s^T\mathbf{v} \tag{4}$$

Here $\mathbf{w}^T\mathbf{X}_s$ is an aggregate time-course corresponding to $\mathbf{w}$ and $\mathbf{v}^T\mathbf{X}_s$ is an aggregate time-course corresponding to $\mathbf{v}$. If $\mathbf{w}$ and $\mathbf{v}$ are made to have unit norm, the dot product of the time-courses is similar to a measure of correlation.

   Now consider an rfMRI dataset for two groups of subjects, with n_1 subjects in group 1 and n_2 subjects in group 2. Analogously to (1), we can seek to maximise the following objective function with respect to $\mathbf{w}$ and $\mathbf{v}$:

$$J_{\text{IDLDA}} = \frac{\left(\frac{1}{n_1}\sum_{s\in C_1} y_s - \frac{1}{n_2}\sum_{s\in C_2} y_s\right)^2}{\sum_{s\in C_1}\left(y_s - \frac{1}{n_1}\sum_{s\in C_1} y_s\right)^2 + \sum_{s\in C_2}\left(y_s - \frac{1}{n_2}\sum_{s\in C_2} y_s\right)^2 + \lambda} \tag{5}$$

The complication in using standard LDA to maximise this function is that we need to maximise two vectors instead of one. However, if we fix $\mathbf{v}$, then:

$$\frac{1}{n_p}\sum_{s\in C_p} y_s = \mathbf{w}^T\frac{1}{n_p}\sum_{s\in C_p} \mathbf{X}_s\mathbf{X}_s^T\mathbf{v} = \mathbf{w}^T\frac{1}{n_p}\sum_{s\in C_p} \mathbf{x}_s = \mathbf{w}^T\boldsymbol{\mu}_p \tag{6}$$

where we have defined $\mathbf{x}_s = \mathbf{X}_s\mathbf{X}_s^T\mathbf{v}$ and $\boldsymbol{\mu}_p = \frac{1}{n_p}\sum_{s\in C_p}\mathbf{x}_s$. This means (5) reduces to (1) and we can use LDA to optimise with respect to $\mathbf{w}$, having held $\mathbf{v}$ constant. Importantly, (5), is invariant to swapping $\mathbf{w}$ and $\mathbf{v}$. Therefore, to maximise (5), we use an iterative approach as follows.

   We initialise $\mathbf{v} = \mathbf{m}_0$ and then use LDA to find $\mathbf{w}$ (defined as $\mathbf{m}_1$ in the algorithm description below). This value of $\mathbf{w}$ is then fixed and $\mathbf{v}$ is found using LDA in the next iteration ($\mathbf{v} = \mathbf{m}_2$), and so on. Due to the symmetry of $\mathbf{w}$ and $\mathbf{v}$, each iteration proceeds in the same way - starting with a fixed vector, $\mathbf{m}_{i-1}$, and then solving for the other, $\mathbf{m}_i$. See the full algorithm description below. This is also shown graphically in Fig. 1. In order to calculate the LDA output $\mathbf{m}_i$ at each iteration, we use an efficient algorithm, based on a singular value decomposition of the constituents of the $\mathbf{S}_W$ matrix.

Algorithm 1. Iterative Dual LDA

1: **for** $(i = 1$ to $k)$ **do**

2:     $\mathbf{x}_s = \mathbf{X}_s \mathbf{X}_s^T \mathbf{m}_{i-1}$ and $\mathbf{S}_W = \sum_p \left(\sum_{s \in C_p} (\mathbf{x}_s - \boldsymbol{\mu}_p)(\mathbf{x}_s - \boldsymbol{\mu}_p)^T \right)$

3:     $\mathbf{m}_i = (\mathbf{S}_W + \lambda \mathbf{I}_{n_v})^{-1} (\boldsymbol{\mu}_1 - \boldsymbol{\mu}_2)$ and $\mathbf{m}_i = \frac{1}{\|\mathbf{m}_i\|} \mathbf{m}_i$

4: **end for**

5: $\mathbf{w} = \mathbf{m}_k$ and $\mathbf{v} = \mathbf{m}_{k-1}$

Our algorithm is comparable to the Dual Regression (DR) approach reported in [1], since $\mathbf{x}_s$ represents a spatial map for subject s, obtained through the dot product of the individual voxel time-courses in $\mathbf{X}_s$ and the aggregate time-course $\mathbf{X}_s^T \mathbf{v}$. However, our algorithm iterates to learn discriminatory information, meaning we do not need to do any ICA decomposition beforehand and can instead initialise $\mathbf{v}$ with a random vector.

After running Iterative Dual LDA (IDLDA) on a training set of subjects, the obtained $\mathbf{w}$ and $\mathbf{v}$ vectors are then used to reduce a test subject's data down to a scalar value using (4). As in standard LDA, any preferred strategy can be chosen for classifying the test subject based on these scalar values.

2.2   Simulated Data

We first tested our algorithm on a simulated dataset that aimed to represent typical rfMRI data. This dataset consisted of 59 healthy subjects and 59 disease subjects, with each subject's data containing 91125 voxels and 180 timepoints. To simulate resting-state connectivity, the 91125 voxels were split equally between 27 brain regions (BRs). Each BR was associated with a unique, intrinsic time-course (TC) that was randomly generated with no autocorrelation. These TCs were stored in a matrix $\mathbf{T}$, of size 27×180. We simulated connectivity between BRs by creating a TC for each BR that was a mixture of its intrinsic TC and the intrinsic TC of all the BRs with which it is connected.

The final resting-state TCs for the set of BRs is given by $\mathbf{R} = \mathbf{MT}$. $\mathbf{R}$ is a 27×180 matrix and $\mathbf{M}$ is a 27×27 mixing matrix that we used to encode the connectivity between regions. Therefore, the rows and columns of $\mathbf{M}$ represent the strength of incoming and outgoing connections respectively. The diagonal elements of $\mathbf{M}$ were all set to 1 while all the off-diagonal elements were set to

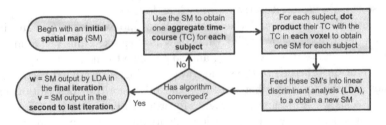

Fig. 1. Flowchart of the proposed Iterative Dual LDA algorithm

random values between 0 and 0.3. The elements of $\mathbf{M}$ were kept consistent across simulation runs and subjects.

For the disease case we assumed that 25 % of the cells in one BR die, and that this results in a 25 % decrease in the intrinsic TC signal in this region, and a 25 % decrease in strength of the incoming and outgoing connections to and from this region (based on decreases in the number of incoming and outgoing synapses/axons connected to functioning cells). When calculating $\mathbf{R}$ for disease subjects, we multiplied the row and column of $\mathbf{M}$ corresponding to the affected region by 0.75. Finally, we added Gaussian noise to the TC of each voxel.

2.3   Parkinson's Disease Data

The real rfMRI dataset we tested our algorithm on was provided to us by the Oxford Parkinson's Disease Centre (OPDC). It consisted of rfMRI scans for 118 subjects, 59 of which were healthy controls (HC) and 59 were PD patients. Data was acquired using Echo Planar Imaging (EPI) with a spatial resolution of $3 \times 3 \times 3.5$ mm and a repetition time of 2 s. The subjects were scanned for 6 min, resulting in a total of 180 time-points.

Preprocessing involved registering to the 2 mm MNI 152 standard space, regression of 24 motion parameters and cleaning using FIX, trained on 50 of the subjects [7]. Other preprocessing steps were followed as described in [5].

3   Results and Discussion

3.1   Simulated Data

We evaluated the algorithm on the simulated data for a variety of noise levels. The noise level is described by g – the standard deviation of the Gaussian noise $\sigma(n)$ divided by the standard deviation of the true resting-state time-course $\sigma(rs)$, $\frac{\sigma(n)}{\sigma(rs)}$. For example, if resting-state activity caused a base-line fMRI signal change of 0.2 %, and the noise caused a base-line change of 1 %, then $g = 5$.

Figure 2(left) shows one slice (containing 9 BRs – arranged in 3×3 blocks) from the final $\mathbf{w}$ and $\mathbf{v}$ images for $g = 5$ when the whole 118 subjects were used as the training set, with $\lambda = 10^9$ and $\mathbf{m}_0 = \mathbf{r}$. Here we use $\mathbf{r}$ to refer to a normalised random vector with each of its elements sampled from a Gaussian distribution. The region highlighted in the $\mathbf{w}$ image in Fig. 2(left) shows the voxels in the BR that we simulated to be affected by disease. Our algorithm clearly picks out these voxels in the $\mathbf{v}$ image and gives a relatively high weighting to these voxels. Furthermore, the objective function monotonically increased with iterations in all cases, converging after 8 iterations for the $g = 5$ dataset.

The reason we chose $\lambda = 10^9$ can be seen in Fig. 2(right). To obtain this graph, for a given λ value, we initialised the algorithm with two different vectors, one being a vector of ones and the other a vector with increased mean in the voxels corresponding to the simulated disease BR. We then calculated the Pearson correlation coefficient (r) between the $\mathbf{w}$ from the first run and the $\mathbf{w}$

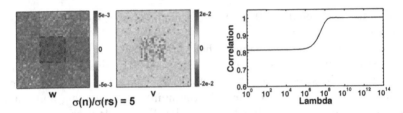

Fig. 2. Left: Final **w** and **v** images (single slice) as output by the algorithm for $\lambda = 10^9$ and $\mathbf{m_0} = \mathbf{r}$ with $g = 5$. Right: Correlation between output vectors corresponding to two runs initialised with different $\mathbf{m_0}$.

from the second run. The same was done for **v** and the smaller of the two r's was recorded. The correlation approximately equals one at around $\lambda = 10^9$, hence we used this value. We also found that there was a relationship between the number of voxels and the λ at which the algorithm becomes desensitised to initialisation. The plot for this is shown in Fig. 3(left). In general, based on projected training samples, this λ corresponded to under-regularisation. This is promising since it provides a lower-bound for choosing λ, but still leaves room for optimising it.

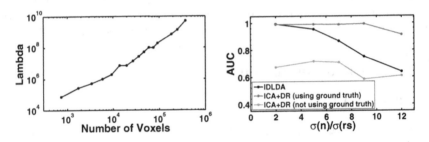

Fig. 3. Left: λ at which the algorithm stops being sensitive to initialisation (using a cut off of $r = 0.99$) as a function of number of voxels in the dataset. Right: Leave-one-out AUC as a function of noise level for $\lambda = 10^9$ and $\mathbf{m_0} = \mathbf{r}$.

To assess the classification performance of the algorithm, we re-simulated the data and used a leave-one-out (LOO) cross-validation with $\lambda = 10^9$, and $\mathbf{m_0} = \mathbf{r}$. The classification performance was evaluated by calculating the area-under-curve (AUC) of the receiver operator characteristic (ROC) curve. The ROC curve was obtained using the normalised test sample values. The normalisation was calculated using ((LOO subject value of y) - (training group 2 mean of y)) divided by (difference of training group means). The classification accuracy as a function of noise level is shown in Fig. 3(right). The figure shows that the algorithm performs well, in the region of 1-0.85, at low to moderate noise levels.

We applied the ICA+DR approach reported in [8] to the simulated data for comparison. However, DR requires the manual selection of the discriminating component, thus needing knowledge of the ground truth. For an upper bound on performance we used our prior knowledge of the ground truth and selected the ICA component that corresponded to the simulated disease region. For a lower bound we selected a different ICA component chosen at random. The AUC values for these are shown in Fig. 3(right). At low to medium noise levels the performance of IDLDA is close to the upper bound, moving towards the lower bound for high noise levels.

3.2 Parkinson's Disease Data

Initially, we applied the algorithm to the OPDC dataset using the full 118 subjects as the training set, $\lambda = 10^{13}$ (the reason for this choice of λ is explained later on) and $\mathbf{m}_0 = \mathbf{r}$. The algorithm monotonically increased the objective function, reaching convergence after 11 iterations for this parameter set. The $\mathbf{w}$ and $\mathbf{v}$ image outputs are shown in Fig. 4. We ran the algorithm a few times with different $\mathbf{m}_0$ and it converged to the same $\mathbf{w}$ and $\mathbf{v}$ each time. The $\mathbf{w}$ image does not contain any obvious structure while the $\mathbf{v}$ image has large weightings in superior and inferior-posterior gray-matter voxels. Regions with large weightings in $\mathbf{w}$ may be interpreted as having the most altered functional connectivity with heavily weighted voxels in $\mathbf{v}$.

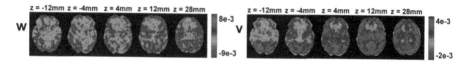

Fig. 4. Output $\mathbf{w}$ and $\mathbf{v}$ images when training using $\lambda = 10^{13}$ and $\mathbf{m}_0 = \mathbf{r}$.

We again assessed the classification performance using a LOO cross-validation and the AUC metric from the corresponding ROC curve. The parameters we used were $\lambda = 10^{13}$ and $\mathbf{m}_0 = \mathbf{r}$. We also used $\lambda = 10^{11}$ (AUC = 0.71), 10^{12} (AUC = 0.71), and 10^{14} (AUC = 0.69) in LOO cross-validation but $\lambda = 10^{13}$ (AUC = 0.75) gave the better classification performance hence we report results for this value. We also calculated the AUC after each iteration and this plot is shown in Fig. 5(left). The AUC increases from 0.56 to 0.75 from the first to the last iteration, which suggests the iterative framework does well to learn discriminatory aspects of the data. The ROC curve at the last iteration is shown in 5(right).

For comparison, we applied the ICA+DR-based discrimination method to our OPDC dataset, using the Basal-Ganglia (BG) component for discrimination as in [8]. The threshold free cluster enhancement output (TFCE) output was thresholded over a range of values and we present the ROC's corresponding to the best AUC in Fig. 5(right). ICA+DR 1 and ICA+DR 2 correspond to including only BG plus noise components, and all independent components in the design matrix in DR, respectively. Our algorithm performs better with an AUC of 0.75 compared to an AUC of 0.67 for ICA+DR 2.

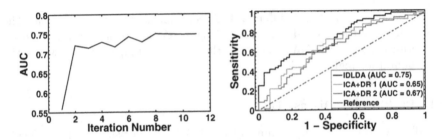

Fig. 5. Left: LOO AUC at each iteration for $\lambda = 10^{13}$ and $\mathbf{m}_0 = \mathbf{r}$. Right: ROC curve for IDLDA at the final iteration, with ROC curves from ICA+DR for comparison.

4   Conclusion

We proposed a novel algorithm for rfMRI classification, based on LDA, which we call Iterative Dual LDA. On simulated data this method effectively picks out voxels affected by disease across a range of noise levels. On a real PD dataset, leave-one-out cross-validation gave an AUC of 0.75, better than a recently reported ICA-based discrimination when applied to the same dataset. Currently the only choice a user of our algorithm has to make is the value of λ, but in future work we will explore strategies for automatically choosing λ such that the generalisation error is minimised.

Acknowledgements. This work was supported by EPSRC and MRC [grant number EP/L016052/1], and the NIHR Oxford Biomedical Research Centre.

References

1. Beckmann, C., Mackay, C., Filippini, N., et al.: Group comparison of resting-state FMRI data using multi-subject ICA and dual regression. In: OHBM (2009)
2. Beckmann, C., Smith, S.: Probabilistic ICA for functional magnetic resonance imaging. IEEE Trans. Med. Imaging **23**, 137–152 (2004)
3. Castellanos, F., Martino, A.D., Craddock, R., et al.: Clinical applications of the functional connectome. NeuroImage **80**, 527–540 (2013)
4. Fisher, R.: The use of multiple measurements in taxonomic problems. Ann. Eugenics **7**, 179–188 (1936)
5. Griffanti, L., Rolinski, M., Szewczyck-Krolikowski, K., et al.: Challenges in the reproducibility of clinical studies with resting state fMRI: an example in early Parkinson's disease. NeuroImage **124**, 704–713 (2016)
6. Rosazza, C., Minati, L.: Resting-state brain networks: literature review and clinical applications. Neurol. Sci. **32**, 773–785 (2011)
7. Salimi-Khorshidi, G., Douaud, G., Beckmann, C., et al.: Automatic denoising of functional MRI data: combining independent component analysis and hierarchical fusion of classifiers. NeuroImage **90**, 449–468 (2014)
8. Szewczyk-Krolikowski, K., Menke, R., Rolinski, M., et al.: Functional connectivity in the basal ganglia network differentiates PD patients from controls. Neuorology **83**, 208–214 (2014)

Mitosis Detection in Intestinal Crypt Images with Hough Forest and Conditional Random Fields

Gerda Bortsova[1,2], Michael Sterr[3], Lichao Wang[1,2], Fausto Milletari[2], Nassir Navab[2,4], Anika Böttcher[3], Heiko Lickert[3], Fabian Theis[1,5(✉)], and Tingying Peng[1,2,5(✉)]

[1] Institute of Computational Biology, Helmholtz Zentrum München, Oberschleißheim, Germany
`fabian.theis@helmholtz-muenchen.de,`
`tingying.peng@tum.de`
[2] Computer Aided Medical Procedures, Technische Universität München, Munich, Germany
[3] Institute of Diabetes and Regeneration Research, Helmholtz Zentrum München, Munich, Germany
[4] Computer Aided Medical Procedures, Johns Hopkins University, Baltimore, USA
[5] Chair of Mathematical Modelling of Bioloigcal Systems, Technische Universität München, Munich, Germany

Abstract. Intestinal enteroendocrine cells secrete hormones that are vital for the regulation of glucose metabolism but their differentiation from intestinal stem cells is not fully understood. Asymmetric stem cell divisions have been linked to intestinal stem cell homeostasis and secretory fate commitment. We monitored cell divisions using 4D live cell imaging of cultured intestinal crypts to characterize division modes by means of measurable features such as orientation or shape. A statistical analysis of these measurements requires annotation of mitosis events, which is currently a tedious and time-consuming task that has to be performed manually. To assist data processing, we developed a learning based method to automatically detect mitosis events. The method contains a dual-phase framework for joint detection of dividing cells (mothers) and their progeny (daughters). In the first phase we detect mother and daughters independently using Hough Forest whilst in the second phase we associate mother and daughters by modelling their joint probability as Conditional Random Field (CRF). The method has been evaluated on 32 movies and has achieved an AUC of 72 %, which can be used in conjunction with manual correction and dramatically speed up the processing pipeline.

Keywords: Mitosis detection · Hough forest · Conditional random field

1 Introduction

The intestinal epithelium is the most vigorously renewing adult tissue in mammals. The intestinal stem cells (ISCs) located at the bottom of the crypts fuel this process [1]. Under normal conditions, ISCs are maintained by symmetric self-renewal and undergo

© Springer International Publishing AG 2016
L. Wang et al. (Eds.): MLMI 2016, LNCS 10019, pp. 287–295, 2016.
DOI: 10.1007/978-3-319-47157-0_35

neutral competition to contact their supporting niche cells. Upon loss of short range niche signals, ISCs can be under differentiation [2]. Nevertheless, asymmetric modes of ISC division, contributing to ISC homeostasis and secretory progenitor commitment, are under debate [3]. The differentiation of the secretory lineage is of particular interest, since it comprises the enteroendocrine cells, which secrete various hormones, involved in energy and glucose homeostasis [4]. In recent years, the role of enteroendocrine cells in development and treatment of diabetes is increasingly recognized, but the exact mechanism of their differentiation remains unclear.

In order to investigate the mechanisms underlying enteroendocrine differentiations, we monitor dynamic cell division and differentiation of murine intestinal crypt using confocal microscope. Based on these live cell movies, we can correlate cell division modes to specific image features. For example, symmetrically divided daughter cells have a very similar cell shape and appearance, whilst asymmetrically divided daughter cells, by contrast, tend to have different sizes, shapes and appearance. Particularly, in a typical asymmetric division case, only one daughter cell touches the crypt outer membrane (as shown in Fig. 1).

So far, these live cell movies are inspected manually, which is laborious and time-consuming. Hence we aim to develop an automatic processing pipeline to accelerate the analysis, in which the key component is an automatic detection of cell division (mitosis) for these movies.

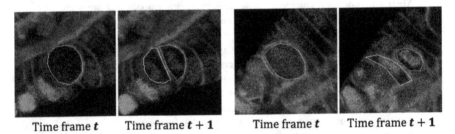

| Time frame t | Time frame $t+1$ | Time frame t | Time frame $t+1$ |

Fig. 1. Exemplary symmetric (left image pair) and asymmetric cell divisions (right pair). Cell membranes are visualized in red channel and nuclei are shown in green channel. Mothers are outlined with yellow contour, daughters with white and blue. The symmetrically divided daughters have similar shape and appearance, whilst the asymmetrically divided daughters have different appearance. (Color figure online)

2   Problem Definition

Unlike "mitosis detection" of histology images where mitotic cells are identified based on one single static image [5], our goal is to detect "mitosis" as a dynamic process, i.e., to identify both mother cell right before the division and daughter cell pair right after the division (Fig. 1).

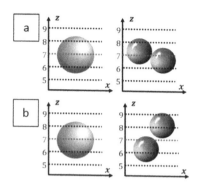

Fig. 2. Daughters may stay on the same z-plane as their mother (a) or move to other planes (b).

The first challenge that we are facing is the time resolution in our movie is rather low (15 min between frames; higher time resolution often results in cell death). With this temporal resolution, one cannot see all the stages of the division (e.g. elongation of the cell) but rather an instant mother to daughter cell splitting between two consecutive frames (also shown in Fig. 1). Compared to mother cells which usually have a characteristic round shape, daughter cells are much less distinguishable from other normal cells and also have larger variability of their shape and appearance, which makes the identification of daughter cells difficult. Besides, the time gap also results in a significant frame-to-frame cell movement as well as variations in their shape and appearance.

Another significant challenge is the poor z-axis resolution ($\approx$25 times smaller than in x and y) of our dataset which makes 3D cell detection almost impossible as daughter cells can be viewed well mostly at one z-plane. Cell divisions, however, do happen in 3D, so the daughters may stay on the same z-plane with their mother, and may migrate to other z-planes (Fig. 2). In the latter case it is difficult to confidently track daughter cells even for a human expert. Hence, we don't consider this case in our detection, and focus only on the case when the mother and both daughters are visible in the same z-plane, which makes our detection essentially 2D. Since our ultimate goal is to quantify the ratio of symmetric and asymmetric cell divisions in crypt, ignoring out-of-plane cell division is not a problem, as the ratio should stay the same when large amount of movies are analysed.

Rapid frame-to-frame cell movement and low z-resolution create a situation where roughly in half of the cases a mother cell is identified but at least one of its two daughters cannot be confidently traced. Such a case is not considered as a complete "mitosis event" for us (as we need both mother and daughter pair).

3 Methods

In this paper, we propose a dual-phase scheme for mitosis detection (shown in Fig. 3). The input to the algorithm is two consecutive time frames belonging to the same z-plane. The goal of the first phase is to obtain two probability maps: the probability of location of a mother on the first frame and a daughter pair on the following one. The method to obtain these maps is described in Sect. 3.1. In the second phase we use a joint probability distribution modelled by Conditional Random Field (CRF) in order to detect mitosis events by matching candidate mother and daughter pair. This is explained in details in Sect. 3.2.

The Framework

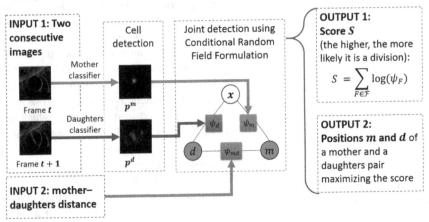

Fig. 3. The dual-phase mitosis detection scheme.

3.1 Cell Detection with Hough Forest

Cell detection is an important and classic research topic in automatic bioimage processing. Among proposed learning-based methods, one approach treats cell detection as a classification problem and trains a classifier to identify cell centroids (e.g. [6]). The classifiers are applied either densely on images or on candidate regions found by e.g. blob detectors or other classifiers [7]. This approach could be problematic in case of a small dataset, i.e. number of positive samples would be also small and hence lead to a high overfitting risk. Another approach is to formulate the problem as regression problem and learn a distance map to a closest cell's centre [8]. Regression solves the problem of having several detections per cell which classic classification might have and hence achieves better performance. A similar method that has this advantage is Hough forest [9], which also learn displacement vectors to object's centre. Compared to classic classification forest, Hough forest does not only split based on information gain, but also splits to increase the uniformity of the displacement vectors of the positive points (negative points do not participate in the voting). Therefore, Hough forest implicitly enforces shape constraints on objects and conveniently provides both segmentation of an object and its centre. Furthermore, unlike regression forest, Hough forest is easily extended to multiclass (which is the case of our problem as we need to detect two kinds of cells: mother and daughter). Although being previously used for many computer vision problems, Hough forest, to our best knowledge, hasn't been used for cell detection so far.

The class distribution of our learning problem is highly imbalanced as the foreground points (positive) constitute less than 0.5 % of all points. Instead of creating a balanced training dataset which the variability of negative class is under-represented, we weight the class frequencies n^l by calculating a probability of assigning a sample in leaf l to class c with inverse prior class probabilities p^{prior}:

$$p_c^l = \frac{n_c^l / p_c^{prior}}{\sum_{i \in C} n_i^l / p_i^{prior}}$$

In classification splits, a splitting function minimizing Shannon entropy is chosen:

$$\mathbb{H}(p^l) = \sum_{c \in C} p_c^l \log p_c^l$$

In vote uniformity splits, a sum of Euclidean distances of the votes $\mathcal{V}(l)$ from the mean vote $\mu_{\mathcal{V}(l)}$ is minimized:

$$VS(l) = \sum_{v_i \in \mathcal{V}(l)} \left\| v_i - \mu_{\mathcal{V}(l)} \right\|$$

3.2 Joint Detection of Mother and Daughters Using CRF

Conditional Random Fields (CRF) were successfully used for joint object detection problems such as human pose estimation [10] or anatomical landmarks detection [11]. This is because that individual object detection might produce many false positives or generate impossible object configuration, enforcement of constraints on geometrical relationships between objects by CRF usually improves the performance. In our problem, daughter cell detection is inherently challenging, as they are not easy to be distinguished from normal cells and have large shape variability. Hence we use the geometrical constraints on daughter cells (our observation is that daughters are usually not too far away from their mother) to reduce their false detection rate.

Our CRF has two random variables: one denoting a position of the mother cell centre (M) and the other denoting a position of the daughter pair centre (D) (see Fig. 3). A feature vector X denotes our Hough maps from individual cell detection. Hence, the joint probability of a location of a mother at a candidate point m and a daughter pair at d follows Gibbs distribution:

$$p(D = d, M = m | X = x) = \frac{1}{Z} \psi_m(m|x) \psi_d(d|x) \psi_{md}(m, d|x) \tag{1}$$

The unary potentials depend on Hough maps from mother and daughter detection:

$$\psi_m(m|x) = \exp(w_m h_m(m)), \psi_d(d|x) = \exp(w_d h_d(d)) \tag{2}$$

The binary potential depends on the Euclidean distance between m and d:

$$\psi_{md}(m, d|x) = \exp(w_d \mathcal{N}(\|m - d\| | \mu, \sigma)) \tag{3}$$

The distance is converted to a probability by modeling distance as a normal distribution. Mean and standard deviation of mother-daughter distances are calculated from the training set.

We use the mitosis score S to select good mitosis candidates. It is based on logarithm of the CRF probability distribution:

$$log(p(m, d|x)) = -logZ + w_m h_m(m|x) + w_d h_d(d|x) + w_{md}p_{dist}(m, d|x)$$
$$S = w_m h_m(m|x) + w_d h_d(d|x) + w_{md}p_{dist}$$

(4)

The normalizing constant Z is omitted due to the fact that it is the same over a neighborhood in the images. Hence the mitosis score turns out to be a simple weighted sum of Hough scores and the probability of distance. In some works in joint object detection the weights of potentials are empirically chosen [12]. However, weighting can greatly affect the results and tuning it manually is usually difficult. A better approach is to learn the weights [11]. In our work, the weights of the CRF potentials are learned using logistic regression.

In order to obtain the maximum a posterior (MAP) estimation of the cell positions in a neighbourhood of an image, we try all possible combinations of mother centre position candidates and daughters centre position candidates by thresholding respective Hough maps, and take one with a highest score. Note that the positions with the highest score are also the ones with the highest probability.

4   Results

4.1   Experiment and Dataset Description

Crypts, isolated from the small intestine of Foxa2-Venus fusion; mT/mG mice, were cultured in matrigel for 4 days prior to live cell imaging. Crypts were then imaged using a HC PL APO 20x/0.75 IMM CORR CS2 objective (Leica) on a confocal laser scanning microscope (Sp5, Leica) in bidirectional mode (400 Hz), with $2 \times$ line averaging per channel at a resolution of 1024×1024 pixels in x-y direction and a z-step size of 3.99 μm. The resulting voxel size is 0.15 μm $\times$ 0.15 μm $\times$ 3.99 μm and the time resolution is approximately 15 min. Venus and tdTomato fluorescence were detected simultaneously. We annotated 505 images from 32 different movies, which consists of 424 mother and 233 pair of daughter cells (233 mitosis events).

4.2   Evaluation of Cell Detection

Firstly, we would like to evaluate our Hough forest based cell detection method, by comparing our Hough forest detection (splitting based on both information gain and voting uniformity, denoted as HF), classification forest detection (splitting based on information gain only) with a subsequent centroid Hough voting (CF+HV), and classification forest detection without any centroid voting (CF). A detected cell centre is considered a true positive (TP) if it is located inside a contour of a segmented cell. In case if there are multiple detections within one contour, one is considered as a TP and all the others are counted as false positives (FP). Any detection that does not fall into a contour of a cell of a given class (mother or daughter) is considered to be FP. Contours without any matching detections are false negatives (FN).

Both the first and second methods generate a Hough voting map of the objective centres, i.e. the centre of a mother cell and the centre of a daughter cell pair (although in the second experiment we do not attempt to increase the voting uniformity in the leaves, but we still store the displacement vectors associated with positive sampling points and hence create Hough maps). Cell detections are obtained by non-maximum suppression of the Hough maps followed by thresholding. The purpose of the comparison of these two approaches is to understand how much the explicit vote uniformity optimization is contributing to the performance. In the third experiment we obtained detections by applying connected components algorithm on segmentations produced by the classification forest and extracting components' centres. This experiment is to evaluate the effectiveness of shape enforcement by Hough voting to filter out the false positive points (the predicted positive points that do not accumulate high amount of votes are very likely to be false positive). All three compared methods are computed with 8 trees with maximum height of 19. At each split we evaluate 500 features and 50 thresholds for each feature, minimum number of samples per leaf is set to 10. We use Haar-like features that are computed on the fly with integral images.

All three methods are evaluated by the Precision-Recall curve and the area under the curve (AUC) for both mother detection (Fig. 4, left) and daughter detection (Fig. 4, right). Each point on the curve is the average of 5-fold cross-validation. The training and testing images are sampled on different movies. The curves were obtained by varying threshold on Hough maps (first and second experiments) and on connected components (third experiment).

As shown in Fig. 4, the performance of daughter detection is not as good as that of mother. This is expected as daughter detection is much more challenging due to a number of factors, such as less distinguishing appearance, larger shape variability as well as a much smaller training set (only half of mothers).

As for the comparison of different methods, classic classification forest approach gives substantially worse results (mother AUC: 32.5 %, daughter AUC: 11.4 %) as compared to the other two methods. It is also expected, as classification alone is not robust against touching cells and can also result in fragmented foreground where either only parts of a cell are presented or they are not in a corrected spatial ordering. Hough forest resolves these issues by implicitly controlling cell shapes using centroid voting.

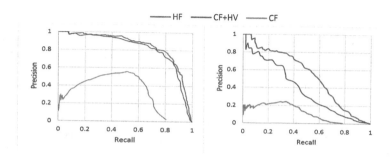

Fig. 4. Precision-Recall curves of mother cell detection (left) and daughter pair detection (right) with three compared methods.

Particularly, optimisation of vote uniformity in Hough forest leads to a further improvement compared to only casting non-optimised votes of training samples in classification forest plus Hough voting (mother AUC: 84.6 % vs. 82.1 %, daughter AUC: 53.9 % vs. 38.4 %).

4.3 Evaluation of Mitosis Detection

The performance of the mitosis detector is also evaluated using Precision-Recall curve. Based on a similar principle as the cell detector, a TP mitosis event is counted only when the detected mother and daughter pair positions are both inside their corresponding ground truth segmented contours. In case of multiple detections per mitosis event, one is considered as TP and the rest are FP. Other detection cases are FP, and unmatched contours are FN.

As explained in Sect. 3.2, our joint detection takes into an account three components: detection for mother, detection of daughter pair, both in the form of Hough voting map at candidate positions, as well as an Euclidean distance between these positions that converted into a probability by assuming Gaussian distribution. We evaluate the contribution of each component using weights learned from training data (Eq. 4). Figure 5 plots the Precision-Recall curve of the mitosis detection, again by 32-folds cross-validation (leave one movie out). It illustrates that the full model with all three components achieves the best accuracy (AUC: 72.4 %). By contrast, performance of reduced models where only two components are considered is lower (mother+daughter: 66.5 %, daughter+distance: 61.3 %, mother+distance: 30.8 %).

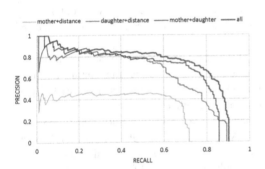

Fig. 5. Mitosis detection with CRF.

5 Discussion

At present, our proposed dual-phase detection framework achieves a mitosis detection accuracy of 72.4 % (AUC), which is very exciting for this challenging problem. The detection accuracy is expected be further improved by providing more annotations, particularly in terms of daughter cells, which have a larger variability in appearance. With current performance, we can already use our automatic mitosis detection algorithm as a pre-processing step and false detections can be manually corrected. Compared to pure manual annotation in which every frame has to be inspected, this pre-processing can dramatically accelerate the analysis process by narrowing manual assessment down to a very small subset of images. For example, if we take 80 % recall (detects 80 % true mitosis events, we would detect 230 events with 70 % precision, that is, around 460 frames (2 frames per event) need to be manually inspected, which is less than 5 % of original workload (32 movies, each contains three central z-planes where mitosis events are concentrated and 60–140 frames per plane).

Our present detection algorithm provides us only with the centre of a daughter pair and the corresponding segmentation from Hough forest is not very accurate, as daughters are not separated. This is not sufficient to automatically extract features from daughter cells (such as their size, shape and orientations). So the next step is to develop new processing algorithms to recover more accurate daughter cell segmentation.

References

1. Barker, N.: Adult intestinal stem cells: critical drivers of epithelial homeostasis and regeneration. Nat. Rev. Mol. Cell Biol. **15**, 19–33 (2014)
2. Snippert, H.J., et al.: Intestinal crypt homeostasis results from neutral competition between symmetrically dividing Lgr5 stem cells. Cell **143**, 134–144 (2010)
3. Simons, B.D., Clevers, H.: Stem cell self-renewal in intestinal crypt. Exp. Cell Res. **317**, 2719–2724 (2011)
4. Parker, H.E., et al.: The role of gut endocrine cells in control of metabolism and appetite. Exp. Physiol. **99**, 1116–1120 (2014)
5. Cireşan, D.C., Giusti, A., Gambardella, L.M., Schmidhuber, J.: Mitosis detection in breast cancer histology images with deep neural networks. In: Mori, K., Sakuma, I., Sato, Y., Barillot, C., Navab, N. (eds.) MICCAI 2013, Part II. LNCS, vol. 8150, pp. 411–418. Springer, Heidelberg (2013)
6. Chen, T., Chefd'hotel, C.: Deep learning based automatic immune cell detection for immunohistochemistry images. In: Wu, G., Zhang, D., Zhou, L. (eds.) MLMI 2014. LNCS, vol. 8679, pp. 17–24. Springer, Heidelberg (2014)
7. Arteta, C., Lempitsky, V., Noble, J., Zisserman, A.: Learning to detect cells using non-overlapping extremal regions. In: Ayache, N., Delingette, H., Golland, P., Mori, K. (eds.) MICCAI 2012, Part I. LNCS, vol. 7510, pp. 348–356. Springer, Heidelberg (2012)
8. Kainz, P., Urschler, M., Schulter, S., Wohlhart, P., Lepetit, V.: You should use regression to detect cells. MICCAI 2015, Part III. LNCS, vol. 9351, pp. 276–283. Springer, Heidelberg (2015). doi:10.1007/978-3-319-24574-4_33
9. Gall, J., et al.: Hough forests for object detection, tracking, and action recognition. IEEE Trans. Pattern Anal. Mach. Intell. **33**, 2188–2202 (2011)
10. Felzenszwalb, P.F., Huttenlocher, D.P.: Pictorial structures for object recognition. Int. J. Comput. Vis. **61**, 55–79 (2005)
11. Wang, L., et al.: Anatomic-landmark detection using graphical context modelling. In: ISBI (2015)
12. Wang, H., et al.: Landmark detection and coupled patch registration for cardiac motion tracking. In: SPIE (2013)

Comparison of Multi-resolution Analysis Patterns for Texture Classification of Breast Tumors Based on DCE-MRI

Alexia Tzalavra[1(⊠)], Kalliopi Dalakleidi[1], Evangelia I. Zacharaki[2],
Nikolaos Tsiaparas[1], Fotios Constantinidis[3], Nikos Paragios[2],
and Konstantina S. Nikita[1]

[1] School of Electrical and Computer Engineering,
National Technical University of Athens, Athens, Greece
{atzalavra,kdalakeidi,ntsiapar,
nkinita}@biosim.ntua.gr
[2] CentraleSupélec, Inria, Université Paris-Saclay, Saint-Aubin, France
{evangelia.zacharaki,
nikos.paragios}@centralesupelec.fr
[3] NHS Greater Glasgow and Clyde, Glasgow, UK
Fotios.Constantinidis@ggc.scot.nhs.uk

Abstract. Although Fourier and Wavelet Transform have been widely used for texture classification methods in medical images, the discrimination performance of FDCT has not been investigated so far in respect to breast cancer detection. In this paper, three multi-resolution transforms, namely the Discrete Wavelet Transform (DWT), the Stationary Wavelet Transform (SWT) and the Fast Discrete Curvelet Transform (FDCT) were comparatively assessed with respect to their ability to discriminate between malignant and benign breast tumors in Dynamic Contrast-Enhanced Magnetic Resonance Images (DCE-MRI). The mean and entropy of the detail sub-images for each decomposition scheme were used as texture features, which were subsequently fed as input into several classifiers. FDCT features fed to a Linear Discriminant Analysis (LDA) classifier produced the highest overall classification performance (93.18 % Accuracy).

Keywords: Breast tumor diagnosis · DCE-MRI · Texture · Wavelet · Classification

1 Introduction

Breast cancer is a primary cause of mortality and morbidity in women. It is commonly conceded that early diagnosis can be the key to increased survival rates and also to more specific and less aggressive therapy options. Breast magnetic resonance (MR) imaging has emerged as a promising modality for breast cancer detection [1]. Dynamic contrast-enhanced MR imaging (DCE-MRI) involves assessing the changes in signal intensity over time. This follows the intravenous injection of a paramagnetic contrast agent [2].

© Springer International Publishing AG 2016
L. Wang et al. (Eds.): MLMI 2016, LNCS 10019, pp. 296–304, 2016.
DOI: 10.1007/978-3-319-47157-0_36

Several machine learning approaches have been proposed to analyze DCE-MRI data for breast tumor diagnosis. The implemented methods vary not only regarding the features extracted but also regarding the classification techniques used. A wide range of features have been explored in breast tumor Computer Aided Diagnosis (CAD) systems. Dynamic features [3, 4] have been used to characterize the temporal enhancement pattern of a tumor, while architectural features [3, 4] have been extracted to characterize the morphology of the tumor. Moreover, kinetic [5, 6] and texture features [7, 8] have been used to distinguish between malignant and benign tumors. More specifically, Yao et al. [8] computed textural features based on the co-occurrence matrix and also extracted frequency features by applying the discrete wavelet transform (DWT) on the texture temporal sequences of the breast tumors in order to classify them. Shannon et al. [9] applied textural kinetics to capture spatiotemporal changes in breast lesion texture in order to distinguish malignant from benign lesions. Furthermore, spatiotemporal features have proved to exhibit high performance in charactering breast tumors. Zheng et al. [10] used spatiotemporal enhancement patterns involving Fourier transformation and Gabor filters to analyze breast tumors. Gal et al. [11] extracted spatiotemporal features from a parametric model of contrast enhancement. Tzalavra et al. [12] extracted textural features from SWT detail sub-images in DCE-MRI data.

Furthermore, several classification methods have been used in breast tumor CAD systems. More specifically, Twellman et al. [13] presented a classification technique using artificial neural networks. Zheng et al. [10] assessed the diagnostic performance of the features they extracted for differentiating between benign and malignant tumors using linear discriminant analysis (LDA). Yao et al. [8] used support vector machines (SVM) for breast tumor classification.

The DWT has been widely used in several texture classification methods in medical images [14, 15] due to its multi-resolution characteristics. The Stationary Wavelet Transform (SWT), a modified time-invariant version of DWT, has been used in texture classification tasks [16]. The FDCT has been effectively used for characterizing carotid atherosclerotic plaque from B-mode ultrasound and discriminating between symptomatic and asymptomatic cases [17].

The purpose of this paper was to investigate the efficiency of multi-resolution wavelet methods to characterize the texture of breast tumors on DCE-MRI data. Three different decomposition schemes, namely the DWT, SWT and FDCT were implemented in order to characterize the spatial enhancement of the breast tissue. A set of classifiers were used for evaluating each decomposition scheme's ability to discriminate between benign and malignant tumors. More specifically, the following classifiers were compared in terms of classification accuracy: Bagging, K-means, Decision Table, Logistic Model Trees, Multilayer Perceptron, Naïve Bayes and LDA.

2 Multi-resolution Image Analysis

Images usually contain information at multiple resolutions. Therefore, multi-resolution analysis has emerged as a useful framework for many image analysis tasks. The approach followed in this study, consists of the following main steps: tumor segmentation, normalization across subjects, feature extraction from the tumor region and tumor classification into malignant or benign. In this study, tumor segmentation was manually performed by an expert radiologist. The manually segmented breast tumors are first spatially normalized using Principal Component Analysis (PCA), as described in [10], in order to eliminate scale variations. Fourier transform is subsequently applied to capture the temporal enhancement properties, hence to kinetic information. Then 3D wavelet transforms were applied to capture the spatiotemporal characteristics of the tumor. Specially, the FDCT method allows capturing both spatial and temporal characteristics, as described in Sect. 3.2 below. Texture features from the resulting images were extracted and introduced into different classifiers for tumor classification.

Discrete Wavelet Transform. The two dimensional DWT is an effective tool to analyze images in a multi-scale framework [18]. The DWT is implemented via iterative linear filtering and critical down-sampling on the original image yielding three high-frequency directional sub-bands at each scale level and also one low-frequency sub-band usually known as image approximation. Directional sub-bands are sub-images exhibiting image details according to horizontal, vertical and diagonal orientations [19, 20].

Stationary Wavelet Transform. The SWT [21] is a translation-invariance modification of the DWT. More specifically, no down-sampling is performed in SWT. Instead, up-sampling of the low-pass and high-pass filters is carried out.

Fast Discrete Curvelet Transform. The FDCT [22, 23] involves initially the application of a 2D FFT to the image and then the windowing in a parallelogram of finite support for each scale and angle. The final result is obtained with the application of the 2D inverse FFT. FDCT [22] is more fast and accurate and less redundant than Discrete Curvelet Transforms (DCT).

3 Materials and Methods

3.1 DCE MRI Data

The images used in this study were provided by the University of Pennsylvania. They were acquired from patients with breast tumors in a 1.5 T scanner (Siemens Sonata) or a 3 T scanner (Siemens Trio). In total, there were 44 subjects used, including 23 malignant and 21 benign cases. All of the samples were histologically verified. The boundary of the suspicious tumors was outlined on the images by a radiologist with expertise in breast imaging. Examples of benign and malignant tumors are shown in Fig. 1.

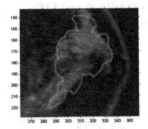 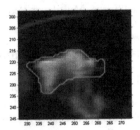

Fig. 1. Examples of a manually segmented malignant (right) and a benign (left) tumor

3.2   Extraction of Texture Features

This section briefly describes the extraction of the texture features for each of the decomposition schemes.

The maximum value of decomposition of each of the investigated schemes equals to $min(log_2N, log_2M)$, where N is the number of rows and M is the number of columns of the image. In our experiments N = M = 150, thus the maximum level of decomposition equals to 7. The statistics estimated from each detail sub-image were the mean and entropy of the absolute value of the detail sub-images, which both commonly have been used as texture descriptors.

DWT and SWT: Several basic functions from different wavelet families were used, including Haar (haar), Daubechies (db), symlets (sym), coiflets (coif), and biorthogonal (bior). The 3-level decomposition scheme resulted in 9 detail sub-images for each time instance; hence totally 27 detail sub-images and consequently 54 texture features were obtained. The approximation sub-images were not used for texture analysis because they are the rough estimate of the original image. Figures 2 and 3 show examples of DWT and SWT detail sub-images.

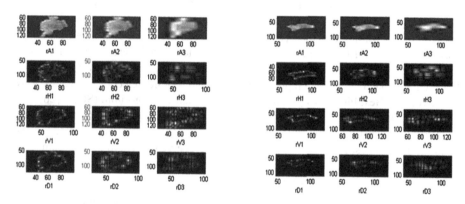

Fig. 2. Examples of DWT sub images for 3 levels of decomposition for a malignant (right) and a benign (left) tumor (corresponding to images in Fig. 1(a) and (b)). The images in the first row correspond to the approximation images. For the images in rows 2–4, each column corresponds to the detail sub-images of the levels 1–3 respectively

FDCT: For the production of the detail sub images 4 decomposition scales were used. The number of angles for the second level was set to 16 (multiple of 4) and complex valued curvelets were used for the coefficients at the first level. For each level only the first half of the total coefficients was considered because curvelets produce symmetric coefficients for angles θ and $\theta + \pi$. The total number of curvelet coefficients obtained was 150, leading to 300 texture features.

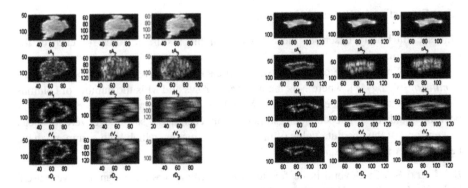

Fig. 3. Examples of SWT sub images for 3 levels of decomposition for a malignant (right) and a benign (left) tumor (corresponding to images in Fig. 1(a) and (b)). The images in the first row correspond to the approximation images. For the images in rows 2–4, each column corresponds to the detail sub-images of the levels 1–3 respectively

3.3 Classification

In order to classify the breast DCE-MRI tumors into benign and malignant, 6 classification algorithms in combination with 3 feature selection methods, provided by the WEKA 3 Data Mining Software [24], were used. The performance of these classifiers was compared with LDA. All classifiers were evaluated with the leave-one-out method.

Feature selection can be applied in two different ways, the wrapper approach and the filter approach. For the wrapper approach, two feature selection strategies were employed, the Best First (BF) [25] and the Simple Genetic Algorithm (SGA) [26], and were combined with the classifiers used later on for classification. For the filter approach, Information Gain (IG) [27] was used as the evaluation criterion of the features. The 10 best features according to the average value of information gain from the 44 leave-one-out iterations were then used for classification.

The following classifiers were used:

(a) Bagging is a meta-classifier based on the bagging approach. The initial training set D of size N_1 is used to generate m new training sets D_i, each of size N_2, by sampling from D uniformly and with replacement. The m base classifiers of the ensemble are trained with these m new training sets. Then, the m base classifiers are tested on a test set and their classification results are combined by voting.

(b) K-means clustering [28] aims to partition n observations into k clusters in which each observation belongs to the cluster with the nearest mean.

(c) A decision table majority classifier [29] consists of a schema which is a set of features that are included in the table and a body consisting of labeled instances from the space defined by the features in the schema. Given an unlabeled instance, a decision table classifier searches for exact matches in the decision table using only the features in the schema. If no instances are found the majority class of the classifier is returned, otherwise the majority class of all matching instances is returned.

(d) Logistic Model Trees [30] are constructed by growing a standard classification tree, building logistic regression models for all nodes, pruning some of the sub trees using a pruning criterion, and then combining the logistic models along a path into a single model.

(e) Multilayer Perceptron is a neural network [31] with one or more hidden layers that uses back-propagation to estimate the weights of the network. All nodes of the network use the sigmoid transfer function.

(f) Naïve Bayes [32] implements the probabilistic Naïve Bayes classifier, which is a specialized form of a Bayesian network, termed naïve because it relies on two important simplifying assumptions: firstly, that the predictive attributes are conditionally independent given the class, and, secondly that no hidden or latent attributes influence the prediction process.

(g) Linear Discriminant Analysis classifier [33] is based on the fact that distributions, which have a greater variance between the two classes and smaller variance within each class, are easier to separate.

4 Results

Table 1 shows the classification results for all the above mentioned classifiers and all feature sets for each of the multi-resolution methods.

Table 1. Classification results for multi-resolution schemes: DWT, SWT, FDCT: ACC: accuracy, SN: sensitivity, SP: specificity.

Multiresolution scheme	Classification performance (%)			
	Algorithm	Accuracy	Sensitivity	Specificity
DWT (db4, L = 3)	BF-Naïve Bayes	84.09	73.91	95.24
	BF-Multilayer Perceptron	77.27	69.57	85.71
	IG-Bagging	79.54	78.26	80.95
	BF-K-means	77.27	56.52	**100.00**
	BF-Decision Table	72.73	69.57	76.19
	BF-Logistic Model Trees	79.55	73.91	85.71
	LDA	**86.36**	**91.30**	80.95
SWT (sym9, L = 3)	BF-Naive Bayes	81.82	69.57	**95.24**
	BF-Multilayer Perceptron	79.55	78.26	80.95
	SGA-Bagging	79.55	73.91	85.71
	BF-K-means	70.45	47.83	**95.24**
	BF-Decision Table	86.36	78.26	**95.24**
	BF-Logistic Model Trees	77.27	73.91	80.95
	LDA	**91.00**	**100.00**	85.71
FDCT (4 scales)	BF-Naive Bayes	86.36	82.61	90.48
	BF-Multilayer Perceptron	86.36	82.61	90.48
	Bagging	77.27	73.91	80.95
	IG-K-means	84.09	69.57	**100**
	BF-Decision Table	81.82	78.26	85.71
	IG-Logistic Model Trees	81.82	78.26	85.71
	LDA	**93.18**	**100.00**	85.71

The highest accuracy and sensitivity scores for all methods are obtained with LDA. More specifically, for FDCT, LDA yielded an accuracy of 93.18 % and a sensitivity of 100 %. Additionally, the meta-classifier based on K-means for the DWT and FDCT datasets yields the highest specificity value of 100 %.

5 Conclusion

In this work, we investigated the possibility of using multi-resolution wavelet schemes to characterize the texture of breast tumors in DCE-MRI. Texture features were extracted from each scheme and fed into several classifiers. The experimental results illustrated high accuracy rates in breast tumor classification using FDCT and LDA as a classifier. Therefore, it can be concluded that curvelets can be key to breast tumor detection.

A main limitation of the method is its dependency on tumor boundary segmentation, currently performed manually. This limitation can be overcome by incorporating an automatic segmentation technique [34] making the method more robust and reproducible. Also, the refinement of the rough manual segmentation prior to feature extraction is possible to increase lesion classification accuracy, as shown in prior work [10]. Additional studies, systematically applying new multi-resolution schemes and more classifiers to larger populations, are expected to verify our findings. Finally, the use of automatic segmentation could result to ameliorated classification results.

Acknowledgements. The authors wish to thank Dr. Sarah Englander and Dr. Mitchell Schnall from University of Pennsylvania, USA, who supported the collection of the data. It should also be noted that K. V. Dalakleidi was supported by a scholarship for Ph.D. studies from the Hellenic State Scholarships Foundation "IKY fellowships of excellence for post-graduate studies in Greece-Siemens Program". This work has been partially supported from the European Research Council Grant 259112.

References

1. http://www.breastcancer.org/symptoms/understand_bc/statistics
2. Orel, S.G., Schnall, M.D.: MR imaging of the breast for the detection, diagnosis, and staging of breast cancer. Radiology **220**, 13–30 (2001)
3. Schnall, M.D., et al.: Diagnostic architectural and dynamic features at breast MR imaging: multicenter study. Radiology **238**, 42–53 (2006)
4. Gilhuijs, K.G.A., et al.: Computerized analysis of breast lesions in three dimensions using dynamic magnetic-resonance imaging. Med. Phys. **25**, 1647–1654 (1998)
5. Chen, W., Giger, M.L., Bick, U., Newstead, G.M.: Automatic identification and classification of characteristic kinetic curves of breast lesions on DCE-MRI. Med. Phys. **33**, 1076–1082 (2006)
6. Lee, S.H., et al.: Optimal clustering of kinetic patterns on malignant breast lesions: comparison between K-means clustering and three-time-points method in dynamic contrast-enhanced MRI. In: Engineering in Medicine and Biology Society (2007)

7. Gibbs, P., Turnbull, L.W.: Textural analysis of contrast-enhanced MR images of the breast. Magn. Reson. Med. **50**, 92–98 (2003)
8. Yao, J., Chen, J., Chow, C.: Breast tumor analysis in dynamic contrast enhanced MRI using texture features and wavelet transform. IEEE J. Sel. Top. Signal Process. **3**(1), 94–100 (2009)
9. Agner, S.C., et al.: Textural kinetics: a novel dynamic contrast-enhanced (DCE)-MRI feature for breast lesion classification. J. Digit. Imaging **24**(3), 446–463 (2010)
10. Zheng, Y., et al.: STEP: spatiotemporal enhancement pattern for MR-based breast tumor diagnosis. Med. Phys. **36**(7), 3192–3204 (2009)
11. Gal, Y., Mehnert, A., Bradley, A., Kennedy, D., Crozier, S.: New spatiotemporal features for improved discrimination of benign and malignant lesions in dynamic contrast-enhanced magnetic resonance imaging of the breast. J. Comput. Assist. Tomogr. **35**(5), 645–652 (2011)
12. Tzalavra, A.G., Zacharaki, E.I., Tsiaparas, N.N., Constantinidis, F., Nikita, K.S.: A multiresolution analysis framework for breast tumor classification based on DCE-MRI. In: 2014 IEEE International Conference on Imaging Systems and Techniques (IST) Proceedings, pp. 246–250 (2014)
13. Twellmann, T., Lichte, O., Nattkemper, T.W.: An adaptive tissue characterization network for model-free visualization of dynamic contrast-enhanced magnetic resonance image data. IEEE Trans. Med. Imaging **24**(10), 1256–1266 (2005)
14. Mojsilovic, M., Popovic, M.V., Neskovic, A.N., Popovic, A.D.: Wavelet image extension for analysis and classification of infracted myocardial tissue. IEEE Trans. Biomed. Eng. **44**(9), 856–866 (1997)
15. Chen, D.R., Chang, R.F., Kuo, W.J., Chen, M.C., Huang, Y.L.: Diagnosis of breast tumors with sonographic texture analysis using wavelet transform and neural networks. Ultrasound Med. Biol. **28**(10), 1301–1310 (2002)
16. Tsiaparas, N.N., Golemati, S., Andreadis, I., Stoitsis, J.S., Valavanis, I., Nikita, K.S.: Comparison of multiresolution features for texture classification of carotid atherosclerosis from B-Mode ultrasound. IEEE Trans. Inf Technol. Biomed. **15**(11), 130–137 (2011)
17. Tsiaparas, N.N., Golemati, S., Andreadis, I., Stoitsis, J., Valavanis, I., Nikita, K.S.: Assessment of carotid atherosclerosis from B-mode ultrasound images using directional multiscale texture features. Measur. Sci. Technol. **23**(11), 114004 (2012)
18. Mallat, S.: Theory for multiresolution signal decomposition: the wavelet representation. IEEE Trans. Pattern Anal. Mach. Intell. **11**(7), 674–693 (1989)
19. Furht, B.: Discrete Wavelet Transform (DWT). Encyclopedia of Multimedia. Springer, New York (2008)
20. The Wavelet Tutorial, Part IV. http://users.rowan.edu/~polikar/WAVELETS/WTpart4.html
21. Kumar, B.S., Nagaraj, S.: Discrete and stationary wavelet decomposition for IMAGE resolution enhancement. Int. J. Eng. Trends Technol. (IJETT) **4**(7), 2885–2889 (2013)
22. Candès, E., Demanet, L., Donoho, D., Ying, L.: Fast discrete curvelet transforms. Multiscale Model. Simul. **5**(3), 861–899 (2006)
23. Candes, E.J., Donoho, D.L.: Curvelets, multiresolution representation, and scaling laws. In: SPIE Proceedings, vol. 4119 (2000)
24. Witten, I.H., Frank, E., Hall, M.A.: Data Mining: Practical Machine Learning Tools and Techniques. Morgan Kaufmann, San Francisco (2011)
25. Pearl, J.: Heuristics: Intelligent Search Strategies for Computer Problem Solving. Addison-Wesley, Reading (1984)
26. Goldberg, D.: Genetic Algorithms in Search, Optimization and Machine Learning. Addison-Wesley, Boston (1989)

27. Manning, C.D., Raghavan, P., Schuetze, H.: An Introduction to Information Retrieval. Cambridge University Press, Cambridge (2008)
28. Hartigan, J.A.: Clustering Algorithms. Wiley, New York (1975)
29. Kohavi, R.: The power of decision tables. In: Lavrač, N., Wrobel, S. (eds.) ECML 1995. LNCS, vol. 912, pp. 174–189. Springer, Heidelberg (1995)
30. Landwehr, N., Hall, M., Frank, E.: Logistic model trees. Mach. Learn. **95**(1–2), 161–205 (2005)
31. Haykin, S.: Neural Networks: A Comprehensive Foundation. Prentice Hall, Upper Saddle River (1999)
32. John, G.H., Langley, P.: Estimating continuous distributions in Bayesian classifiers. In: Eleventh Conference on Uncertainty in Artificial Intelligence, San Mateo, pp. 338–345 (1995)
33. Lachenbruch, P.A.: Discriminant Analysis. Hafner, New York (1975)
34. Zhan, T., Renping, Y., Zheng, Y., Zhan, Y., Xiao, L., Wei, Z.: Multimodal spatial-based segmentation framework for white matter lesions in multi-sequence magnetic resonance images. Biomed. Signal Process. Control **31**, 52–62 (2017)

Novel Morphological Features for Non-mass-like Breast Lesion Classification on DCE-MRI

Mohammad Razavi[1]([✉]), Lei Wang[1,5], Tao Tan[2], Nico Karssemeijer[2], Lars Linsen[3], Udo Frese[4], Horst K. Hahn[1], and Gabriel Zachmann[4]

[1] Fraunhofer MEVIS - Institute for Medical Image Computing, Bremen, Germany
mrazavi@iat.uni-bremen.de
[2] Radboud University Medical Center, Nijmegen, The Netherlands
[3] Jacobs University Bremen, Bremen, Germany
[4] University of Bremen, Bremen, Germany
[5] Surpath Medical GmbH, Würzburg, Germany

Abstract. For both visual analysis and computer assisted diagnosis systems in breast MRI reading, the delineation and diagnosis of ductal carcinoma in situ (DCIS) is among the most challenging tasks. Recent studies show that kinetic features derived from dynamic contrast enhanced MRI (DCE-MRI) are less effective in discriminating malignant non-masses against benign ones due to their similar kinetic characteristics. Adding shape descriptors can improve the differentiation accuracy. In this work, we propose a set of novel morphological features using the sphere packing technique, aiming to discriminate non-masses based on their shapes. The feature extraction, selection and the classification modules are integrated into a computer-aided diagnosis (CAD) system. The evaluation was performed on a data set of 106 non-masses extracted from 86 patients, which achieved an accuracy of 90.56 %, precision of 90.3 %, and area under the receiver operating characteristic (ROC) curve (AUC) of 0.94 for the differentiation of benign and malignant types.

1 Introduction

Dynamic contrast enhanced MRI (DCE-MRI) has been widely used in breast cancer screening of high risk patients, preoperative staging, and post-treatment follow-up, for its high sensitivity. According to the BI-RADS lexicon, based on the morphological characteristics, the lesions are classified into mass-like, non-mass-like, and foci [1]. The diagnosis of breast cancer in its intraductal stage might help to prevent it from becoming invasive cancer [2]. However, the delineation and diagnosis of non-masses, most notably DCIS, is challenging in breast MRI reading even for human observers [2,3]. Clinical evidences show that the kinetic parameters have the potential to distinguish benign and malignant in masses more effectively, but fail to demonstrate usefulness in discriminating the non-masses [3]. Therefore, the computer-aided diagnosis (CAD) tools strongly relying on kinetic features often fail in classifying non-masses. In terms of sensitivity and specificity in non-masses, no previous trials achieved a performance

© Springer International Publishing AG 2016
L. Wang et al. (Eds.): MLMI 2016, LNCS 10019, pp. 305–312, 2016.
DOI: 10.1007/978-3-319-47157-0_37

matching CAD approaches for solid masses [2]. To achieve better performance, there is a demand for prominent morphological features depicting the lesion shapes and distributions [1].

Recently, a few CAD systems focusing on differentiating non-masses in MRI have been reported [4,5]. Chen et al. [4] combines the kinetic features derived from characteristic kinetic curves (CKCs), morphological and texture features, which were tested with a collection of both mass and non-mass lesions and yield an AUC of 0.85. Hoffmann et al. [5] evaluated the discriminative power of a set of morphological and kinetic descriptors separately, and the Zernike velocity moments, capturing the joint spatiotemporal behaviors of the lesions, to diagnose a collection of non-mass-like breast lesions. However, none of the features exceeds an AUC value of 0.8. Goto et al. [6] directly compared the diagnostic performance of DCE-MRI (early enhancement) with that of high-spatial-resolution MRI (morphologic features) for the first time. They claimed that in the majority of cases breast lesions were correctly diagnosed merely based on certain morphologic features, which makes those features more important than early enhancement for differentiating malignant breast lesions from benign. The accuracy of 95 % and 87 % were achieved for masses and non-masses respectively.

In this work, we propose three novel morphological features, describing lesion shapes based on the already existing sphere packing algorithm [7], in combination with Zernike descriptors [8]. These features lead to a more precise shape based delineation of malignant and benign lesions and thus a higher discrimination accuracy. Beside introduction of novel morphological features, the contribution of this paper lies in the feature extraction and selection of the features and the evaluation of their performance in discriminating benign and malignant non-mass-like lesions. All these feature types are integrated as modules into a CAD framework implemented on MeVisLab platform[1]. The processing pipeline depicting each individual module is shown in Fig. 1. To test the performance of the introduced features, we conducted several experiments using a data set including 86 patients with 106 non-mass-like lesions, among which 68 were pathologically confirmed malignant, and 38 were benign findings. We evaluated the classifier performance using the mentioned features with a Random Forest (RF) classifier

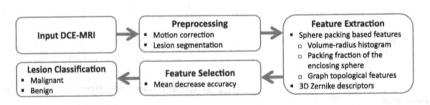

Fig. 1. The integrated framework comprising preprocessing, feature extraction and selection, and lesion analysis modules.

---

[1] MeVisLab: Medical image processing and visualization platform: http://www.mevislab.de [Accessed on 16 March 2016].

in a 10-fold cross-validation scheme, and we achieved an accuracy of 90.56 %, precision of 90.3 %, and the area under the ROC curve (AUC) value of 0.94.

2   Materials and Methods

2.1   Imaging Technique and Data Set

The DCE-MRI images were acquired on a 1.5T scanner (Magnetom Vision, Siemens, Erlangen) in Nijmegen, Netherlands. A dedicated breast coil (CP Breast Array, Siemens, Erlangen) was used in prone patient placement. The pixel spacing differed between volumes with values ranging from 0.625 mm to 0.722 mm. The slice thickness was 1.3 mm, and the volume size was $512 \times 256 \times 120$ voxels. TR and TE were 6.80 s and 4.00 s, respectively, at a 20° flip angle. All patients were histologically confirmed by needle aspiration/excision biopsy or surgical removal. Subsequently, the amount of malignant lesions were 68, most of which were diagnosed as DCIS. The rest were diagnosed as invasive ductal carcinoma (IDC), invasive lobular carcinoma (ILC), lobular carcinoma in situ (LCIS) and metastasis. On the other hand, benign histologic findings were found in 38 lesions including fibrocystic changes (FCC), adenosis and hyperplasia. One experienced radiologist retrospectively reviewed the histologic reports and identified the reported lesions. All the lesions were manually segmented with a computer-assistant tool using region-growing and manual correction.

2.2   Feature Extraction

A total of four morphological features are proposed, including three novel shape descriptors based on the already existing data structure generated by sphere packing algorithm, plus the Zernike descriptors. These features are able to efficiently describe the shape and distribution properties of the lesions.

Features Based on Sphere Packing. The morphological features that we explored are extracted using the data structures generated by the sphere packing technique [7], which is a new and promising data representation for several fundamental problems in computer graphics and virtual reality, such as collision detection and deformable object simulation. The algorithm iteratively fills the lesion with a fixed number of non-overlapping spheres starting with the one with the largest possible radius, under the condition that they should completely locate inside the lesion. Next, all the components of the spheres (3D coordinates and radius) are normalized by scaling down to unit length with respect to their minimum and maximum values of the components. Once each lesion is packed by the aforementioned spheres, the following morphological features are extracted.

(a) Volume-radius histogram: A histogram in which the radius ranges of internal spheres lie on the x-axis with an arbitrary number of bins and the y-axis is the sum of the spheres volumes with the radius falling into a bin. The

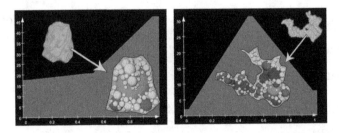

Fig. 2. The volume-radius histogram of two lesions packed with 200 spheres. In benign lesions **(left)** most of their space is filled with sizable spheres; in malignant lesions **(right)**, medium-sized ones occupy most of the internal space.

sphere packing initially occupies as much volume from the lesion as possible with the biggest possible sphere. Therefore, in benign lesions (with a more regular or round shape), the majority of the lesion space is occupied by a few number of sizable spheres and the rest by considerably smaller ones. In contrast, in malignant lesions, most of the volume is occupied with medium-sized spheres (Fig. 2).

(b) Packing fraction of enclosing sphere: For each lesion, all the internal spheres generated by the sphere packing algorithm were enclosed by a bigger sphere or ball and the occupied fraction of that is calculated as a feature. It is dimensionless and always less in unit range. Several strategies can be applied to define the center point's location of the aforementioned sphere, such as mean centering of coordinates, placing it between the two most distant spheres, in the center of the largest internal sphere, and the center of the smallest enclosing ball [9]. In benign lesions (which often have a regular and round shape) the enclosing sphere is more occupied and has less empty gaps than the malignant ones. This fraction is closer to one for benign and is near zero for malignant lesions.

(c) Graph topological features: Graph analysis can assist characterizing the complex structures, leading to a better realization of relations that exist between their components [10]. In this work, it is adapted to characterize the spatial arrangement of the lesion's internal spheres. We constructed the graphs, in which the center points of embedded spheres are considered as nodes, and spatial relationship between them as edges with weights according to their distance. Several structures, including Prim's and Kruskal's minimum spanning trees, relative neighborhood, Gabriel, and β-skeleton graphs were examined to gain the best accuracy (Fig. 3). Finally, the Gabriel graph showed the highest. Furthermore, spatial constraints such as maximum neighbors (K-Max) were employed to form sub-graphs. We used several cluster validity indices, such as graph compactness indices, edge density, structure linearity [11], Dunn's Index, Davies Bouldin index, MinMaxCut, graph's cohesion [12], modularization quality, global silhouette index, Jaccard Coefficient, Folkes, Mallows, Hubert, and Arabie's indices [13] to extract the global and local graph-based geometrical features. The feature vector is formed by the values of all the aforementioned indices.

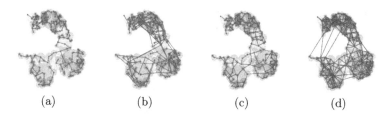

(a)   (b)   (c)   (d)

Fig. 3. Kruskal's **(a)** and Prim's **(b)** minimum spanning trees, relative neighborhood **(c)**, and Gabriel **(d)** graph structures obtained by connecting 200 internal spheres.

3D Zernike Descriptors. Moment-based descriptors have been broadly used for object recognition [8] and shape matching [14] to provide a compact numerical expression of the spatial features. We extracted 3D Zernike descriptors using an extension of spherical-harmonics-based descriptors, presented by Novotni and Klein [15], which captures object coherence in the radial direction.

3   Results and Evaluations

To examine the performance of the proposed features, the first evaluation was conducted without applying any feature selection. We adopted all 106 findings comprising 68 malignant and 38 benign lesions. Each lesion was packed with 4000 spheres. The parameter tuning for the aforementioned features was performed by parameter sweeping of values in a multi-dimensional parameter space and applying the following classification on the feature vectors of each combination to get the best parameter values of the highest accuracy (see Table 1).

Table 1. Feature types and their parameter space, plus the optimized values and number of their output features.

Feature extraction module	Parameters	Best value	No. Features
Volume-radius histogram	Number of bins	50	50
Packing fraction of the enclosing ball	Center point's location	Mean centering	1
Graph morphological features	K-Max, Graph type	No. nodes, Gabriel	19
Zernike descriptors	Maximum order	15	72

For validation of the extracted features, binary classifiers - including Random Forest, Naive Bayes, AdaBoost, and Support Vector Machine (SVM) - were trained with a total of 142 features acquired from the above mentioned methods. For each classifier, a stratified 10-fold cross-validation scheme was applied on the lesions in the data set. The classification power, expressed as AUC is listed in Table 2. The best results were achieved with the RF classifier.

Table 2. The TP and FP rates, precision, and AUC values from classification results of different lesion types using four different classifiers (ben. is benign and mal. is malignant). Here the RF classifier outperforms the other three.

Classifier type	TP Rate		FP Rate		Precision		AUC	
	ben.	mal.	ben.	mal.	ben.	mal.	ben.	mal.
Random forest	0.78	0.91	0.08	0.21	0.83	0.88	0.90	0.90
Naive Bayes	0.86	0.44	0.55	0.13	0.46	0.85	0.66	0.81
AdaBoost	0.65	0.89	0.10	0.34	0.78	0.82	0.83	0.83
Support vector machine	0.68	0.29	0.70	0.31	0.35	0.62	0.48	0.48

3.1 Classification Results with Feature Selection

For the machine learning algorithms, it is important to use feature reduction mechanisms to decrease over-fitting of the training data. Taking advantage of Mean Decrease in Accuracy (MDA) and Mean Decrease GINI (MDG) [16] as variable importance criteria, from a total of 142 features in features set, the top 30 most effective ones were selected for evaluation. Using the RF classifier, MDA ranking showed a higher accuracy than MDG. Among the top features rated by MDA, *volume-radius histogram*, *packed fraction of enclosing ball*, *graph features*, and *Zernike descriptors* features gained the highest order respectively. It should be mentioned that, among those features, only three graph features of *linear structure*, *new compactness index Cp^**, and *Dunn's index* [13] (Eq. 1) appeared on the top 30 MDA features.

$$Dunn(C) = \frac{d(C_i, C_j)}{\text{diam}(C_h)}, \qquad Cp^* = \frac{\sum_{i=1}^{N-1} \sum_{j=i+1}^{N} \text{sim}(v_i, v_j)}{N(N-1)/2} \qquad (1)$$

Furthermore, applying the Principal Component Analysis (PCA) feature selection was investigated to reduce the dimensionality even more and find the best correlation between the features. However, no improvement was seen in the evaluation results. Table 3 shows the classification results of the RF using 10-FCV before and after applying MDA, MDG, PCA over MDA, and PCA over MDG.

Table 3. The classification results of the RF using 10-FCV before and after applying MDA and MDG rankings, plus PCA on them (ben. is benign and mal. is malignant).

Feature selection	No. features	TP Rate		FP Rate		Precision		Accuracy		AUC	
		ben.	mal.	ben.	mal.	ben.	mal.	ben.	mal.	ben.	mal.
No selection	142	0.789	0.912	0.088	0.211	0.833	0.886	13.2 %	86.79 %	0.907	0.907
MDG	30	0.816	0.956	0.044	0.184	0.912	0.903	9.43 %	90.56 %	0.935	0.935
MDA	30	0.816	0.956	0.044	0.184	0.912	0.903	9.43 %	90.56 %	0.94	0.94
PCA on MDG	5	0.763	0.941	0.059	0.237	0.879	0.877	12.26 %	87.73 %	0.935	0.935
PCA on MDA	5	0.816	0.926	0.074	0.184	0.861	0.900	11.32 %	88.67 %	0.936	0.936

4   Conclusion and Discussion

This paper focuses on utilizing the sphere packing (non-overlapping and non-uniform radii) to develop a set of novel morphological features to classify breast non-mass-like lesions. Under the assumption that malignant lesions tend to have irregular shapes and margins compared to benign lesions (which have more regular and round shape), the sphere packing based features can effectively capture the shape differences and thus increase the discrimination accuracy. All the proposed features are translation, rotation, and scaling invariant, since they either are coordinate free features, or because we normalized the data at first.

To our knowledge, this is the first time that such an object representation has been investigated for classifying non-mass lesions in MRI. One advantage of sphere packing is that it can describe volumetric shapes more concisely than a voxel representation or mesh surface. In addition, it allows for deriving additional meta-representations (e.g. proximity graphs and skeletons), which we investigated in this work too. Among many other insights, we discovered that the volume-radius histogram is a particularly efficient shape descriptor to classify non-mass breast lesions into benign and malignant.

To reduce the redundancy of the extracted features, we investigated the application of two feature selection techniques: MDA and PCA to decrease the overfitting of the data. The classification performance of these features was tested with a data set of 106 non-mass-like lesions collected from 86 patients. Two experiments comparing the performance with and without feature selection were conducted. The classification accuracy, using different classifiers was evaluated. The best AUC value of 0.94 was achieved when using MDA selected features with a RF classifier and 10-FCV scheme. The experiment demonstrated the discriminative power of our proposed features and their potential to increase the diagnostic accuracy of a CAD system. In the future, we will focus on further improving the calculation efficiency of these features and also investigate more features based on the sphere packing.

We acknowledge that there are limitations in our study. Firstly, to the best of our knowledge, there is no validated data set for non-masses publicly available that we can perform a benchmark on and compare the results with others. Therefore, we used aforementioned data set that were labeled meticulously by radiologists, which makes it the best-suited data set for our work. Secondly, we are aware that the evaluation using the 10-FCV method might cause some overfitting on the data. Nevertheless the 10-FCV is generally even more reliable than other current methods, such as leaveone out CV and Bootstrap, as it has a lower variance. Reducing the number of features to 30 finals using MDA leads to very low over-fitting and unbiased results at the end.

References

1. Jansen, S.A., Shimauchi, A., Zak, L., Fan, X., Karczmar, G.S., Newstead, G.M.: The diverse pathology and kinetics of mass, nonmass, and focus enhancement on MR imaging of the breast. J. MRI **33**(6), 1382–1389 (2011)

2. Kuhl, C.K., Schrading, S., Bieling, H.B., Wardelmann, E., Leutner, C.C., Koenig, R., Kuhn, W., Schild, H.H.: MRI for diagnosis of pure ductal carcinoma in situ: a prospective observational study. Lancet **370**(9586), 485–492 (2007)

3. Jansen, S.A., Fan, X., Karczmar, G.S., Abe, H., Schmidt, R.A., Giger, M., Newstead, G.M.: DCEMRI of breast lesions: is kinetic analysis equally effective for both mass and nonmass-like enhancement? Med. Phys. **35**(7), 3102–3109 (2008)

4. Chen, W., Giger, M.L., Newstead, G.M., Bick, U., Jansen, S.A., Li, H., Lan, L.: Computerized assessment of breast lesion malignancy using DCE-MRI: robustness study on two independent clinical datasets from two manufacturers. Acad. Radiol. **17**(7), 822–829 (2010)

5. Hoffmann, S., Shutler, J.D., Lobbes, M., Burgeth, B., Meyer-Bäse, A.: Automated analysis of non-mass-enhancing lesions in breast MRI based on morphological, kinetic, and spatio-temporal moments and joint segmentation-motion compensation technique. EURASIP J. Adv. Sig. Process. **2013**(1), 1–10 (2013)

6. Goto, M., Ito, H., Akazawa, K., Kubota, T., Kizu, O., Yamada, K., Nishimura, T.: Diagnosis of breast tumors by contrast-enhanced MR imaging: comparison between the diagnostic performance of dynamic enhancement patterns and morphologic features. J. Magn. Reson. Imaging **25**(1), 104–112 (2007)

7. Weller, R., Zachmann, G.: Protosphere: a GPU-assisted prototype guided sphere packing algorithm for arbitrary objects. In: ACM SIGGRAPH ASIA, p. 8 (2010)

8. Chen, Z., Sun, S.-K.: A Zernike moment phase-based descriptor for local image representation and matching. IEEE Trans. Image Process. **19**(1), 205–219 (2010)

9. Gärtner, B.: Fast and robust smallest enclosing balls. In: Nešetřil, J. (ed.) ESA 1999. LNCS, vol. 1643, pp. 325–338. Springer, Heidelberg (1999)

10. Ali, S., Veltri, R., Epstein, J.A., Christudass, C., Madabhushi, A.: Cell cluster graph for prediction of biochemical recurrence in prostate cancer patients from tissue microarrays. In: SPIE Medical Imaging, p. 86760H. International Society for Optics and Photonics (2013)

11. Botafogo, R.A., Rivlin, E., Shneiderman, B.: Structural analysis of hypertexts: identifying hierarchies and useful metrics. ACM Trans. Inf. Syst. (TOIS) **10**(2), 142–180 (1992)

12. Raidou, R.G., Van Der Heide, U., Dinh, C.V., Ghobadi, G., Kallehauge, J.F., Breeuwer, M., Vilanova, A.: Visual analytics for the exploration of tumor tissue characterization. Comput. Graph. Forum **34**, 11–20 (2015). Wiley Online Library

13. Boutin, F., Hascoet, M.: Cluster validity indices for graph partitioning. In: 2004 Proceedings of Eighth International Conference on Information Visualisation, IV 2004, pp. 376–381. IEEE (2004)

14. Ricard, J., Coeurjolly, D., Baskurt, A.: Generalizations of angular radial transform for 2D and 3D shape retrieval. Pattern Recogn. Lett. **26**(14), 2174–2186 (2005)

15. Novotni, M., Klein, R.: Shape retrieval using 3D Zernike descriptors. Comput. Aided Des. **36**(11), 1047–1062 (2004)

16. Calle, M.L., Urrea, V.: Letter to the editor: stability of random forest importance measures. Briefings Bioinform. **12**, 86–89 (2010)

Fast Neuroimaging-Based Retrieval for Alzheimer's Disease Analysis

Xiaofeng Zhu, Kim-Han Thung, Jun Zhang, and Dinggang Shen[✉]

Department of Radiology and BRIC, University of North Carolina at Chapel Hill,
Chapel Hill, USA
dgshen@med.unc.edu

Abstract. This paper proposes a framework of fast neuroimaging-based retrieval and AD analysis, by three key steps: (1) *landmark detection*, which efficiently extracts landmark-based neuroimaging features without the need of nonlinear registration in testing stage; (2) *landmark selection*, which removes redundant/noisy landmarks via proposing a feature selection method that considers structural information among landmarks; and (3) *hashing*, which converts high-dimensional features of subjects into binary codes, for efficiently conducting approximate nearest neighbor search and diagnosis of AD. We have conducted experiments on Alzheimer's Disease Neuroimaging Initiative (ADNI) dataset, and demonstrated that our framework could achieve higher performance than the comparison methods, in terms of accuracy and speed (at least 100 times faster).

1 Introduction

Recent studies have demonstrated that neuroimaging data are useful for neurodegenerative disease analysis [2,7]. For example, Magnetic Resonance (MR) image is able to show different soft tissues in the brain with good contrast, and thus gives us important information about brain atrophy resulting from neurodegeneration. In addition, MR image is also non-invasive and safe. As a result, studies have been using MR images to devise biomarkers for AD (and its related disease stages) identification [8,10,17].

Conventional methods of AD diagnosis using neuroimaging data (*e.g.,* MR images), like ROI-based methods [16,17] and voxel-based methods [3], involve a time-consuming nonlinear registration process to register all the images into the same common space, before performing further analysis. For example, Zhang *et al.* [11] reported that the time cost of nonlinear registration in the seminal works, such as HAMMER [6] and FSL [13], are around 30 min and at least 3 min, respectively. Such time cost makes the conventional methods impractical for real-time neuroimaging analysis in clinical study. In addition, rather than predicting categorical labels, the clinician is also interested in retrieving similar subjects of each new subject, to assist diagnosis. This is unfortunately unaccounted for by the conventional methods, which only provide the diagnosis label prediction.

© Springer International Publishing AG 2016
L. Wang et al. (Eds.): MLMI 2016, LNCS 10019, pp. 313–321, 2016.
DOI: 10.1007/978-3-319-47157-0_38

In this paper, we overcome the aforementioned issues by proposing a framework of fast neuroimaging-based retrieval and AD analysis, which consists of three key elements: (1) *landmark detection* [12], which avoids time-consuming process of nonlinear registration, as needed in conventional ROI-based and voxel-based methods, in testing stage. We first identify the discriminative landmarks in the MR images, via group comparison in the training set. Then, we construct a regression-forest-based landmark detection model to efficiently predict the landmarks of testing MR images. In this way, the neuroimaging features of testing MR images can be extracted without involving the process of non-linear registration and thus enabling to conduct real-time neuroimaging-based retrieval and AD analysis. (2) *landmark selection*, which removes redundant/noisy landmarks by proposing a novel feature selection method. We first arrange the feature vector of each landmark side by side to obtain a feature matrix for each subject. Then, we consider structural information among landmarks and possible noise in the feature vector of each landmark, to devise a novel landmark selection model. (3) *hashing*, which converts the high-dimensional feature vector of each subject into a short binary code. After landmark selection, the features of the selected landmarks within one subject are concatenated into a long vector, where the dimension is still too high (more than 20,000 in our experiments) to train a stable classifier. Hashing is able to convert long-dimensional vector into short binary codes while preserving their neighborhood relationship. By representing each subject by a short binary code vector, we can effectively retrieve the neighboring MR images of a testing image for AD retrieval and analysis.

2   Proposed Framework

Figure 1 shows the flowchart of the proposed framework, which consists of 2 stages, *i.e.*, training stage and testing stage, respectively. We describe details in the following.

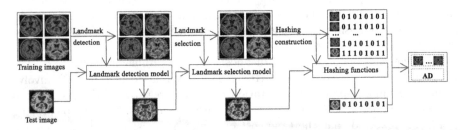

Fig. 1. The flowchart of the proposed framework of fast neuroimaging-based AD analysis. The blue arrows and the red arrows, respectively, represent training stage and testing stage. It is noteworthy that training stage involves three main sequential steps, *i.e.*, landmark detection, landmark selection, and hashing. (Color figure online)

2.1   Landmark Detection

We employ the method in [11] to define AD-related landmarks in MR images and learn a regression-forest-based landmark detection model. We first nonlinearly register all the training MR images to a template image, where the voxels with their corresponding local morphological features significantly different between two groups (*i.e.*, AD and normal control (NC)) are identified as landmarks. Then, we map the landmarks in the template to the training images (through the deformation fields estimated by nonlinear registrations), to obtain the landmarks of all the training images. Using the detected landmarks, we construct a regression-forest-based landmark detection model, where the Low-Energy Pattern (LEP) features [12] of the subject voxels and their corresponding displacements to the detected landmarks are used as input and output of the model, respectively. Note that all these time-consuming processes are done offline. In testing stage, we use the learnt landmark detection model to find the landmarks of testing MR images, which is extremely fast, as no time-consuming process (*i.e.*, either nonlinear registration or regression-forest training) is involved.

2.2   Landmark Selection

After landmark detection, Zhang *et al.* [11] uses the morphological (*i.e.*, LEP) features of all the landmarks to train a classifier (*i.e.*, Support Vector Machine (SVM)) for predicting categorical labels of subjects. As the number of landmarks is about 1741, and the number of features for each landmark is 50, the total number of features for each subject is very high, *i.e.*, over 80,000, while there are only few hundreds of subjects available. Obviously, there is a "High Dimension Low Subject Size" (HDLSS) issue, which makes conventional machine learning techniques like SVM unstable. Moreover, as the landmarks are detected based on group comparison, which does not consider correlations among landmarks, for such large number of landmarks, it is highly possible that the detected landmarks are redundant or not discriminative to the classifier. Thus, we perform landmark selection to remove redundant and noisy landmarks.

To this end, we propose a novel landmark selection method that integrates subspace learning and 2D feature selection in a unified framework. Firstly, we represent each subject as a 2D feature matrix, by concatenating the LEP features of all the landmarks in one subject side by side, rather than concatenating all the features into a long vector (as in [11]). In this way, we preserve the spatial information among landmarks, which helps us in identifying redundant (*e.g.*, by checking the correlation among landmarks) and noisy landmarks (*e.g.*, by checking the discriminative power of the landmarks in classification task). We then convert the high-dimensional LEP features of the landmarks into target-like (*i.e.*, clinical-status-like) features, and jointly select the discriminative landmarks of all the subjects.

Let us denote $\mathbf{X}_i \in \mathbb{R}^{l \times d}$ as the feature matrix of the i-th subject, where l is the number of landmarks, and d is the dimension of LEP features for each landmark. The corresponding clinical status of i-th subject is denoted as $\mathbf{y}_i \in \mathbb{R}^{c \times 1}$, where c is the number of possible clinical statuses. Assuming linear relationship between $\mathbf{X}_i$ and $\mathbf{y}_i$ and n number of subjects, we formulate our landmark detection algorithm as

$$\min_{\mathbf{S},\mathbf{R}} \sum_{i=1}^{n} \|\mathbf{y}_i^T - \mathbf{s}_i^T \mathbf{X}_i \mathbf{R}\|_F^2 + \gamma \|\mathbf{S}\|_{2,1}, s.t., \mathbf{R}^T \mathbf{R} = \mathbf{I}, \qquad (1)$$

where $\mathbf{S} = [\mathbf{s}_1, ..., \mathbf{s}_n] \in \mathbb{R}^{l \times n}$ and $\mathbf{R} \in \mathbb{R}^{d \times c}$ are coefficient matrices, and γ is the tuning parameter. $\mathbf{s}_i \in \mathbb{R}^{l \times 1}$ is a sparse vector, which is used to select landmarks for i-th subject, and linearly combines the selected landmarks into a single vector (i.e., $\mathbf{s}_i^T \mathbf{X}_i$ is a d dimensional row vector). To select common landmarks for all the subjects, we use group sparsity regularizer (i.e., $l_{2,1}$-norm) on $\mathbf{S}$, i.e., $\|\mathbf{S}\|_{2,1} = \sum_i^l \sqrt{\sum_j^n s_{ij}^2}$. The group sparsity regularizer (i.e., the second term in Eq. (1)) encourages all-zero-value rows in $\mathbf{S}$, to jointly select discriminative landmarks for all the subjects. In addition, we would like to select landmarks not based on the original high-dimensional (and possibly noisy) feature space spanned by the landmarks, but rather based on a low-dimensional and target-like feature space, via the transformation matrix $\mathbf{R}$. Specifically, $\mathbf{R}$ maps a high-dimensional feature vector of each landmark (i.e., a d-dimensional row vector of $\mathbf{X}_i$) into a c-dimensional target-like feature space ($\mathbf{X}_i \mathbf{R} \in \mathbb{R}^{l \times c}$). It is noteworthy that the inequality $c \ll d$ always holds in AD study. With this, the orthogonal constraint on $\mathbf{R}$ enables to output unrelated low-dimensional vectors, thus actually conducting subspace learning.

After optimal condition is met, an index of selected landmarks can be obtained through all-non-zero rows of $\mathbf{S}$.

2.3   Hashing Construction

After landmark selection, we represent each subject using a long feature vector, which is the concatenation of LEP features of the selected landmarks. The dimension of such a feature vector is still too high to construct an effective and efficient classification model. In addition, unlike conventional neuroimaging analysis methods that only focus on classification task, we are also interested in efficiently retrieving similar subjects, which can assist the clinician to conduct AD analysis. Both of these issues can be addressed through hashing, which involves converting high-dimensional data into short binary codes [14,15], while preserving the neighborhood relationship among subjects in the original data space as much as possible. Specifically, the neighboring subjects of each testing subject can efficiently be found by first representing them with short binary codes and then comparing their binary codes (i.e., calculating the Hamming distance between this testing subject and its neighbors) in the memory of PC. We can also obtain the diagnosis label of this testing subject with the majority voting rule on the labels of its neighboring subjects.

To this end, we employ the hashing framework in [18], which includes two key steps, i.e., probabilistic representation step and hash function learning step.

In the probabilistic representation step, we employ a probabilistic method to represent high-dimensional data using low-dimensional probabilistic representation. This step is aimed to resolve the HDLSS issue while preserving the local structures of the data, which are the most important factors in constructing effective hashing method [18]. In the hash function learning step, we encode the probabilistic representations (of all the subjects) using a dictionary, and then binarize the resulting coding coefficients as final hash codes. As described in [18], the dictionary and the binarization threshold are learnt jointly.

Probabilistic Representation. Let $\tilde{\mathbf{x}}_i$ denotes the long feature vector of the i-th subject after landmark selection, and $\tilde{\mathbf{X}} = [\tilde{\mathbf{x}}_1 \cdots \tilde{\mathbf{x}}_n]$ is the feature matrix. We first partition $\tilde{\mathbf{X}}$ into m clusters and then compute the probability of each subject belonging to each cluster by calculating the Euclidean distance between the subject and the centroid of the cluster. Considering the fact that a subject $\tilde{\mathbf{x}}_i$ can only be members of several neighboring clusters, the Probabilistic Representation (PR) of a subject, $\mathbf{p}_i = [p_{i,1} \cdots p_{i,k} \cdots p_{i,m}]$ ($p_{i,k}$ denotes the probability of i-th subject belonging to k-th cluster), should be sparse. Therefore, we only preserve the first few largest probabilities in $\mathbf{p}_i$, and set the remaining minor probabilities to 0. Finally, we denote the PR of $\tilde{\mathbf{x}}_i$ after sparsity thresholding as $\tilde{\mathbf{p}}_i = [\tilde{p}_{i,1} \cdots \tilde{p}_{i,m}]^T$. $\tilde{\mathbf{p}}_i$ is a sparse vector, and it can well characterize the original spatial location of $\tilde{\mathbf{x}}_i$ in $\tilde{\mathbf{X}}$. In this way, similar subjects should have similar PR vectors, and therefore $\tilde{\mathbf{p}}_i$ is a good representation of $\tilde{\mathbf{x}}_i$ for effective hashing.

Hash Function Learning. Let $\tilde{\mathbf{P}} = [\tilde{\mathbf{p}}_1, \tilde{\mathbf{p}}_2, \cdots, \tilde{\mathbf{p}}_n] \in \mathbb{R}^{m \times n}$ be the set of PRs of all training subjects in $\tilde{\mathbf{X}}$. The hash function can then be learnt from $\tilde{\mathbf{P}}$ by using:

$$\min_{\mathbf{\Phi}, \mathbf{\Lambda}} \|\tilde{\mathbf{P}} - \mathbf{\Phi}\mathbf{\Lambda}\|_F^2 + \lambda \sum_{i=1}^{n} \|\boldsymbol{\alpha}_i - \boldsymbol{\mu}\|^2, \ s.t. \ \|\boldsymbol{\phi}_j\|^2 = 1 \tag{2}$$

where $\mathbf{\Phi} \in \mathbb{R}^{m \times a}$ is called the encoding dictionary and each atom $\boldsymbol{\phi}_j \in \mathbb{R}^m$ in $\mathbf{\Phi}$ has unit ℓ_2-norm; $\mathbf{\Lambda} = [\boldsymbol{\alpha}_1, ..., \boldsymbol{\alpha}_n] \in \mathbb{R}^{a \times n}$ is the coding matrix of $\tilde{\mathbf{P}}$ using dictionary $\mathbf{\Phi}$, with $\boldsymbol{\alpha}_i$ being the coding vector of $\tilde{\mathbf{p}}_i$; $\boldsymbol{\mu} = \frac{1}{n}\sum_{i=1}^{n} \boldsymbol{\alpha}_i$ is the mean of all coding vectors; λ is a tuning parameter; and a is the number of atoms or the code length.

We alternatively optimize $\mathbf{\Phi}$ and $\mathbf{\Lambda}$ to solve Eq. (2). First, we randomly initialize $\mathbf{\Phi}$ and solve for $\mathbf{\Lambda}$ to yield the following analytical solution to each $\boldsymbol{\alpha}_i$ in $\mathbf{\Lambda}$:

$$\boldsymbol{\alpha}_i = \mathbf{T}\tilde{\mathbf{p}}_i + \boldsymbol{\beta} \tag{3}$$

where $\begin{cases} \mathbf{T} = (\mathbf{\Phi}^T\mathbf{\Phi} + \lambda\mathbf{I})^{-1}\mathbf{\Phi}^T \\ \boldsymbol{\beta} = \lambda(\mathbf{\Phi}^T\mathbf{\Phi} + \lambda\mathbf{I})^{-1}(\mathbf{\Phi}^T\mathbf{\Phi})^{-1}\mathbf{\Phi}^T\mathbf{z} \end{cases}$, $\mathbf{I}$ is the identity matrix, and $\mathbf{z} = \frac{1}{n}\sum_{i=1}^{n}\tilde{\mathbf{p}}_i$ is the mean of all PR vectors $\tilde{\mathbf{p}}_i$. Equation (3) defines our hash functions; that is, the real-valued hash code of $\tilde{\mathbf{p}}_i$ is obtained by projecting it onto $\mathbf{T}$ with a shift $\boldsymbol{\beta}$.

With all $\boldsymbol{\alpha}_i$ available, the mean vector $\boldsymbol{\mu} = \frac{1}{n}\sum_{i=1}^{n}\boldsymbol{\alpha}_i$ can be readily computed. We then binarize $\boldsymbol{\alpha}_i$ as follows:

$$\begin{cases} \mathbf{b}_i(j) = 1 \ \ if \ \ \boldsymbol{\alpha}_i(j) \geq \boldsymbol{\mu}_i(j) \\ \mathbf{b}_i(j) = 0 \ \ if \ \ \boldsymbol{\alpha}_i(j) < \boldsymbol{\mu}_i(j) \end{cases} \tag{4}$$

That is, the mean value is used as the threshold for binarization. Note that in our model, the mean $\boldsymbol{\mu}$ is actually optimized jointly with dictionary $\boldsymbol{\Phi}$, which directly determines the hash transform matrix $\mathbf{T}$ and shift $\boldsymbol{\beta}$. Arranging all the binary codes together will form the hash matrix of PR matrix $\tilde{\mathbf{X}}$, $i.e.$, $\mathbf{B} = [\mathbf{b}_1, ..., \mathbf{b}_n]$.

2.4   Testing Stage

Given a testing subject $\hat{\mathbf{x}}$, we detect its landmarks using the learnt landmark detection model, remove redundant/noisy landmarks via keeping the indices of selected landmarks, extract LEP features from the selected landmarks, compute the corresponding PR vector and its real-valued code using Eq. 3, and binarize the code using Eq. (4). Finally, the Hamming distance between the binarized code of $\hat{\mathbf{x}}$ and $\mathbf{B}$ is computed to find the nearest neighboring subjects of $\hat{\mathbf{x}}$. The associated labels of the neighboring subjects are then ensembled to obtain the categorical label of $\hat{\mathbf{x}}$, via the majority voting rule.

3   Experiments

To evaluate the proposed framework, we conducted experiments using two disjoint subsets of Alzheimer's Disease Neuroimaging Initiative (ADNI) dataset. Specifically, we used 199 ADs and 229 age-matched NCs from ADNI-1 as training data, while used 159 ADs and 201 age-matched NCs from ADNI-2 as testing data. To obtain more robust results, we employed 10 repetitions of 10-fold cross validation on the training (ADNI-1) data, to use only subset ($i.e.$, 9 out of 10 folds) of the training data to train the model in each experiment, and testing the model using testing (ADNI-2) data. In each experiment, we conducted nested 5-fold cross-validations, in the grid searching range of $\{10^{-5}, ..., 10^{5}\}$, to determine the parameter values of the models ($e.g.$, γ in Eq. (1), and λ in Eq. (2)).

We only evaluate the proposed landmark selection model and the hashing method of our framework, as the landmark detection model used in this work is the same as [11]. Using the landmark detection model in [11], we obtained 1500 landmarks for each MR image, and 50-dimensional LEP features for each landmark, to conduct the following experiments.

3.1   Experimental Results of Landmark Selection

To evaluate our landmark selection model, we conducted landmark selection (via Eq. (1)) using the training set via 10-fold cross-validation for 10 times. Using the results of this experiment, we knew how frequent each landmark was selected.

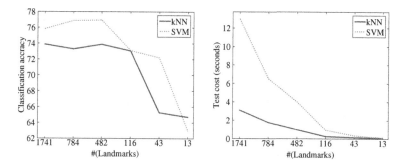

Fig. 2. The classification accuracy (left) and testing cost (right), using different number of selected landmarks, based on k Nearest Neighbors (kNN) and Support Vector Machine (SVM) classification method.

By setting different thresholds for this frequency values, we can select different number of landmarks. We then used LEP features for all the selected landmarks to train classifiers and reported the results in Fig. 2, in terms of average classification accuracy and testing cost (in time). The numbers in the horizontal axis of Fig. 2, from right to left, are respectively corresponding to the number of landmarks which is at least 100 % (13 landmarks), 95 % (43 landmarks), 90 % (116 landmarks), 85 % (482 landmarks), and 80 % (784 landmarks) being selected in the aforementioned experiment using Eq. (1). From Fig. 2, we found that testing cost is proportional to the number of landmarks used, while the classification accuracy is maximum when around 482 to 784 landmarks are used. Considering the tradeoff between accuracy and testing cost, we chose to use 482 landmarks to represent each subject for the next step.

3.2 Experimental Results of Hashing

In this section, we evaluated our hashing method by comparing its AD diagnosis performance with other state-of-the-art hashing methods, such as Anchor Graph Hashing (AGH) [5], ITerative Quantization (ITQ) [1], Spectral Hashing (SpH) [9], and Locality-Sensitive Hashing (LSH) [4]. Figure 3 shows that our hashing method consistently outperforms other comparison hashing methods, in terms of classification accuracy, using different number of bit lengths.

Figure 3 also includes kNN and SVM results using all the original landmark features (*i.e.,* 75,000-dimensional LEP features), which are 73.89 % and 75.83 % respectively for classification accuracy, and 12.86 (seconds) and 3.05 (seconds) respectively for testing cost. We found that the classification accuracies of three hashing methods (*i.e.,* AGH, ITQ and proposed) with moderate code length (*i.e.,* from 28 bits to 52 bits) are generally better than kNN and SVM, while they are faster than them for more than 100 times.

We also checked whether the top 10 nearest neighbors of all testing subjects have the same diagnosis labels with testing subjects. The results showed that

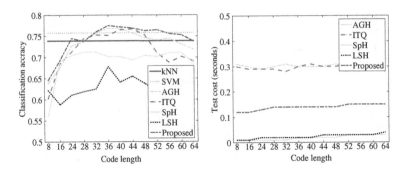

Fig. 3. The classification accuracy (left) and testing cost (right), of all methods.

most hashing methods (including ours, AGH, ITQ, and SpH) with code length 36, on average achieved around 79.05 % of accuracy, compared to 68.29 % for kNN.

4   Conclusion

In this paper, we propose a framework of fast neuroimaging-based retrieval and AD analysis, which includes three main steps, *i.e.,* landmark detection, landmark selection, and hashing construction, respectively. Experimental results using the ADNI dataset showed that the proposed framework achieved higher classification accuracy and faster retrieval results, compared to traditional classification methods, such as kNN and SVM. In our future work, we will design new hashing techniques to further improve the performance of neuroimaging-based retrieval and AD analysis diagnosis.

Acknowledgements. This work was supported in part by NIH grants (EB006733, EB008374, EB009634, MH100217, AG041721, AG042599). Xiaofeng Zhu was supported in part by the National Natural Science Foundation of China under grants 61573270 and 61263035.

References

1. Gong, Y., Lazebnik, S., Gordo, A., Perronnin, F.: Iterative quantization: a procrustean approach to learning binary codes for large-scale image retrieval. IEEE Trans. Pattern Anal. Mach. Intell. **35**(12), 2916–2929 (2013)
2. Huang, L., Jin, Y., Gao, Y., Thung, K., Shen, D., Alzheimer's Disease Neuroimaging Initiative: Longitudinal clinical score prediction in Alzheimers disease with soft-split sparse regression based random forest. Neurobiol. Aging **46**, 180–191 (2016)
3. Hutton, C., De Vita, E., Ashburner, J., Deichmann, R., Turner, R.: Voxel-based cortical thickness measurements in MRI. Neuroimage **40**(4), 1701–1710 (2008)
4. Kulis, B., Grauman, K.: Kernelized locality-sensitive hashing for scalable image search. In: ICCV, pp. 2130–2137 (2009)

5. Liu, W., Wang, J., Kumar, S., Chang, S.F.: Hashing with graphs. In: ICML, pp. 1–8 (2011)
6. Shen, D., Davatzikos, C.: HAMMER: hierarchical attribute matching mechanism for elastic registration. IEEE Trans. Med. Imaging **21**(11), 1421–1439 (2002)
7. Thung, K., Wee, C., Yap, P., Shen, D.: Neurodegenerative disease diagnosis using incomplete multi-modality data via matrix shrinkage and completion. NeuroImage **91**, 386–400 (2014)
8. Thung, K., Wee, C., Yap, P., Shen, D.: Identification of progressive mild cognitive impairment patients using incomplete longitudinal MRI scans. Brain Struct. Funct. 1–17 (2015)
9. Weiss, Y., Torralba, A., Fergus, R.: Spectral hashing. In: NIPS, pp. 1753–1760 (2009)
10. Zhang, C., Qin, Y., Zhu, X., Zhang, J., Zhang, S.: Clustering-based missing value imputation for data preprocessing. In: INDIN, pp. 1081–1086 (2006)
11. Zhang, J., Gao, Y., Gao, Y., Munsell, B., Shen, D.: Detecting anatomical landmarks for fast Alzheimer's disease diagnosis. IEEE Trans. Med. Imaging **PP**(99), 1 (2016)
12. Zhang, J., Liang, J., Zhao, H.: Local energy pattern for texture classification using self-adaptive quantization thresholds. IEEE Trans. Image Process. **22**(1), 31–42 (2013)
13. Zhang, Y., Brady, M., Smith, S.: Segmentation of brain MR images through a hidden Markov random field model and the expectation-maximization algorithm. IEEE Trans. Med. Imaging **20**(1), 45–57 (2001)
14. Zhu, X., Huang, Z., Cheng, H., Cui, J., Shen, H.T.: Sparse hashing for fast multimedia search. ACM Trans. Inf. Syst. **31**(2), 9 (2013)
15. Zhu, X., Huang, Z., Shen, H.T., Zhao, X.: Linear cross-modal hashing for efficient multimedia search. In: ACM Multimedia, pp. 143–152 (2013)
16. Zhu, X., Suk, H.-I., Shen, D.: A novel multi-relation regularization method for regression and classification in AD diagnosis. In: Golland, P., Hata, N., Barillot, C., Hornegger, J., Howe, R. (eds.) MICCAI 2014. LNCS, vol. 8675, pp. 401–408. Springer, Heidelberg (2014). doi:10.1007/978-3-319-10443-0_51
17. Zhu, X., Suk, H.I., Wang, L., Lee, S.W., Shen, D., et al.: A novel relational regularization feature selection method for joint regression and classification in AD diagnosis. Med. Image Anal. (2015)
18. Zhu, X., Zhang, L., Huang, Z.: A sparse embedding and least variance encoding approach to hashing. IEEE Trans. Image Process. **23**(9), 3737–3750 (2014)

Author Index

Printed in the United States
By Bookmasters